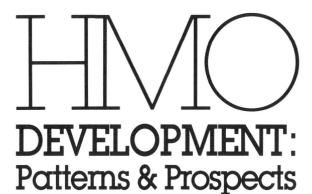

HMO
DEVELOPMENT:
Patterns & Prospects

a comparative analysis of HMOs

Odin W. Anderson, Ph.D
Terry E. Herold, M.A.
Bruce W. Butler, M.B.A.
Claire H. Kohrman, M.A.
Ellen M. Morrison, M.A.

pluribus press inc.

DIVISION OF TEACH EM INC

University of Chicago, Center for Health Administration Studies
Continuing CHAS Research Series—No. 33

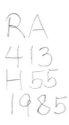

89   88   87   86   85   5   4   3   2   1

Library of Congress Catalog Card Number:
84-61462

International Standard Book Number:
0-931028-57-4

Pluribus Press, Inc., Division of Teach'em, Inc.
160 East Illinois Street
Chicago, IL 60611

Center for Health Administration Studies
University of Chicago
5720 South Woodlawn
Chicago, IL 60637

Printed in the United States of America

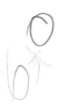

Contents

Tables

Preface

This study investigated the factors affecting the introduction and development of HMOs in Minneapolis-St. Paul and in Chicago. The project focused on market characteristics, sources of community support and resistance, and organizational and managerial factors. Three types of data were collected in both sites: 1) longitudinal data describing the sociodemographic, economic, and health system characteristics of the market areas, 2) intensive interviews with health care and community leaders who were influential in the development of the health systems and alternative delivery systems, and 3) organizational case histories of the HMOs themselves. This study provides both a conceptual and an empirical basis for understanding the factors that affect the introduction and growth of alternative delivery systems. A wealth of data was collected for understanding the potential role of these initiatives in cost containment and in the emergence of a competitive health services market. The methodology developed on this project can be readily applied in other market areas to inventory and evaluate the factors that affect the potential of competitive delivery system alternatives at the individual, organizational, and health care system levels. Thus, the findings of this study will be of interest to a wide audience.

Acknowledgements

The magnitude of this study, in two cities four hundred miles apart, with fifteen health maintenance organizations, calls for many acknowledgements. We are particularly grateful to three sources of funds for the research project. The Henry J. Kaiser Family Foundation, Menlo Park, California; The Chicago Community Trust; and the Blue Cross/Blue Shield Plan of Illinois. The Kaiser Family Foundation supported the Minneapolis-St. Paul site of the project, and part of the Chicago site in cooperation with the agencies mentioned. The Center for Health Administration Studies Graduate School of Business, University of Chicago; the base of operations for the project, also contributed financial support directly and indirectly.

The research project required a great deal of cooperation from the fifteen health maintenance organizations in the two metropolitan areas. We are particularly appreciative of the information provided us in interviews with their directors and staffs, and for their assistance in sharing background and developmental materials from their records. It required no small amount of their staff time.

Then, we should thank the 325 people we interviewed personally in the two metropolitan areas—141 in Minneapolis-St. Paul and 184 in Chicago—representing insurers, hospitals, consumer groups, legislature and regulatory agencies, physicians, employers and unions. There were hardly any refusals. Inter-Study; Paul Ellwood, M.D., its president; and his staff were very helpful in briefing us on the Minneapolis-St. Paul situation and suggesting appropriate people to interview. The Chicago Hospital Council also provided invaluable material and staff support in the execution of the Chicago employer survey.

As the Principal Investigator, I wish to thank my stellar staff who worked long hours and who helped me conceptualize the project, work out a research design and strategy, and complete the extensive field work. All of them fit admirably in the mosaic of the division of labor required of a research project of this kind. I, therefore, wish to mention Lu Ann Aday, Ph.D., Co-Principal Investigator and Senior Research Associate and Associate Director for Research; Terry Herold, Project Director; Bruce Butler, Assistant Project Director; Claire Kohrman, Research Project Analyst; Ellen Morrison, Project Assistant; and the project's able Research Assistants—Lynn Seermon, Stuart Friedman, Marilyn Schlein, and Nancy Grab. L. Robert Burns and James Morone, Project Specialists, also provided invaluable conceptual and empirical input in the early stages of the project. Always in the background offering counsel and support was Ronald M. Andersen, Ph.D., Professor of Sociology, Graduate School of Business and Department of Sociology and Director for the Center for Health Administration Studies.

For typing numerous drafts, we are indebted to Dorothy Frazier, Annette Twells, Joyce Van Grondelle and June Veenstra.

Odin W. Anderson, Ph.D.
Emeritus Professor of Sociology
Graduate School of Business and
The Department of Sociology
University of Chicago
  and
Professor of Sociology
Department of Sociology
University of Wisconsin-Madison
June, 1984

Introduction

Group practice prepayment plans as a method of financing and delivering personal health services are peculiar to the United States. Insurance for personal health services is also peculiar to the United States certainly as regards its dominance as the major means of paying for day-to-day services. Group practice prepayment emerged in part as a reaction to the seeming looseness of the relationship between providers, insurers, and the member-patients. Ostensibly no one was in charge or perhaps all were in charge. The rapid rise of prices and expenditures for personal health services during the early 1970s stimulated interest in and growth of health maintenance organizations and prepaid-group-practice plans as a means of controlling the pace of rising expenditures, which the mainstream Blue Cross-Blue Shield plans and the private insurance companies seemed incapable of doing.

The emerging faith in group practice prepayment has resulted in the creation of several variants resting under the umbrella term of health maintenance organization (HMO). Only in the United States has this manner of activity been possible, because the open system of the voluntary hospital and the privately practicing physician, literally force-fed by a seemingly inexhaustible source of funding from employers, employees, and government over the past thirty years, led consumers, business and industry, and providers to support and develop parallel agencies called HMOs.

A health maintenance organization is a formally organized system of health care delivery that combines the delivery and

---

The introduction was written by Odin W. Anderson and Terry E. Herold.

financing functions and provides comprehensive services to an enrolled membership for a fixed, prepaid fee (Zelten, 1979). The term HMO is applied to a variety of organizational forms (Zelten, 1979; Wolinsky, 1980). While the term HMO is relatively new, health care organizations meeting this definition can be traced to the nineteenth century in the United States (Luft, 1981b).

HMOs followed the establishment and rapid growth of main-line health insurance plans as early as the 1940s and 1950s. Well-known examples include the Medical Bureaus in the state of Washington; the Kaiser Permanente Foundation on the West Coast; the Health Insurance Plan of Greater New York; and consumer cooperatives in Seattle, WA, St. Paul, MN, and Washington, D.C. The objectives of these early HMOs were mixed, but the primary one was to create a rational structure—combining providers, management, and budget in one organization with a known population to be served. It would seem that saving money was an incidental objective. The automobile analogy might not be a Cadillac but a Malibu. No one, though, proposed the Volkswagen Beetle as a model.

Given the private ownership of hospitals, the privately practicing physician in solo or group practice, and the various sources of funds for both daily operations and capital formation, the American pluralistic system provided a seedbed for the emergence of this dynamic diversity greased by the entrepreneurial style of American business, which also spills over to the personal health services. These services, however, are clothed with the public interest, so HMOs became ambiguous in how they were to survive in the market and at the same time be community-oriented institutions in competition with other forms of health service delivery.

One should remember that HMO variants evolved from a private practice model. Physicians had gradually joined together at such medical facilities as the Mayo Clinic in Rochester, MN, the Crile Clinic in Boston, and the Ochsner Clinic in New Orleans. Later, venturesome physicians and others built on this concept by adding prepayment. This kind of venture was exceedingly controversial in the mainstream medical community. Nevertheless, they took root as a natural method to incorporate the many medical specialties emerging, to stabilize a source of patients and funding, and to enable the public to have an orderly method of paying for services before illness struck.

In those early days, say thirty years ago, seemingly idiosyncratic factors fostered the emergence of group practice prepayment. Disparate beginnings converged into a movement, and sponsorships came from physician groups themselves, mainline insurance companies, corporations set up specifically for that purpose, and large hospitals. The key ingredient was capital—direct or indirect. The Health Maintenance Organization Act of 1973 helped to publicize the concept considerably, since it had some support in the Congress through the Nixon, Ford, Carter, and Reagan administrations. This is not to say that financial support for start-up costs was generous, nor is it easy to evaluate the impact of the act on HMO growth, but clearly the concept became better known to politicians, employers, and the general public.

Since the early 1970s, HMOs have developed in a variety of regions and communities. Impressionistically, certain community and regional characteristics are more amenable to HMO growth than others. Seattle, Rochester, MN, New York, Denver, San Francisco, Boston, and Minneapolis-St. Paul come to mind. Other areas, now in an early stage, are Chicago, Milwaukee, and Madison, WI.

RESEARCH ISSUES

Initial interest in HMOs (and their organizational precursors) centered on their ability to improve health care access and coverage. Current interest in HMOs centers on their ability to contain costs. In many ways, this shift in interest parallels that in national health care policy during the past three decades. While policy interest in HMOs shifted, research interest in HMOs focused on their performance (Luft, 1981a). Ironically, while federal policy initiatives in the late 1970s concentrated on introducing HMOs and on facilitating their growth, research conducted during this period did not include these issues.

The necessary ingredients for successful HMO introduction and growth have not been identified. Previous research has focused on microlevel determinants and indicators of HMO performance rather than on factors that affect the ability of HMOs to demonstrate significant impact. In addition to microlevel issues of performance, it is necessary to understand both internal and external factors affecting the growth and impact of HMOs. Because HMOs operate within the broad context of a community and a health care market, influential individuals and organizations can affect their acceptance and development. Furthermore, because HMOs are highly interdependent, they require the expertise and resources of all the parties involved in the health care system—physicians, hospitals, insurers, employers, consumers, and regulators. The overall impact that these parties have on the introduction and development of HMOs and the manner by which diverse interests can be accommodated in this process has not been fully documented.

Once HMOs are established and become viable, they affect the health care markets in which they operate. Few studies have focused on the impact of HMOs on other parties involved in health care. Although many claims have been made concerning the macrolevel effects of HMOs, systematic research has not documented the actual range of effects—positive or negative.

In recent years, policy makers, practitioners, and researchers have become increasingly interested in the concept of competition in health care markets. Strategies for increasing competition have occupied prominent positions in national health policy under recent administrations. Unfortunately, most of the proposals advanced to increase competition have been based on abstract theory rather than on careful observation of existing health care markets.

HMOs have occupied a central role in many proposals to encourage competition, but the changes wrought by HMOs in the structure and operation of the health care market are not fully understood. Few investigations have centered on the role of HMOs as competitive forces in the health care market or on the perception of competition by the principal parties in the health care market.

This study investigated these important unresolved topics. The issues chosen for investigation are relevant to policy makers, plan designers, implementors, managers, and health services researchers; and they complement existing research in the field. This study provides documentation of 1) the factors that affect the introduction and growth of HMOs; 2) the impact of HMOs on other parties involved in the health care system; and 3) the role of HMOs as a change agent in the health care system, particularly in introducing competitive forces. These research objectives are clearly related, and together they yield a comprehensive understanding of the development and impact of HMOs.

CONCEPTUAL FRAMEWORK

The conceptual framework that guided this study integrated basic tenets of the health systems and organizational approaches in health services research (Anderson and Kravits, 1968; Anderson, 1972; Shortell and Kaluzny, 1983). HMOs operate and adapt as one part of the whole health care system. An analysis of the development and impact of HMOs requires an understanding of the structure, operation, and development of the larger system. The whole health care system defines the potential for HMOs in terms of resource availability and a market for their services. Within this system, the internal structure and management of HMOs affects their growth and impact.

This study's conceptual framework recognizes the dynamic interplay between environmental and organizational variables in the development of HMOs. HMOs adapt to the health care markets where they operate and, in turn, affect other health care actors and organizations. The detailed methodology of this study follows in appendix A.

A major focus of this study is the integration of HMOs into the health care system. Hence, the study is developmental and historical in perspective. This approach recognizes the importance of the temporal dimension in the development of HMOs and the market for their services. It recognizes that certain factors may be differentially important at various times in the development sequence.

Finally, to fully understand the range and combination of factors affecting HMO development and impact, HMOs are examined within two health care markets displaying diverse characteristics. By observing HMOs in several health care markets, additional insights can be gained regarding the variability of factors under different environmental conditions. A comparative focus is important when analyzing the impact of HMOs on other components of the health care system. In addition, generalizations of HMO experiences can be better evaluated when more than one health care market is studied.

RESEARCH SITES

This study examines HMOs in two very different health care markets—Minneapolis-St. Paul and Chicago. Viewing HMOs in these two areas affords a better understanding of the developmental influences and system impacts that are common to all HMO markets and those that are market-specific.

The Minneapolis-St. Paul area has been declared an exemplar of HMO development in recent years. Their health care market has been seen as an example of the emerging role of competition, and HMOs were given much of the credit (Enthoven, 1980; Christianson and McClure, 1979). By 1981, seven HMOs had enrolled approximately 24 percent of the population. Recently, two HMOs merged, leaving six, an indication of the desire to expand and to hold their market positions. Also, all of the HMO organizational forms, from the staff model to the independent practice association (IPA) model, have been represented. This area has become, therefore, a natural experiment.

On the other hand, the HMO market in Chicago has displayed markedly slower development. By 1981, seven HMOs had enrolled approximately 3.5 percent of the metropolitan population. Several studies have been conducted to understand why HMO growth has proceeded at such a different rate there (ICF, 1980). Chicago has been an excellent study site because its HMOs appear to be approaching a takeoff point.

HMOs Surveyed (year of establishment, model)

Minneapolis-St. Paul:
  Group Health Plan (1957, staff)
  Ramsey Health Plan [now, Coordinated Health Care] (1972, network)
  MedCenter Health Plan (1972, network)
  Nicollet-Eitel Health Plan (1973, group)
  SHARE Health Plan (1973, staff/network)
  HMO Minnesota (1974, network/IPA)
  Physicians Health Plan (1975, IPA)

Chicago:
  Union Health Service (1955, staff)
  Anchor Organization for Health Maintenance (1971, staff)
  Intergroup [now, Maxicare/Intergroup] (1972, network)
  Michael Reese Health Plan (1972, group/staff)
  Co-Care [now, HMO Illinois] (1972, network)
  NorthCare [now, PruCare] (1975, group)
  Roosevelt Health Plan [now, Chicago HMO] (1976, network)
  Cooperative Health Plan (1982, IPA)

The Twin Cities' style of problem solving is consensual; Chicago's style is confrontational, arriving at a fairly low common denominator of compromise. Even so, both areas accept the operating premise that "nothing of importance is done in Chicago [or the Twin Cities] without its first being discovered what interests will be affected and how they will be affected and without the losses that will accrue to some being weighed carefully against the gains that will accrue to others. It is easy for Americans to take this kind of thing for granted, but there are cities—London, for example—where great decisions are made with little understanding of the consequences for those interests which are not plainly visible to the decision-makers" (Banfield, 1961).

In both the Twin Cities and Chicago, interest groups are plainly visible and vocal. Indeed, the political culture is open enough that this can be so. In the Twin Cities, however, as required by the consensus approach, public policy decision making is much more structured than in Chicago. The reason for this stems from the ethnic characteristics of early settlers, both American and foreign-born, in the two areas and, it would seem, the differences in population concentrations that facilitate or inhibit routine or spontaneous interactions between the groups that are part and parcel of the American political process.

Minneapolis-St. Paul: Homogeneity and consensus

The Twin Cities area was first settled by New Englanders and upstate New Yorkers, who opened this large and productive area to agriculture and commerce and established the legal system and political process. They were accustomed to a very local type of democracy and to nonprofessional politicians, who did not make a career of politics. They were also moralistic in their attitudes of the public good and were willing to work through government, if necessary, but hardly exclusively, in the public interest (Elazar, 1970). Still, public policy issues emanated from private and respected interest groups or consortia of them to be taken up in the official political process if so indicated. There was and is very little political corruption. By the turn of the century, these early American-born settlers from the Northeast were engulfed by Norwegians, Swedes, and Germans. Fortunately, the Scandinavians and Germans fit easily into the social and political matrix established by the early American-born settlers. The later settlers were accustomed to and insisted upon democratic political participation, and before long their names appeared on the rosters of political parties. In fact, the Scandinavians, who started the dairy industry and the grain fields, were the major force behind the establishment of the Farmer-Labor party as a protest against large business monopolies, railroads, and farm machinery manufacturers, and also distant Washington, which the party felt was controlled by big business. Big business and big government influenced the price of freight and the price of farm produce (Blegen, 1975; Nye, 1959; Gieske, 1979).

According to Nye, "the progressive [another name for Farmer-Laborites] wished to extend the power of the state in two ways: negatively, to use the power of government to limit and regulate capital and business, and positively, to use it to promote and protect the public social and economic welfare" (Nye, 1959). These farmers were also pragmatists. "The Midwest farmer wanted, as he always had, a good market with high prices, control of his own government, more currency, easier credit, and good times. The intellectual's Utopia was a trifle too complicated for him to take in all at once" (Nye, 1959). Ownership of his own land was a fundamental value.

In 1930, 59 percent of the population of the Twin Cities area were Swedes, Norwegians, and Germans, foreign-born or of foreign-born parents. Twenty-seven percent were Swedes; 19 percent were Norwegians; and 13 percent were Germans (Schmid, 1937). Thus, there is clear evidence of the preponderance of these ethnic groups. Although they were upwardly mobile, they had not yet reached top-level positions in business and industry. Their names were more likely to appear in politics, but there was turnover. They did not seem to remain professional politicians like the Irish in Chicago.

In the early 1940s, a voluntary association of citizens concerned with local problems was gradually created. The Citizens League had its beginnings in an older generation of civic and political leadership in Minneapolis. Younger persons in locally based business and industry were moving into leadership positions. For about ten years they met informally, usually for lunch at the YMCA, to discuss public issues. They were organized loosely without staff in a network that was called Good Government Groups (Citizens League, 1976).

In 1951, a report of the Citizens League stimulated by Hubert Humphrey, mayor of Minneapolis, pointed to a revival of public life. In all probability, this revival followed the singled-minded national objective of winning World War II; communities across the United States began to look at local problems. Minneapolis became a prime example. There was then an effort to strengthen the capacity "to provide careful, objective research on important local problems" (Citizens League, 1976).

Apparently, similar moves were in motion in Seattle and Cleveland, for discussions were held with similar groups there. In 1951, the Citizens League was formed in Minneapolis. It was guaranteed $30,000 a year for three years by local firms, and the first staff was hired in early 1952. It is interesting to note that an early function of the league was to review and rate candidates for local political office. Given the desired nonpartisan nature of the league, this became difficult to do well and credibly. This created factions rather than consensus and was quickly dropped. More in line with the purpose of the Citizens League, the emphasis while building membership was on "retailing" information to the community. They sponsored large public meetings (2,700 came to hear Frank Lloyd Wright in 1956), publications, and radio and television programs. Gradually, as the league got deeper into issues, its role changed to that of a "wholesaler" to specific persons working on public affairs issues in other organizations. Also, the league acted as a community sounding board for proposals initiated by local government, such as, "Should the new library be located at Fourth and Nicollet?"

Apparently, in 1962 there was a breakthrough for the league as an agency for policy discussions by citizens when it reviewed the proposal of the school board for the first major building program since the 1920s. The league rejected the notion of rehabilitation of old buildings and proposed instead a replacement program involving closing and demolishing whole schools. The Minneapolis community rejected the proposal of the school board and accepted the one from the league.

Eventually the Citizens League expanded to involve the whole Twin Cities area. Currently the league has around three thousand individual members with dues of $25 a year per family or $15 per individual. There is a renewal rate of 90 percent. Around $240,000 a year is contributed by six hundred local business firms. As is true of all voluntary groups, which try to address the public interest, "it is a struggle to get enough diversity" of membership from a cross-section of society (Citizens League, 1976). The creation of consensus is helped considerably, however, by the homogeneous population, the occupational structure, and the relatively high educational and income level of the area. One observer was moved to quip, "The Twin Cities is a middle class area with middle class problems" (Morone, 1982). Still, the league cannot implement its own recommendations directly. It contributes ideas, but it has no official status nor the financial resources necessary for implementation. Nevertheless, it has credibility and influence because it is an organization with a network of ties throughout the community. This is a prime example, it would seem, of pluralism at its best, a structured rather than a chaotic one.

The other overall community agency, a product of the political system (the state government) and established after the Citizens League (in 1967), is the Metropolitan Council. It may seem reasonable to assume that one needed to follow the other; the league to anticipate overall community issues, the council to help implement policy recommendations from the league. Life being what it is, i.e., complicated, the differentiation in function may not be that clear, but the blurred outlines are there nevertheless.

As is typical of metropolises in the Midwest, there is a fantastic variety of local government units. In 1977, there were a total of 273 governments in the Twin Cities. If the twenty-three housing and redevelopment authorities are counted, the total number of "governments" approaches three hundred. In the Chicago area, the situation is essentially the same (Karlen, 1958). The Twin Cities, however, have succeeded in establishing an official umbrella agency that transcends these many local government units to act on problems that are regional rather than local, such as sewage disposal, water supply, a network of urban highways, and recreational land.

Since the inception of the Metropolitan Council in 1967, its role and authority have evolved to the point where the council has been able to establish metropolitan policies for a wide range of public services. Further, it has acquired the power to enforce certain policies on the other 272 governments in the metropolitan area. "This evolution of the Metropolitan Council's responsibilities has been unprecedented in American local government" (Harrigan and Johnson, 1978).

Within the context of the organizations and activities of the Citizens League and the Metropolitan Council there were other developments as well, if not influenced directly by the league and the council, certainly indicating that other voluntary agencies of one kind or another were expressions of the problem-solving style indigenous to the area. It is to be noted that the hospital planning process began formally as early as 1962 with the formation of the St. Paul Planning Council (Citizens League, 1977). The Planning Agency for Hospitals of Metropolitan Minneapolis was created in 1964. The two agencies developed a joint staff in 1966 and in 1969 consolidated to form the Metropolitan Hospital Planning Agency.

The Metropolitan Council's role in health planning began in 1968 with a federal grant to develop a comprehensive health planning program as envisaged by the federal Comprehensive Health Planning Act of 1966. The Metropolitan Hospital Planning Agency, the Health and Welfare Planning Councils, and the Citizens League participated. The Metropolitan Council was designated as the so-called B Agency. To satisfy the Comprehensive Health Planning Act, the council established an advisory body called the Metropolitan Health Board. A major function of the board was to develop the section of the Metropolitan Development Guide that was the Metropolitan Council's regional policy plan for the future provision of health services, facilities, and personnel. This first plan was jointly formulated by the council and health board with participation from providers and consumers in the area, the public and private sectors, and the official health services. In the meantime, the Minnesota legislature enacted a certificate-of-need law for hospitals in 1971, thus giving official sanction to emerging voluntary actions. This collectively formulated regional plan emphasized containing the expansion of acute hospital and nursing home services, expanding primary care services based on needs identified by each county, and encouraging the growth of HMOs. This type of locally initiated planning continued until the National Health Planning and Resources Development Act of 1974. Under this law the Metropolitan Council was conditionally named as the Health Systems Agency (HSA) for the seven-county area. Full designation was accorded in 1978.

It should be noted that in the Twin Cities there were no competing applicants or major conflicts, as in Chicago, regarding the formation and control of the HSA. There was no polarization of factions, reflecting the consensual character of the area. The HSA in the Twin Cities was regarded as a legitimate political actor from the beginning. Under state law, the Metropolitan Health Board functions primarily as the Metropolitan Council's health planning arm and chief advisor in health matters. Responsibility is shared with the Minnesota Certificate of Need Act of 1971.

As to operating style, the importance of this style can hardly be overemphasized. Morone observed that the members of the Metropolitan Health Board had developed an extremely active system of formal and informal connections. Issues are discussed in detail over the telephone or at lunch, and the board and staff members know each other well (Morone, 1982). There are heavy time commitments and few reported less than twenty hours a week of his or her time devoted to board problems. Thus, the members are very sophisticated, very knowledgable consumers. Some seemed more like professionals than volunteers.

One indication of this level of sophistication, both in the board members and the politicians in the Minnesota legislature, is that the legislature has abolished the certificate-of-need law, which was passed in 1971 (before the Health Planning Act of 1974), effective in 1984, pending the language of the current revisions being discussed in Congress regarding the future of the federal Health Planning Act. Minnesota thereby intends to test the competitive concept as far as possible.

We have held off until near the end to assess the influence of a very specific goal-directed agency, InterStudy, headed by Paul Ellwood, M.D. Ellwood, a pediatrician, was a staff member of the Sister Kenny Institute for Rehabilitation. Through the rehabilitation process, he developed the belief that personal health services needed to be integrated into one service component rather than "fragmented," as in the mainline delivery system. He was, and is, very wary of regulation as well, and in a short time he became a leading theoretician and proponent of HMOs and competitive options to increase efficiency and contain costs. In the 1970s, he singlehandedly used the Twin Cities area as a proving ground for HMOs and the competitive options concept. He did so by going to the employers from whom most of the money through fringe benefits was coming. He addressed meetings of business and industry leaders one after another. His approach was low-key and analytical, a missionary who did not look and behave like one. InterStudy became an agency to collect data and operate as a think tank, supposedly neutral on the side of the competitive concept and HMOs. Ellwood helped several young people become HMO administrators in the Twin Cities. His influence was immeasurable. It is interesting to speculate what would have happened in the Twin Cities and to the HMO competitive concept had he not been there. The same can be said of Walter McClure, who was brought in on Ellwood's staff. McClure now has his own health policy agency near the University of Minnesota campus. The juxtaposition of the problem-solving style of the Twin Cities and Ellwood, a native of California, is one of those rare combinations of circumstances, and Ellwood was aware of it, as is evident in his training and method of operation.

Chicago: Diversity and confrontation

While prepaid-group-practice plans in Chicago can be traced as far back as the Great Depression, the move toward HMOs in the Chicago area started later than the Twin Cities. Now it is gathering momentum. HMOs in Chicago operate in a very different context from those in the Twin Cities. This fact shows that the HMO and the competitive option concept is not peculiar to a particular part of the country. The Twin Cities and Chicago areas share basically the same personal health services delivery structure characteristic of the entire United States—voluntary hospitals and private practicing physicians, solo and group, funded by health insurance and federal and state governments. Expenditures have been rising rapidly everywhere, and employers are clearly restive. The differences are a matter of degree. The perceived problems are the same, but the style of meeting these problems differs. Both areas share in the pluralistic interest group political process, but the Twin Cities' is structured and consensual, as has been described. The Chicago process is adversarial and confrontational.

The history of the Chicago area began as early settlers, of old American or Anglo-Saxon descent, developed the region as a transportation hub and manufacturing center. Unlike the Twin Cities, these early settlers were engulfed by a variety of immigrants from all of Europe. The population was a conglomeration, exacerbated by racial prejudice against the increasing numbers of blacks after World War I and spearheaded politically by the Irish, with their extended family propensities rippling over into the political machine. The Chicago development was unmanageable and hence wide-open and heady. From this matrix evolved Chicago's style of problem solving.

Perhaps most illustrative of the differences between the

Twin Cities and Chicago is the volume and, by some criteria, the kind of historical and political literature on the two metropolitan areas. Literature about the Twin Cities is self-conscious, consistent, and abundant, as revealed in the foregoing section. It was easy to construct a historical and current matrix there, but not so for Chicago. Literature about Chicago is fragmented and difficult to put together. One person who grasped the essence of Chicago in one ringing phrase was a poet, Carl Sandburg who called it, the "city of the big shoulders." But the city seems to be much more complex than during Sandburg's time. Writers have been fascinated by the political and psychological presence of Richard J. Daley and by the race riots following the assassination of the Reverend Martin Luther King, Jr. as well as the riots during the 1968 Democratic Convention (Gleason, 1970; Royko, 1971). Others have studied bits and pieces of the overall matrix of the city (Banfield, 1961; Greenstone and Peterson, 1973; Janowitz, 1967). Over thirty years ago, Philip Hauser, a demographer, carved out seventy-one Chicago communities (Hauser and Kitagawa, 1953). Mayer, a geographer, and Wade, a historian, compiled a marvelous ecological growth pattern with pictures of the development of Chicago (Mayer and Wade, 1969).

Chicago is bigger both in area and population than the Twin Cities. The Twin Cities metropolitan area has two million people; the Chicago area has seven million. The whole Twin Cities metropolitan area could fit within the city limits of Chicago. Chicago has many more clusters of buyers and decision makers in health services delivery and a hierarchy of business clubs that make it more difficult to facilitate the almost casual interactions that seem to characterize the Twin Cities area. Banfield, a student of urban politics, observed that there are fundamental conflicts of interest and opinions among Chicago's business leaders. Some of these differences are on business grounds alone. What is good for the owners of the downtown hotels is not good for the amphitheatre; what is good for real estate north of the Chicago river is not good for real estate in the Loop, and so on (Banfield, 1961). He continues, "To suppose that these conflicts would be resolved if the top leaders met at lunch is naive." According to Kilian, a journalist, the business establishment breaks down into five groups: utilities, retailers, manufacturers, big conglomerates, and transportation specialists (Kilian, et al., 1979).

Both areas have a multiplicity of governments. The Twin Cities have been able to transcend this complexity by the creation of the Metropolitan Council. The Chicago metropolitan area has no such umbrella agency. The city and the suburbs are especially antagonistic. The area cannot create a central transportation authority for its sprawling population. All issues become highly politicized to lower-common-denominator politics (Karlen, 1958).

The decision-making clusters in the health services delivery system are also numerous—five medical schools, six or so large medical complexes, all struggling now for their own turfs. The area was not able to establish an HSA under the Health Service Planning Act of 1974 without a fight between the mayor's office, which wanted the agency to be controlled by the city council, and the Chicago Community Health Planning Council, which wanted to minimize direct political control. When agency approval by the state came up in early 1976, Governor Walker blocked the Daley administration. The mayor's proposal was criticized by the Governor for lack of consumer representation on the proposed agency's Board of Governors. The board's slate was dominated by city office holders (Kilian, et al., 1979). The Governor also withheld approval from the competing HSA application. The State Commissioner of Health urged the two groups to get together. Finally, the HSA was put under the city council, but it met the stipulations for consumer representation required by the law. In that law, elected politicians are not consumers. Also, the planning area was the city limits of Chicago. The suburbs were not overlapped with natural market areas of city and suburbs. There was a scramble between counties containing suburban areas and the city of Chicago. As stated by a *Chicago Tribune* reporter, "Competition for control of health spending and planning in the nine county Chicago metropolitan area entered a new round this week amid continued controversy and litigation" (Pearre, 1976).

Still, bubbling up in this steaming cauldron were actions symptomatic of the health services delivery problems everywhere. Early in 1972, Illinois inaugurated the Hospital Admission Surveillance Program for Medicaid patients in several major hospitals in Chicago. Contracts for surveillance of admissions were made with the Chicago Medical Society. This agency parallels the one created by the Hennepin County Medical Society in Minneapolis-St. Paul for the same purpose. Both are now contracting with business groups that want some surveillance over the hospital use of their employees (Pearre, 1976).

Also in 1972, the Illinois State Chamber of Commerce sponsored a study that found "inefficient" operation of many hospitals involving vacant beds and duplicated services. The chamber undertook the study at the request of a number of large industries, which felt they paid too much for employee health care benefits (Wolfe, 1972). Later, a certificate-of-need law for hospital beds was recommended. In May 1974, Governor Walker recommended rate regulation for hospitals (Kotulak, 1972). Late in 1975, the Illinois Health Facilities Planning Board conducted a survey of the supply of hospital beds and declared that the Chicago area had an excess over need of 7,675 beds, but shortages were identified on Chicago's south side and sections of south and northwest Cook County. It was estimated that the Chicago metropolitan area had 25,500 beds, so 30 percent were regarded as unnecessary.

Early in 1970, the Chicago Hospital Council, a federation of hospitals in the Chicago area, and its member hospitals sponsored a massive study of the hospital emergency services in the area to assist in classfying hospitals for emergency purposes (Gibson, et al., 1970). The council has also been instrumental in promoting and operating a shared services program in the Chicago area.

Early in the 1970s, Rush-Presbyterian-St. Luke's Medical Center established a prepaid-group-practice plan called Anchor. Likewise, the Michael Reese Hospital and Medical Center established a plan called the Michael Reese Health Plan. Both grew slowly, and in due course, established satellites in the suburbs. A consumer-governed plan started by four homemakers in Evanston in 1974 received a great deal of publicity. Their cause was noble, but their operation was rocky even with grants from Washington. In 1982, they sold the plan to the Prudential Insurance Company. NorthCare, now PruCare, simply did not have the historical tradition of cooperatives nor the kind of market that could sustain that plan—school teachers and civil servants. The CNA Insurance Company established an HMO, but eventually sold out to Maxicare, a California firm specializing in HMO development. These events are described to give an indication of the mixture of local and external sponsorship and ownership of HMOs in Chicago. There are now many HMOs in the Chicago metropolitan area.

The rate review of hospitals started in Illinois a few years ago has since been abandoned. The certificate-of-need law is still intact. Minnesota has or intends to abandon its certificate-of-need law to test competition. Rate setting so far is carried out on a quasi-voluntary nature. Minnesota appears to formulate and execute their policies within a structured framework as described at length previously. Illinois policy formulation is ad hoc, responding to interest group pressures one issue at a time.

So far, it seems that the major umbrella group on the horizon is the business coalition, both in Chicago and in the Midwest region. Unlike the Twin Cities area, however, business and industry do not have the structure to function cooperatively with many, often conflicting, interests.

1

Minneapolis-St. Paul and Chicago

Market conditions have been more favorable to HMO development in Minneapolis-St. Paul than in Chicago. For example, in the Twin Cities one finds greater population growth, more in-migration, and more families with children. The population there is younger, less ethnically diverse, and better educated. There is less unemployment and, among the employed, more white collar workers and a smaller proportion of the labor force in manufacturing. Among providers there are more general practitioners, as well as higher hospital utilization and costs and lower hospital occupancy rates than in Chicago.

To gain a perspective on the development of HMOs in Minneapolis-St. Paul and Chicago, it is necessary to describe the community and health systems characteristics of each area. The environment in which HMOs develop can be categorized according to the following elements: 1) individual and corporate consumers, 2) health care facilities and personnel, and 3) health care financing mechanisms. This chapter presents longitudinal descriptive data relevant to each element to provide a basis for analyzing the relationships between HMOs and their environments in Minneapolis-St. Paul and Chicago. This chapter also presents comparative market area case studies of the Minneapolis-St. Paul and Chicago metropolitan areas and draws heavily on the hypotheses and results generated by other types of studies as well. A brief discussion of each of the major types of previous research follows.

This chapter was written by Bruce W. Butler, Assistant Project Director.

PREVIOUS RESEARCH

Previous research that has addressed the relationship of HMO development to quantifiable environmental characteristics falls into three major categories: multivariate market area analyses, which attempt to identify factors that are positively or negatively related to HMO development in a large number of market areas; HMO enrollment studies, which provide insight into the types of consumers that are more or less likely to join HMOs; and market area case studies, which focus on characteristics of particular markets and attempt either to explain unique patterns of HMO development in those areas or predict the prospects for future growth.

Multivariate market area analyses

Several studies in recent years employed the multivariate market area analysis to explain differential patterns of HMO introduction and/or development across states or cities (McNeil and Schlenker, 1975; Keller, 1981; Luft, 1981; Goldberg and Greenberg, 1981; Morrisey and Ashby, 1981). Results across these studies are not strictly comparable and do not form a clear conclusion, primarily because of differences in study design. Varieties of dependent variables are used, and some of the studies use formal tests of the significance of observed relationships, while others point out monotonic patterns or mean categorical differences. The figure that follows presents a general overview of factors that have been at least tentatively identified as related to HMO introduction or development in one or more of these studies. As is shown in the table, opposite relationships were suggested by different studies for several of the factors.

Enrollment studies

While research efforts in the area of HMO enrollment choice have been much more numerous than in the area of multivariate market area analyses, levels of comparability and contribution to a clear consensus remain limited. In part, this is due to the variety of research questions that have been addressed through enrollment studies, ranging from evaluations of self-selection patterns according to health status to evaluations of possible

Previous Research: Positive (+) or Negative (—) Effects of Market Characteristics on HMO Introduction and Development

	Multivariate Market Area Studies	Enrollment Studies	Market Area Case Studies
Demographic Characteristics			
Population size (HMO introduction)	+		
Population size (HMO growth)	+		
Population size (HMO market share)	—		
Population density	+		
Population growth	+		+
Population mobility	+	+	
Younger population	—		+
Younger larger families		+	
Higher income levels	+/—	—	+
Higher education levels	+		
Prevalence of racial minorities	—		
Employment Characteristics			
Prevalence of manufacturing employment	+/—		—
Prevalence of wholesale/retail employment			—
Prevalence of government employment			+
Prevalence of white collar employment			+
High rates of unionization	+/—		—
High unemployment rates			—
Prevalence of major medical benefits	+		
Health System Characteristics			
Physician density	+		+
Older physicians	+/—		
Younger physicians			+
Hospital bed density	—		+
Hospital occupancy rates	—		—
Hospital expenses	+		+

differences in the appeal of HMOs according to economic status. Conclusions about which there are high levels of agreement, however, are that HMOs have a differentially greater appeal to younger and larger families (Berki and Ashcraft, 1980), to persons with moderately low discretionary incomes, and to persons without a preexisting relationship with a physician (Berki, et al., 1978) or without a preexisting and continuous enrollment in fee-for-service health insurance (Yedidia, 1959). As a proxy for the prevalence of persons without preexisting relationships with physicians or insurers, the prevalence of persons who have recently moved from other areas can be examined. In short, enrollment studies point to family characteristics, population mobility, and income as factors that may affect HMO development.

Market area case studies

Case studies addressing the prospects for HMO development have been conducted for many market areas, including Chicago (ICF, 1980), Philadelphia (ICF, 1980), and Denver (Christianson, 1980). The only major environmental factor considered by the ICF studies was the prevalence of collectively bargained health benefit plans, but Christianson's case study of Denver considered a wide variety of environmental factors thought to affect the prospects of multiple HMO development and subsequent competition in the Denver area. The relationships proposed in these market area case studies are summarized in the figure above.

GEOGRAPHIC UNITS OF ANALYSIS

The geographic unit that is used most extensively in this chapter is the Standard Metropolitan Statistical Area (SMSA). Defined by the U.S. Bureau of the Census, an SMSA is comprised of at least one county containing a central city of 50,000 inhabitants or more, and the contiguous counties, which are socially and economically integrated with the central city. For example, counties from which large numbers of people commute to work in a central city are likely to be included in an SMSA.

Minneapolis-St. Paul

The Twin Cities metropolitan area is centered on Minneapolis on the west bank of the Mississippi River and St. Paul on the east bank. The two cities are included in and surrounded by Hennepin and Ramsey counties, respectively. Other counties containing substantial portions of the metropolitan population include Anoka to the north, Washington to the east, and Dakota to the south. Outlying counties include Scott and Carver to the southwest, Wright to the northwest, Chisago to the northeast, and St. Croix (Wisconsin) to the east. Some cross-commutation may occur with a neighboring SMSA (Eau Claire, Wisconsin) but probably not to the extent that overall social and economic indicators would be disturbed.

The Minneapolis-St. Paul SMSA has undergone significant changes since 1950 to reflect changing development and residence patterns. The original SMSA definition used for the 1950 census included four counties: Hennepin and Ramsey counties, which respectively contain the central cities of Minneapolis and St. Paul, and the suburban Anoka and Dakota counties. In 1958, Washington County was added to the SMSA. This definition was used for both the 1960 and 1970 censuses. In 1973, five additional counties were added: Carver, Chisago, St. Croix (Wisconsin), Scott, and Wright. This definition remained in use for the 1980 census.

The changing SMSA definition presents some problems in the longitudinal analysis of social and economic characteristics. However, 85 percent of the 1980 SMSA population is located in areas which were included in the 1950 SMSA definitions; thus, the social and economic characteristics of the SMSA as a whole have probably not been influenced heavily by the addition of six new counties since 1950.

A second commonly used geographic classification, particularly for local planning and regulatory purposes, is the Health Service Area. The Twin Cities Health Service Area is under the planning jurisdiction of the Metropolitan Health Board. The counties included in this geographic unit are: Anoka, Carver, Dakota, Hennepin, Ramsey, Scott, and Washington. In addition to serving as the unit of analysis for a large body of data collected by planning and regulatory agencies, the Twin Cities Health Service Area is also useful because it has remained stable over time.

Chicago

The Chicago SMSA encompasses 3,724 square miles and includes six counties: Cook, DuPage, Kane, Lake, McHenry, and Will. The city of Chicago is located at the eastern edge of the

SMSA and is surrounded by Lake Michigan on the east and suburban Cook County on all other sides. The other counties in turn surround Cook, with Lake to the north, McHenry to the far northwest, DuPage to the west, Kane to the far west, and Will to the south and southwest. In contrast to the Minneapolis-St. Paul SMSA, the Chicago SMSA definition has remained stable since 1960, when Lake County, Indiana, was dropped from the Chicago SMSA and added to the new Gary-Hammond-East Chicago SMSA. It is worth noting that several complications may arise in using the Chicago SMSA for a unit of market area analysis. For example, extensive commuting may occur between the Chicago SMSA and the contiguous Kenosha (Wisconsin) and Gary-Hammond-East Chicago (Indiana) SMSAs. Also, several cities on the western fringe of the Chicago SMSA, such as Joliet and Aurora, may·be sufficiently large, independent, and distant from Chicago to strain the SMSA concept of social and economic integration with a single central urban area. These cities may actually serve as centers of social and economic activity in their own right, drawing involvement from areas just outside the Chicago SMSA. Despite these complications, however, the great magnitude of social and economic activity wholly contained within the Chicago SMSA ensures that the SMSA retains a high degree of usefulness as a discrete unit of market area analysis.

CHARACTERISTICS OF TWO HEALTH CARE MARKETS

Population size, distribution, and growth

Population serves as the most basic indicator of health services market size. A large SMSA may provide HMOs with an extensive pool of potential consumers, but the market may be so diffuse as to make information transfer difficult. To escape this difficulty, HMOs in large metropolitan areas may seek more manageable market niches that are separated along dimensions of geography, size and type of employer group, socioeconomic status, etc. In contrast, small SMSAs may present HMOs with a more manageable marketing task but offer, of course, a smaller pool of potential consumers. Population growth, especially growth due to in-migration from other areas, is thought to affect HMOs positively due to correlation with the number of persons who are making active choices regarding health care providers and insurance plans. Overall U.S. metropolitan growth rates by decade have been decreasing, from 33.6 percent over 1950 to 1960 to 10.2 percent over 1970 to 1980.

The Minneapolis-St. Paul SMSA is the fifteenth largest in the U.S. Approximately 2.1 million people were distributed fairly evenly across its geographic areas in 1980. With approximately 7.1 million inhabitants in 1980, Chicago is ranked as the third largest SMSA in the country. Its population is fairly centralized, with 74 percent residing in Cook County. Tables 1.1 through 1.6 present population statistics for both areas.

Both the Chicago and Minneapolis-St. Paul SMSAs have experienced population growth rates below the overall U.S. metropolitan rates during all decades for which data was collected, with the one exception of Minneapolis-St. Paul over 1960 to 1970. In all three decades, Minneapolis-St. Paul growth rates were higher than Chicago rates. Rates of in-migration from out-of-state were higher in the Minneapolis-St. Paul SMSA than in the Chicago SMSA.

Age distribution

The age distribution of a market area population is important in that it provides a gross indicator of relative health status and may have some relation to the degree of the population's integration into the health care system. For example, older persons may be more likely to have ongoing relationships with physicians and more stable employment and health insurance coverage, thus decreasing their likelihood of switching health care delivery and financing systems. In addition, age structure variables that indicate a prevalence of families with young children are noteworthy since enrollment choice studies have identified this group as relatively likely to join HMOs.

In the metropolitan U.S., the proportion of persons under age 5 has been declining since 1960, while the proportion of persons age 65 and older has been increasing. Limited data on the median ages of aggregate metropolitan areas is available, but for the U.S. as a whole the median age dropped from 30.2 in 1950 to 27.9 in 1970, and rose to 30.0 in 1980 (table 1.7). The overall pattern is dominated by the well-documented "baby boom" in the 1950s and 1960s, followed by a gradual aging of the population.

Since 1960, median ages for the Minneapolis-St. Paul SMSA

have been lower than for the U.S., while those for the Chicago SMSA have been higher. These differences can be attributed most clearly to the structure of the working-age (18 to 64) population. For Minneapolis-St. Paul, the percentage in the 18 to 44 category is relatively high, but the percentage in the 45 to 64 age category is relatively low; the opposite holds for Chicago. Other factors contributing to the differences in median ages are that the 65-and-older population percentage has increased less rapidly in the Minneapolis-St. Paul SMSA than in Chicago or the metropolitan U.S. and that the percentage of persons under 18, higher than the metropolitan U.S. in both Minneapolis-St. Paul and Chicago, was particularly high for Minneapolis-St. Paul in 1960 and 1970. Thus, the Minneapolis-St. Paul SMSA can be characterized as having a relatively young population with a large proportion of young adults, and the Chicago SMSA can be characterized as having a relatively old population with a larger proportion of older working-age adults.

Racial and ethnic composition

In previous research, ethnic heterogeneity has been suggested as an inhibiting factor to the development of HMOs, particularly staff and group model HMOs with limited delivery sites, because of fragmentation of the health care system into discreet units that serve particular ethnic groups. It has been suggested that racial or ethnic groups, which traditionally have been associated with poorer health status, may be unattractive as target markets for HMOs (Morrisey and Ashby, 1981).

In the metropolitan U.S. as a whole, the black population increased by one percentage point of the population between 1970 and 1980, from 11.6 percent to 12.6 percent (table 1.8). The "other nonwhite" category grew substantially over this period, from 1.4 percent in 1970 to 5.8 percent of the population in 1980. The Hispanic proportion of the metropolitan U.S. population also grew, from 5.8 percent in 1970 to 7.5 percent in 1980.

Compared to the metropolitan U.S. as a whole, Chicago exhibits relatively large nonwhite and Hispanic segments of the population, while Minneapolis-St. Paul exhibit relatively small nonwhite and Hispanic segments. Prevalent European ancestry groups in the Chicago SMSA include German, Irish, Italian, and Polish, while in the Minneapolis-St. Paul SMSA groups with German and Scandinavian ancestry are predominant (table 1.9).

Income and poverty status

The economic status of the population has a variety of potential implications for HMO development. People with higher incomes may be better able to budget for out-of-pocket, fee-for-service health expenditures and therefore be less attracted by the generally more comprehensive coverage of HMOs. Alternatively, high incomes in an area may be indicative of relatively generous wages and fringe benefits. If fee-for-service health insurance benefits are highly comprehensive, developing HMOs may find it easier to compete with established insurers on a premium basis, facilitating their acceptance by employers. People with low incomes might prefer the comprehensive nature of HMOs, but if their employee health benefits are contributory, they might not be able to afford the additional payroll deductions that might be required to enroll. Those with no health benefits at all, as well as the unemployed, might also have difficulty affording HMO premium payments. People with extremely low incomes who are eligible for categorical public sector health care programs present HMOs with a differential segment of the market that they may choose to pursue through contracts with the relevant governmental agencies. Tables 1.10 and 1.11 illustrate some basic indicators of income and poverty status.

Both Minneapolis-St. Paul and Chicago exhibit median family and per capita income levels that are higher than the metropolitan U.S. levels. This may reflect regional variations in wages and costs of living. Trends in income levels in Minneapolis-St. Paul and Chicago have crossed since 1960, with the Chicago metropolitan area exhibiting higher income levels at that time and the Minneapolis-St. Paul metropolitan area exhibiting higher income levels in 1980. The proportions of the population in the poor and near poor categories are consistently lower in the Minneapolis-St. Paul SMSA than in the Chicago SMSA. These proportions have remained fairly stable in the Minneapolis-St. Paul SMSA since 1970. The percentages of families and persons in the poor and near poor categories in the Chicago SMSA rose considerably from 1970 to 1980.

Educational attainment

Multivariate analyses have suggested a tentative relationship between higher levels of educational attainment in a metropolitan area and the likelihood of HMO introduction and development there. This result could be caused by a variety of factors, including a greater willingness to adopt innovations in general, a greater willingness or ability to undertake complex consumer decisions, or the fact that education levels are correlated with several other important variables, such as income and age. Levels of educational attainment in the metropolitan U.S. have risen dramatically since 1960 (table 1.12).

Educational attainment levels in the Minneapolis-St. Paul SMSA are considerably higher than in the Chicago SMSA or the metropolitan U.S. This difference has been increasing for school completion percentages, but it has been decreasing for median years of school completed.

Household and family characteristics

Studies of enrollment patterns have suggested that HMOs have a particularly high appeal to large, young families. Table 1.13 presents data on average household size and the percentage of families with children under 6 years of age and under 18 years of age. For the metropolitan U.S. as a whole, there is a trend since 1960 of decreasing household size and percentage of families with children. Average household size declined from 3.23 in 1960 to 2.73 in 1980, while the percentage of families with children under 18 years old declined from 56.8 percent to 54.3 percent.

Despite an overall decline, the Minneapolis-St. Paul SMSA displayed a consistently larger percentage of families with children under 6 and under 18 than the Chicago SMSA. Average household size was also smaller in Chicago in 1960 and 1970 but was larger than in the Twin Cities in 1980. Thus, the Minneapolis-St. Paul SMSA can be characterized as having a relatively large percentage of families with children. Household size, however, is an imperfect proxy for family size, so it does not exhibit a clear pattern.

Employment patterns

The employed population constitutes the primary market for most HMOs. Marketing to this population is a two-stage process. HMOs must first convince employers of the attractiveness of their services. Employers may then allow HMOs the opportunity of convincing employees likewise. Tables 1.14 through 1.22 present data on employers by size, location, and type in the Twin Cities and Chicago metropolitan areas; the extent and distribution by sector of employment; the extent of unionization; and the extent of eligibility for various types of health insurance benefits. Previous research has suggested that white collar and unionized employment and the prevalence of major medical benefits may be positively related to HMO development, yet the prevalence of large manufacturers may be negatively related to HMO development. Other correlates of the above factors may also be important, including government employment (white collar, unionized) and wholesale/retail employment (relatively low benefit levels). Commuting patterns may be important in defining the relative ease with which HMOs may develop adequate service networks.

In the Minneapolis-St. Paul and Chicago SMSAs, equivalent proportions of private sector employers are located in the counties that contain central cities: 75 percent in Hennepin and Ramsey and 75 percent in Cook. The distribution for employers of 1,000 or more workers is also quite similar in the two SMSAs: 84 percent in Hennepin and Ramsey and 82 percent in Cook. The percentage of workers who both reside and are employed in the central cities declined between 1960 and 1970 in both areas, with a more marked decline in the Minneapolis-St. Paul SMSA. In the Minneapolis-St. Paul SMSA, this decline was partially compensated by an increase in the percentage of workers commuting in from the suburbs. In the Chicago SMSA, commuting in from the suburbs became less prevalent as well, resulting in a stronger shift in employment to the suburbs than was evident in the Minneapolis-St. Paul SMSA.

Manufacturers are the most prevalent employers of 250 or more workers in both SMSAs, but they are more dominant in Chicago than in Minneapolis-St. Paul, where service establishments run a close second. Compared to Chicago, the Minneapolis-St. Paul SMSA has higher percentages of the workforce in white collar occupations, wholesale/retail trade, and government. Labor force participation rates are higher in the Minneapolis-St. Paul SMSA and unemployment rates are lower. Unionization is more extensive in Chicago for all industries combined and for the manufacturing sector, but for nonmanufacturing industries, unionization is slightly more extensive in the Twin Cities for plant workers and less extensive for office workers.

In the Twin Cities SMSA, there is a small segment of plant

workers (4 to 5 percent) who are not eligible for hospitalization insurance, the most basic type of health benefit. Aside from this, health benefits in the Twin Cities appear to be somewhat more generous than in Chicago, with a greater prevalence of major medical and noncontributory plans. There is a much greater prevalence of HMO eligibility in the Twin Cities. In both areas, office workers are more likely to be offered an HMO than are plant workers, but office workers are less likely to be offered a noncontributory HMO.

HEALTH CARE FACILITIES AND PERSONNEL

Health care facilities and personnel constitute the basic resources on which HMOs depend to perform their health services delivery functions. Various characteristics of physicians and hospitals in a particular metropolitan area may affect the course of HMO development, and indicators of hospital utilization may provide some insights into the effect of HMOs on the medical care market.

Physicians

The willingness of physicians to participate in HMOs or to actively oppose HMOs is a potentially important determinant of HMO development. While direct quantitative information linking physician attitudes with HMO development is scarce, previous research has used proxy measures. Physician-to-population ratios are thought to reflect both a greater sensitivity of physicians to the loss of patients to HMOs and a greater willingness to secure their patient base and referral patterns by affiliating with HMOs. Older physicians are thought to be less susceptible to this pressure since they are more likely to have developed secure, stable practices. Younger physicians are thought to be more susceptible to this form of competition and may also be attracted to the relatively low costs of establishing a practice within a group or staff model HMO. Areas where group practice is prevalent are thought to be relatively supportive of HMO development since physicians and patients alike may be more accepting of HMO practice styles. Other important factors that describe the physician community include specialty distribution, board certification, sex distribution, and the prevalence of foreign medical graduates. The number of physicians per 100,000 stood at 192 in both the Minneapolis-St. Paul and Chicago SMSAs in 1980, compared to 185 per 100,000 in the metropolitan U.S. The only difference between the two SMSAs in terms of total physicians per 100,000 is that physician density rose most rapidly between 1970 and 1975 in Chicago, while it rose most rapidly between 1975 and 1980 in the Twin Cities. Despite the similarity between the two SMSAs in terms of total physicians, a breakdown by specialty group yields somewhat different results (table 1.23). The most outstanding differences between the two SMSAs are that there are more general practitioners per 100,000 in the Minneapolis-St. Paul SMSA and more medical specialists per 100,000 in the Chicago SMSA. The prevalence of surgical specialists was equivalent in both SMSAs and is lower than metropolitan U.S. levels, while the prevalence of other specialists was approximately equal in both SMSAs and the metropolitan U.S. The prevalence of hospital-based physicians was equivalent in 1980 in both SMSAs and was substantially higher than metropolitan U.S. levels. In short, both SMSAs have relatively high physician densities, with the Twin Cities differentiated by a relatively high proportion of general practitioners and Chicago by a relatively high proportion of medical specialists.

A comparison of other physician characteristics in the Minneapolis-St. Paul SMSAs indicates that physicians in the Twin Cities are more likely to be board-certified, less likely to be female, less likely to have graduated from a foreign medical school, slightly more likely to be younger, and much more likely to practice in a group setting than physicians in Chicago (table 1.24). The greater prevalence of board-certified physicians in the Twin Cities, despite a low prevalence of specialists relative to general practitioners, may be due to a large number of board-certified family practitioners. Chapter 5 presents details of the role of physicians in the introduction and development of HMOs.

Hospitals

HMO development may be affected by the relative willingness of hospitals to serve as health care delivery resources for HMOs, or possibly by the degree to which HMOs can provide an attractive alternative to high communitywide hospital utilization rates. In previous research, these factors have been proxied by bed-to-population ratios, occupancy rates, and measures of days and discharges per 1,000 persons in various communities. As is shown in the figure on page 20, a favorable environment for HMO development might be characterized by overbedding, low occupancy rates, and high utilization rates, disregarding the potential interactions among these factors. Of these, low occupancy appears to be the most consistent indicator.

Community hospitals are somewhat more centralized within the Twin Cities metropolitan area; 67 percent of Twin Cities area hospitals are located within Minneapolis or St. Paul, while 55 percent of Chicago area hospitals are located within the city of Chicago. Both the Minneapolis-St. Paul SMSA and the Chicago SMSA exhibited 4.9 hospital beds per 1,000 population in 1980, but in the Twin Cities SMSA this level was reached after a decreasing trend while in the Chicago SMSA this level was reached after an increasing trend (table 1.25).

Admissions per 1,000 and days per 1,000 have been declining in the Twin Cities and increasing in Chicago (table 1.26).In 1972, these utilization indicators were higher in the Twin Cities than in Chicago, but the reverse was true by 1980. Average lengths of stay have been quite similar since 1977, with the Chicago SMSA slightly higher previously. Occupancy rates have been lower in the Twin Cities than in Chicago; the Chicago SMSA has exhibited fairly stable occupancy rates, while occupancy rates in the Twin Cities dropped between 1972 and 1975 and rose from 1979 to 1980. Chapter 4 presents details of the role of hospitals in the introduction and development of HMOs.

HMO hospital utilization

Table 1.27 presents data on utilization of hospital days by HMO enrollees. When compared to the total utilization of hospital days in the community, these data offer perspectives on the relative impact that HMOs may have on the market for hospital services. Between 1977 and 1980, HMO hospital days as a percentage of total community hospital days have been increasing rapidly in both the Minneapolis-St. Paul and Chicago metropolitan areas. While not large in absolute terms, the rates of increase —roughly doubling in the Twin Cities and tripling in Chicago— may be signaling the hospital services market that it can expect a larger role for HMOs in the future as HMO enrollment increases,

HMO enrollees age, and HMOs expand their services to the Medicare population.

HEALTH CARE COSTS AND FINANCING

Since HMOs function as health care financing as well as delivery mechanisms, the financial environment of the health care system is potentially relevant to HMO development. For example, high levels of expenditure or high rates of price increase may stimulate purchasers of health care to consider alternatives such as HMOs. In addition, the proportion of health care expenditures in a given area that are mediated by HMOs can provide a measure of how powerful HMOs have become in the market for medical care. This section presents data regarding rates of medical care price increases, overall sources and destinations of funds, extent of private and public third party coverage and expenditures, and community hospital expenses and sources of payment.

Rates of price increase

For people who are interested in managing expenditures within the health care system, the comparison of health care price increases with the price increases of other goods and services provides a useful performance measure. For example, employee benefits managers may compare health insurance premium increases with other price increases faced by the firm. For a more general comparison, the medical care consumer price index (CPI) and the all-item consumer price index can be used. These indicators are presented in table 1.28.

In 1965, the 1957-based medical care CPI was slightly higher for Minneapolis-St. Paul (132.5) than for Chicago (130.0). By 1970, this difference had reversed, with the 1967-based medical care CPI standing at 117.7 for Minneapolis-St. Paul and 119.9 for Chicago. In 1980, this difference had widened to 242.0 for Minneapolis-St. Paul (below the urban U.S. level) to 272.9 for Chicago (above the urban U.S. level). Since 1970, ratios of the medical care CPI to the all-item CPI for the Twin Cities have stood below the urban U.S. ratios, and either at or below the 1.0 level. For Chicago, the opposite is true, with ratios above the 1.0 level and above urban U.S. levels.

Estimates of sources and destinations of funds

Table 1.29 presents estimates of the magnitude of the health care financing systems in the Minneapolis-St. Paul and Chicago metropolitan areas, categorized by sources and destinations of funds. These local estimates were derived from national estimates, with adjustments for particular age distributions in the metropolitan areas. More precise data on particular components of this system, such as Medicare expenditures and total hospital expenses, are available and are discussed in subsequent sections. In some cases, comparisons can be made to assess the validity of the overall estimates. For example, comparison with table 1.36 shows that total expenditures on hospital services may be somewhat underestimated in table 1.29, but that it is fairly reliable guide to general magnitude.

Notable trends between 1965 and 1980 include an expansion of the role of third party reimbursement relative to direct expenditures by consumers, industry, and philanthropy, and an expansion of the role of federal reimbursement relative to private expenditures and state and local government expenditures. The expansion of the federal role is particularly notable with respect to physician reimbursement.

In 1980, the estimated total expenditure for personal health care services in the Minnneapolis-St. Paul SMSA was approximately $2 billion, of which $900 million was devoted to hospital services and $425 million was devoted to physician services. An estimated $1.2 billion of the total was purchased by the private sector, with approximately $540 million purchased by the federal government and approximately $220 million purchased by state and local governments.

The estimated total expenditure for personal health care services in the Chicago SMSA was approximately $6.7 billion for 1980—$3.1 billion to hospitals and $1.4 billion to physicians. Estimated private sector expenditures were roughly $4.1 billion, with $1.8 billion estimated for federal expenditures and $740 million for state and local government expenditures.

Third party coverage: Insurers, Medicare, Medicaid, HMOs

As indicated in the previous section, both the public sector and private sector are responsible for significant components of the health care financing system. This section discusses in greater detail the characteristics of fee-for-service insurance, the Medicare and Medicaid programs, local government expenditures on health and hospitals, and HMOs.

Health insurance premiums and benefit payments in 1978 and 1980 were considerably higher in Illinois than in Minnesota. For example, in 1980 benefit payments per capita in Illinois were $315.86 versus $228.80 in Minnesota. Premium-to-benefit ratios were slightly higher in Minnesota than in Illinois in 1978 and 1980 (table 1.30).

Medicare reimbursement per enrollee in 1970 was higher in Minneapolis-St. Paul than in Chicago for both hospital services reimbursement and medical services reimbursement. By 1979, however, this situation was reversed, with Medicare reimbursement per enrollee in Chicago standing at $1,076.86 for hospital services and $309.12 for medical services, while in Minneapolis-St. Paul reimbursement per enrollee was $822.80 for hospital services and $296.87 for medical services (table 1.31).

Between 1970 and 1980, the proportion of the population on public assistance increased from 5.3 percent to 8.3 percent in the Chicago SMSA, while in the Minneapolis-St. Paul SMSA this proportion increased from 3.6 percent to 4.4 percent (table 1.32). Although the proportion of the population on public assistance is considerably higher in the Chicago area, indicating a greater prevalence of Medicaid recipients, the Medicaid expenditure per enrollee in Illinois was less than half that of Minnesota in 1977 (table 1.33).

Per capita expenditures on health and hospitals by local governments were higher in Chicago than in Minneapolis-St. Paul in 1962, but from 1967 to 1977 local government expenditures were higher in the Twin Cities metropolitan area than in the Chicago area (table 1.34). HMO health care expenditures in 1980 constituted a much larger percentage of total SMSA health care expenditures in Minneapolis-St. Paul than in Chicago. 1980 HMO premium-to-benefit ratios were higher in Chicago than in Minneapolis-St. Paul (table 1.35).

Hospital expenses and sources of payment

Detailed data on the expenses incurred by hospitals are available from annual surveys by the American Hospital Association. Tables 1.36 and 1.37 persent AHA survey data for short-term community (nonfederal, noninstitutional) hospitals. Table

1.38 presents data on sources of payment by discharges collected by community hospital organizations in the Twin Cities and Chicago.

In 1960, 1965, and 1970, per capita hospital expenses were higher in the Minneapolis-St. Paul SMSA than the Chicago SMSA. In 1975 and 1980, however, per capita hospital expenses in the Chicago SMSA rose to levels higher than in Minneapolis-St. Paul—a difference of $47.12 in 1975 and $64.35 in 1980. Similarly, hospital expenses per inpatient day were higher in the Chicago SMSA than in the Minneapolis-St. Paul SMSA in the late 1970s. This gap widened from $23.98 in 1978 to $39.08 in 1980.

Patterns of hospital discharges by source of payment were fairly similar across the two metropolitan areas in 1980, with the exception of higher rates of Medicaid discharges and self-pay discharges in the Chicago area. While HMO discharges were not separated out in surveys, they presumably were a greater factor in the Twin Cities based on differentials in expenditures. In both areas, the percentage of commercial insurer discharges remained about the same between 1974 and 1975 and in 1980. The percentage of Blue Cross discharges declined; the percentage of Medicare discharges increased; and the percentage of self-pay discharges declined. Medicaid discharges increased in the Twin Cities but declined in Chicago.

SUMMARY

Given the results of previous research efforts in the area of quantifiable environmental determinants of HMO development, the preceding description of market characteristics in the Minneapolis-St. Paul and Chicago metropolitan areas allows tentative conclusions to be drawn regarding the relative predisposition of the two areas to HMO development.

Both Minneapolis-St. Paul and Chicago are relatively large SMSAs and have offered HMOs an ample supply of potential enrollees. The Chicago SMSA is so large, in fact, that HMOs may find it necessary to partition the market geographically or by type of employer or consumer to build sufficient consumer familiarity and acceptance.

In light of previous research regarding environmental determinants of HMO development, the discussion highlights a wide variety of differences between the Minneapolis-St. Paul and Chicago metropolitan areas that may have affected the course of HMO development in the two areas. Excluding consideration of other important factors, such as the subjective perceptions of community influentials and the organizational characteristics of the HMOs themselves, the Minneapolis-St. Paul market area can be characterized as having exhibited more characteristics favorable to HMO development than the Chicago market area during the 1970s.

TABLE 1.1 Minneapolis-St. Paul Metropolitan Area Population Distribution

	1950		1960		1970		1980	
Minneapolis-St. Paul SMSA	1,116,509	(100%)	1,482,030	(100%)	1,813,647	(100%)	2,114,256	(100%)
Minneapolis City (b)	521,718	(47%)	482,872	(33%)	434,400	(24%)	370,951	(-18%)
St. Paul City (b)	311,348	(28%)	313,411	(21%)	309,980	(17%)	270,230	(13%)
Anoka County (b)	35,579	(3%)	85,916	(6%)	154,556	(9%)	195,998	(9%)
Carver County (b)	18,155	(a)	21,358	(a)	28,310	(a)	37,046	(2%)
Chicago County	12,669	(a)	13,419	(a)	17,492	(a)	25,717	(1%)
Dakota County (b)	49,019	(4%)	78,303	(5%)	139,808	(8%)	194,111	(9%)
Suburban Hennepin County (b)	154,861	(14%)	359,982	(24%)	525,680	(29%)	570,460	(27%)
Suburban Ramsey County (b)	43,983	(4%)	109,114	(7%)	166,275	(9%)	189,554	(9%)
St. Croix County	25,905	(a)	29,164	(a)	34,354	(a)	43,262	(2%)
Scott County (b)	16,486	(a)	21,909	(a)	32,423	(a)	43,784	(2%)
Washington County (b)	34,544	(a)	52,432	(4%)	82,948	(5%)	113,571	(5%)
Wright County	27,716	(a)	29,935	(a)	38,933	(a)	58,681	(3%)
Seven-County HSA	1,185,694		1,525,297		1,874,380		1,985,705	
Percent Difference Between SMSA and Seven-County HSA Populations	6.2%		2.9%		3.3%		6.5%	

(a) Not included in SMSA total.

(b) Included in seven-county metropolitan area totals.

SOURCE: 18, 21, 24, 26

TABLE 1.2 Minneapolis-St. Paul Metropolitan Area Population Growth Rates

	1950-1960	1960-1970	1970-1980
Metropolitan U.S.	33.6%	16.6%	10.2%
Minneapolis-St. Paul SMSA (a)	28.8%	22.4%	7.6%
Seven-County Metropolitan Area	28.6%	22.9%	5.9%
Minneapolis City	-7.4%	-10.0%	-14.6%
St. Paul City	0.7%	-1.1%	-12.8%
Anoka County	141.5%	79.9%	26.7%
Carver County	17.6%	32.5%	30.8%
Chisago County	5.9%	30.4%	47.0%
Dakota County	59.7%	78.5%	38.8%
Suburban Hennepin County	132.5%	46.0%	8.5%
Suburban Ramsey County	148.1%	52.4%	14.0%
St. Croix County	12.6%	17.8%	25.9%
Scott County	32.9%	48.0%	35.0%
Washington County	51.8%	58.2%	36.8%
Wright County	8.0%	30.1%	50.7%

(a) SMSA definitions at decade-end were used to compute these rates.

SOURCE: 21, 24, 26, 31

TABLE 1.3 Minneapolis-St. Paul Metropolitan Area In-Migration (a)

	1960	1970	1980
Metropolitan U.S.	–	8.9%	–
Minneapolis-St. Paul SMSA	8.0%	8.4%	8.2%
Anoka County	8.6%	7.3%	5.1%
Carver County	3.4%	4.0%	7.7%
Dakota County	6.9%	10.4%	10.1%
Hennepin County	8.6%	8.8%	9.7%
Ramsey County	6.9%	7.4%	6.9%
Scott County	4.5%	6.5%	4.8%
Washington County	8.8%	7.4%	7.5%

(a) Percent of population which resided out-of-state within prior five years.
SOURCE: 21, 22, 24, 26

TABLE 1.4 Chicago Metropolitan Area Population Distribution

	1950	1960	1970	1980
Chicago SMSA	5177868 (100%)	6220913 (100%)	6978947 (100%)	7103624 (100%)
Chicago City	3620962 (70%)	3550404 (57%)	3366957 (48%)	3005072 (42%)
Suburban Cook	887830 (17%)	1579321 (25%)	2125412 (30%)	2248583 (32%)
DuPage	154599 (3%)	313459 (5%)	491882 (7%)	658835 (9%)
Kane	150388 (3%)	208246 (3%)	251005 (4%)	278405 (4%)
Lake	179097 (4%)	293656 (5%)	382638 (5%)	440372 (6%)
McHenry	50656 (1%)	84210 (1%)	111555 (2%)	147897 (2%)
Will	134336 (3%)	191617 (3%)	249498 (4%)	324460 (5%)

SOURCE: 16, 20, 23, 25

TABLE 1.5 Chicago Metropolitan Area Population Growth Rates

	1950–1960	1960–1970	1970–1980
Metropolitan U.S.	33.6%	16.2%	10.2%
Chicago SMSA	20.1%	12.2%	1.8%
Chicago City	−1.9%	−5.2%	−10.8%
Suburban Cook	77.9%	34.6%	5.8%
DuPage	102.8%	56.9%	35.0%
Kane	38.5%	20.5%	10.9%
Lake	64.0%	30.3%	15.1%
McHenry	66.2%	32.5%	32.6%
Will	42.6%	30.2%	30.9%

SOURCE: 19, 20, 22, 23, 25, 31

TABLE 1.6 Chicago Metropolitan Area In-Migration (a)

	1960	1970	1980
Metropolitan U.S.	–	8.9%	–
Chicago SMSA	7.1	6.4	5.9
Cook	6.2	5.1	4.6
Dupage	10.1	11.5	10.0
Kane	7.8	7.6	7.6
Lake	17.8	17.4	13.6
McHenry	7.3	7.5	7.5
Will	7.2	6.1	5.3

(a) Percent of population which migrated from out-of-state within prior five years.

SOURCE: 20, 22, 23, 25

TABLE 1.7 Age Distribution by Metropolitan Area

	1950	1960	1970	1980
MEDIAN AGE				
Chicago SMSA	32.9	31.3	28.4	29.8
Minneapolis-St. Paul SMSA	31.4	28.1	25.7	28.8
United States	30.2	29.4	27.9	30.0
PERCENT UNDER AGE 5				
Chicago SMSA	9.5%	11.5%	8.6%	7.4%
Minneapolis-St. Paul SMSA	10.9%	12.8%	9.3%	7.3%
Metropolitan U.S.	—	11.4%	8.5%	7.1%
PERCENT AGE 5-17				
Chicago SMSA	17.0%	22.3%	25.9%	21.2%
Minneapolis-St. Paul SMSA	17.4%	23.9%	27.0%	21.1%
Metropolitan U.S.	—	23.4%	25.7%	20.7%
PERCENT AGE 18-44				
Chicago SMSA	42.8%	35.8%	35.5%	41.4%
Minneapolis-St. Paul SMSA	41.0%	35.6%	37.3%	44.7%
Metropolitan U.S.	—	36.1%	36.0%	41.8%
PERCENT AGE 45-64				
Chicago SMSA	23.3%	21.8%	21.2%	20.0%
Minneapolis-St. Paul SMSA	22.3%	18.8%	17.6%	17.6%
Metropolitan U.S.	—	20.4%	20.5%	19.7%
PERCENT AGE 65+				
Chicago SMSA	7.4%	8.6%	8.8%	10.0%
Minneapolis-St. Paul SMSA	8.4%	8.8%	8.7%	9.5%
Metropolitan U.S.	—	8.6%	9.3%	10.7%

SOURCE: 15, 16, 17, 18, 19, 20, 21, 22, 23, 24, 25, 26, 31

TABLE 1.8 Racial and Ethnic Composition by Metropolitan Area

	1950	1960	1970	1980
PERCENT WHITE				
Chicago SMSA	89.0%	85.2%	81.3%	73.3%
Minneapolis-St. Paul SMSA	98.6%	98.2%	97.2%	95.0%
Metropolitan U.S.	—	—	87.0%	81.6%
PERCENT BLACK				
Chicago SMSA	10.7%	14.3%	17.6%	20.1%
Minneapolis-St. Paul SMSA	1.1%	1.4%	1.8%	2.4%
Metropolitan U.S.	—	—	11.6%	12.6%
PERCENT OTHER NON-WHITE				
Chicago SMSA	0.3%	0.4%	1.1%	6.6%
Minneapolis-St. Paul SMSA	0.2%	0.5%	1.0%	2.6%
Metropolitan U.S.	—	—	1.4%	5.8%
PERCENT HISPANIC				
Chicago SMSA	—	—	4.7%	8.2%
Minneapolis-St. Paul SMSA	—	—	1.5%	1.1%
Metropolitan U.S.	—	—	5.8%	7.5%

SOURCE : 16, 17, 18, 20, 21, 22, 23, 24, 31

TABLE 1.9 Selected Ancestry Groups, 1980

	Named as a single ancestry group	Named as one of multiple ancestry groups
ENGLISH		
Chicago SMSA	2.9%	7.4%
Minneapolis-St. Paul SMSA	2.8%	10.9%
GERMAN		
Chicago SMSA	7.1%	14.7%
Minneapolis-St. Paul SMSA	13.5%	27.9%
IRISH		
Chicago SMSA	4.3%	11.4%
Minneapolis-St. Paul SMSA	2.7%	14.8%
ITALIAN		
Chicago SMSA	3.8%	3.5%
Minneapolis-St. Paul SMSA	0.6%	1.4%
POLISH		
Chicago SMSA	6.1%	5.1%
Minneapolis-St. Paul SMSA	1.6%	3.8%
SWEDISH/NORWEGIAN		
Chicago SMSA	1.3%	--
Minneapolis-St. Paul SMSA	8.6%	--

SOURCE: 25, 26

TABLE 1.10 Income by Metropolitan Area

	1960	1970	1980
PER CAPITA INCOME			
Chicago SMSA	$2451	$3827	$8568
Minneapolis-St. Paul SMSA	$2198	$3621	$8666
Metropolitan U.S.	-	$3352	$7771
MEDIAN FAMILY INCOME			
Chicago SMSA	$7342	$11,391	$24,539
Minneapolis-St. Paul SMSA	$6840	$11,682	$24,646
Metropolitan U.S.	$6324	$10,474	-

SOURCE: 19, 20, 21, 22, 23, 24, 25, 26, 31

TABLE 1.11 Poverty Status by Metropolitan Area

	1970	1980
FAMILIES BELOW POVERTY LEVEL		
Chicago SMSA	6.8%	8.8%
Minneapolis-St. Paul SMSA	4.6%	4.9%
Metropolitan U.S.	8.5%	—
FAMILIES BELOW 125% OF POVERTY LEVEL		
Chicago SMSA	9.3%	11.2%
Minneapolis U.S.-St. Paul SMSA	6.9%	6.8%
Metropolian U.S.	12.0%	—
PERSONS BELOW POVERTY LEVEL		
Chicago SMSA	9.3%	11.3%
Minneapolis-St.Paul SMSA	6.7%	6.8%
Metropolitan U.S.	11.2%	—
PERSONS BELOW 125% OF POVERTY LEVEL		
Chicago SMSA	12.4%	14.4%
Minneapolis-St. Paul SMSA	9.4%	9.4%
Metropolitan U.S.	15.4%	—

SOURCE: 22, 23, 24, 25, 26

TABLE 1.12 Educational Attainment by Metropolitan Area

	1950	1960	1970	1980
MEDIAN SCHOOL YEARS COMPLETED, POPULATION OVER AGE 25				
Chicago SMSA	9.9	10.9	12.1	12.5
Minneapolis-St. Paul SMSA	11.2	12.1	12.4	12.8
Metropolitan U.S.	–	11.1	12.2	–
PERCENT OF POPULATION OVER AGE 25 WITH 12 OR MORE YEARS OF SCHOOL				
Chicago SMSA	36.4%	42.1%	53.9%	65.0%
Minneapolis-St. Paul SMSA	44.7%	52.6%	66.1%	80.0%
Metropolitan U.S.	–	44.2%	55.3%	–
PERCENT OF POPULATION OVER AGE 25 WITH 16 OR MORE YEARS OF SCHOOL				
Chicago SMSA	6.7%	8.4%	11.7%	15.9%
Minneapolis-St. Paul SMSA	8.1%	10.4%	14.8%	21.8%
Metropolitan U.S.	–	8.8%	12.0%	–

SOURCE: 15, 16, 17, 19, 20, 21, 22, 23, 24, 25, 26

TABLE 1.13 Household and Family Characteristics by Metropolitan Area

	1960	1970	1980
	----	----	----
AVERAGE HOUSEHOLD SIZE			

Chicago SMSA	3.20	3.14	2.79
Minneapolis-St. Paul SMSA	3.28	3.18	2.71
Metropolitan U.S.	3.23	3.09	2.73
PERCENT OF FAMILIES WITH			
CHILDREN UNDER 18 YEARS OLD			

Chicago SMSA	55.3%	55.3%	52.1%
Minneapolis-St. Paul SMSA	59.2%	59.8%	55.4%
Metropolitan U.S.	56.8%	55.9%	54.3%
PERCENT OF FAMILIES WITH			
CHILDREN UNDER 6 YEARS OLD			

Chicago SMSA	30.6%	26.7%	22.7%
Minneapolis-St. Paul SMSA	35.3%	31.1%	24.1%
Metropolitan U.S.	31.0%	26.4%	–

SOURCE: 19, 20, 21, 22, 23, 24, 25, 26, 31

TABLE 1.14 Minneapolis-St. Paul Private Sector Employers by Size and County, 1980

	Total Establishments	250-499 Employees	500-999 Employees	1000+ Employees
Minneapolis-St. Paul SMSA	44,097 (100%)	298 (100%)	100 (100%)	84 (100%)
Anoka County	2,566 (6%)	17 (6%)	0 (0%)	9 (11%)
Carver County	626 (1%)	1 (0.3%)	1 (1%)	0 (0%)
Chisago County	463 (1%)	2 (1%)	1 (1%)	0 (0%)
Dakota County	3,107 (7%)	19 (6%)	5 (5%)	2 (2%)
Hennepin County	24,006 (54%)	187 (63%)	60 (60%)	48 (57%)
Ramsey County	9,252 (21%)	63 (21%)	30 (30%)	23 (27%)
St. Croix County	768 (2%)	2 (1%)	1 (1%)	0 (0%)
Scott County	875 (2%)	3 (1%)	1 (1%)	0 (0%)
Washington County	1,456 (3%)	3 (1%)	1 (1%)	2 (2%)
Wright County	978 (2%)	1 (0.3%)	0 (0%)	0 (0%)

SOURCE: 27

TABLE 1.15 Chicago SMSA Private Sector Employers by Size and County, 1980

TABLE 4.15   CHICAGO SMSA PRIVATE SECTOR EMPLOYERS BY SIZE AND COUNTY, 1980

	Total Establishments	250-499 Employees	500-999 Employees	1000+ Employees
Chicago SMSA	133,340 (100%)	922 (100%)	369 (100%)	231 (100%)
Cook	99,941 (75%)	741 (80%)	293 (79%)	189 (82%)
DuPage	13,490 (10%)	72 (8%)	26 (7%)	20 (9%)
Kane	5,450 (4%)	34 (4%)	18 (5%)	7 (3%)
Lake	7,647 (6%)	40 (4%)	16 (4%)	9 (4%)
McHenry	2,856 (2%)	11 (1%)	9 (2%)	1 (1%)
Will	4,226 (3%)	24 (3%)	7 (2%)	5 (2%)

SOURCE: 27

TABLE 1.16 Composition of Private Industry in the Minneapolis-St. Paul SMSA (a)

	1962	1970	1980
All Establishments with 250 or More Employees	211 (100%)	338 (100%)	482 (100%)
Manufacturing Establishments	88 (42%)	134 (40%)	180 (37%)
Wholesale/Retail Establishments	45 (21%)	73 (22%)	86 (18%)
Personal and Business Service Establishments	54 (26%)	92 (27%)	166 (34%)
Other Establishments	24 (11%)	39 (12%)	50 (10%)

(a) Establishments with 250 or more employees.

SOURCE: 27

TABLE 1.17 Composition of Private Industry in the Chicago SMSA (a)

	1962	1970	1980
All Establishments with 250 or More Employees	1123 (100%)	1441 (100%)	1522 (100%)
Manufacturing Establishments	635 (57%)	744 (51%)	689 (45%)
Wholesale/Retail Establishments	175 (16%)	253 (18%)	206 (14%)
Personal and Business Service Establishments	231 (21%)	330 (23%)	443 (29%)
Other Establishments	82 (7%)	114 (8%)	184 (12%)

(a) Establishments with 250 or more employees.

SOURCE: 27

TABLE 1.18 Commuting Patterns

	1960	1970
18A Work and Residence Location		
Live and work in Central City		
Chicago	50.4%	35.4%
Minneapolis-St. Paul	51.5%	31.9%
Metropolitan U.S.	43.8%	-
Live in outer SMSA, work in Central City		
Chicago	13.2%	12.7%
Minneapolis-St. Paul	20.6%	23.5%
Metropolitan U.S.	15.5%	-
Live in Central city, work in Outer SMSA		
Chicago	3.6%	7.3%
Minneapolis-St. Paul	3.6%	7.8%
Metropolitan U.S.	4.9%	-
Live and Work in outer SMSA		
Chicago	14.8%	35.1%
Minneapolis-St. Paul	18.9%	30.5%
Metropolitan U.S.	27.1%	-
Live in SMSA, work outside SMSA		
Chicago	1.5%	2.0%
Minneapolis-St. Paul	1.5%	1.5%
Metropolitan U.S.	3.9%	-
Not Reported		
Chicago	6.5%	7.5%
Minneapolis St. Paul	3.9%	4.8%
Metro U.S.	4.8%	-

18.B Mean Travel Time to Work (minutes)	1980
Chicago	28.2
Minneapolis-St. Paul	20.1

SOURCE : 19, 20, 21, 22, 23, 24

TABLE 1.19 Employment Patterns by Metropolitan Area

LABOR FORCE PARTICIPATION RATE	1950	1960	1970	1980
Chicago SMSA	57.9%	58.9%	61.3%	65.1%
Minneapolis-St. Paul SMSA	56.3%	58.8%	64.3%	70.4%
Metropolitan U.S.	-	55.7%	58.2%	-
UNEMPLOYMENT RATE				
Chicago SMSA	4.2%	4.3%	3.5%	6.8%
Minneapolis-St. Paul SMSA	3.6%	3.8%	3.2%	4.0%
Metropolitan U.S.	-	5.0%	4.3%	6.9%
PERCENT OF WORKFORCE EMPLOYED				
IN WHITE COLLAR OCCUPATIONS				
Chicago SMSA	44.3%	45.5%	52.9%	55.1%
Minneapolis-St. Paul SMSA	49.4%	51.9%	56.7%	61.1%
Metropolitan U.S.	-	45.6%	52.3%	-
PERCENT OF WORKFORCE EMPLOYED				
IN MANUFACTURING				
Chicago SMSA	37.5%	34.2%	31.7%	27.3%
Minneapolis-St. Paul SMSA	25.2%	26.0%	24.7%	23.6%
Metropolitan U.S.	-	29.0%	26.1%	-
PERCENT OF WORKFORCE EMPLOYED				
IN WHOLESALE RETAIL TRADE				
Chicago SMSA	20.1%	18.0%	20.8%	21.7%
Minneapolis-St. Paul SMSA	24.2%	20.4%	22.8%	22.1%
Metropolitan U.S.	-	18.6%	20.6%	
PERCENT OF WORKFORCE EMPLOYED				
BY GOVERNMENT				
Chicago SMSA	7.6%	8.2%	11.7%	13.6%
Minneapolis-St. Paul SMSA	10.0%	11.4%	14.4%	14.1%
Metropolitan U.S.	-	15.4%	17.7%	17.9%

SOURCE : 16, 17, 18, 19, 20, 21, 22, 23, 24, 25, 26

TABLE 1.20 Unionization by State and Metropolitan Area

20 A   PERCENT OF NON-AGRICULTURAL WORKERS IN UNIONS, BY STATE

	1970	1980
Illinois	37.3%	30.6%
Minnesota	31.9%	26.2%
United States	30.8%	25.2%

20B   PERCENT OF WORKERS IN UNIONIZED ESTABLISHMENTS, MINNEAPOLIS--ST PAUL (a)

	1975	1978	1981
All Industries			
Plant Workers	71	68%	68%
Office Workers	11	9%	6%
Manufacturing			
Plant Workers	72	66%	64%
Office Workers	1	3%	2%
Non-Manufacturing			
Plant Workers	-	69%	73%
Office Workers	-	13%	9%
Transportation & Utilities			
Plant Workers	97	98%	99%
Office Workers	51	60%	58%

20C PERCENT OF WORKERS IN UNIONIZED ESTABLISHMENTS, CHICAGO (a)

	1974	1977	1980
All Industries			
Plant Workers	72	68	71%
Office Workers	13	11	12%
Manufacturing			
Plant Workers	74	68	71%
Office Workers	12	7	8%
Non-Manufacturing			
Plant Workers	-	68	70%
Office Workers	-	13	14%
Transportation and Utilities			
Plant Workers	97	98	94%
Office Workers	68	70	72%

(a) Percentage of workers employed in establishments where the majority of
    workers in the listed categories were under contract; limited to
    establishments with 100 or more workers.

SOURCE: 32, 34

TABLE 1.21 Health Benefits Eligibility in the Twin Cities Metropolitan Area (a)

	1972	1975	1978	1981
HOSPITALIZATION INSURANCE				
Plant Workers	96	96	95%	96%
Office Workers	99	99	99%	99%
NON-CONTRIBUTORY HOSPITALIZATION INSURANCE				
Plant Workers	81	82	81%	84%
Office Workers	56	56	57%	57%
MAJOR MEDICAL INSURANCE				
Plant Workers	77	83	86%	94%
Office Workers	95	98	99%	99%
NON-CONTRIBUTORY MAJOR MEDICAL INSURANCE				
Plant Workers	58	62	66%	75%
Office Workers	51	54	54%	54%
HMOs				
Plant Workers	–	–	–	46%
Office Workers	–	–	–	64%
NON-CONTRIBUTORY HMOs				
Plant Workers	–	–	–	30%
Office Workers	–	–	–	28%

(a) Percent of full-time workers eligible, employers of 100 or larger.

SOURCE: 34

TABLE 1.22 Health Benefits Eligibility in the Chicago Metropolitan Area (a)

	1971	1974	1977	1980
HOSPITALIZATION INSURANCE				
Plant Workers	99%	99%	99%	99%
Office Workers	98%	99%	98%	99%
NON-CONTRIBUTORY HOSPITALIZATION INSURANCE				
Plant Workers	74%	74%	76%	77%
Office Workers	48%	54%	57%	57%
MAJOR MEDICAL INSURANCE				
Plant Workers	76%	82%	91%	92%
Office Workers	92%	95%	95%	97%
NON-CONTRIBUTORY MAJOR MEDICAL INSURANCE				
Plant Workers	52%	59%	67%	69%
Office Workers	41%	49%	50%	53%
HMOs				
Plant Workers	–	–	–	22%
Office Workers	–	–	–	38%
NON-CONTRIBUTORY HMOs				
Plant Workers	–	–	–	10%
Office Workers	–	–	–	9%

(a) Percent of workers eligible, employers of 100 or larger.

SOURCE: 34

TABLE 1.23   Physicians by Specialty and Metropolitan Area

	1965	1970	1975	1980
TOTAL PHYSICIANS				
Physicians per 100,000				
Chicago SMSA	147	144	159	192
Cook County	162	159	206	210
Minneapolis-St. Paul SMSA	149	142	152	192
Hennepin County	187	184	223	283
Ramsey County	150	146	166	223
Metropolitan U.S.	-	-	160	185
OFFICE-BASED PHYSICIANS				
General Practitioners Per 100,000				
Chicago SMSA	37	24	21	20
Cook County	39	25	21	21
Minneapolis-St. Paul SMSA	32	26	25	29
Hennepin County	33	28	27	33
Ramsey County	38	29	27	33
Metropolitan U.S.	-	-	20	19
Medical Specialists Per 100,000				
Chicago SMSA	23	24	30	41
Cook County	25	25	32	43
Minneapolis-St. Paul SMSA	21	22	26	36
Hennepin County	26	29	40	54
Ramsey County	24	29	29	46
Metropolitan U.S.	-	-	31	40
Surgical Specialists Per 100,000				
Chicago SMSA	29	29	31	37
Cook County	31	29	32	38
Minneapolis-St. Paul SMSA	32	31	31	37
Hennepin County	41	40	46	54
Ramsey County	33	33	38	46
Metropolitan U.S.	-	-	37	41
Other Specialists Per 100,000				
Chicago SMSA	15	19	23	35
Cook County	17	20	24	36
Minneapolis-St. Paul SMSA	17	22	25	33
Hennepin County	21	29	55	50
Ramsey County	20	21	28	36
Metropolitan U.S.	-	-	26	34
HOSPITAL-BASED PHYSICIANS				
Chicago SMSA	41	49	52	59
Cook County	50	59	67	71
Minneapolis-St. Paul SMSA	46	42	45	58
Hennepin County	65	58	73	94
Ramsey County	34	39	46	61
Metropolitan U.S.	-	-	45	49

SOURCE: 7

TABLE 1.24 Selected Physician Characteristics by Metropolitan Area, 1975

	1975
PERCENT BOARD CERTIFIED	----
Chicago SMSA	39%
Minneapolis-St. Paul SMSA	50%

PERCENT FEMALE

| Chicago SMSA | 14% |
| Minneapolis-St. Paul SMSA | 9% |

PERCENT FOREIGN MEDICAL GRADUATES (NON-U.S./CANADA)

| Chicago SMSA | 30% |
| Minneapolis-St. Paul SMSA | 7% |

AGE DISTRIBUTION

Chicago SMSA	
Less than 35	33%
35-44	24%
45-64	31%
65 and over	12%

Minneapolis-St. Paul SMSA	
Less than 35	34%
35-44	26%
45-64	31%
65 and over	9%

	1980
PERCENT OF PHYSICIANS PRACTICING	----
IN A GROUP SETTING	
Minnesota	71%
Illinois	24%
United States	21%

SOURCE: 33

TABLE 1.25   Hospital Facilities by Metropolitan Area (a)

	1960	1965	1970	1975	1980
Hospitals					
Chicago SMSA	108	115	111	112	103
Chicago City	71	70	67	66	57
Minneapolis-St. Paul SMSA	32	32	34	38	36
Minneapolis	14	14	14	12	14
St. Paul	12	12	12	11	10
Beds per 1000					
Chicago SMSA	4.0	4.3	4.5	4.9	4.9
Minneapolis-St. Paul SMSA	5.3	5.4	5.6	5.4	4.9
Metropolitan U.S.	-	-	-	4.5	4.4

(a) Short-term, non-federal, non-institutional (prisons, colleges, etc.) hospitals.

SOURCE: 1,3,4,5

TABLE 1.26 Hospital Utilization by Metropolitan Area

	1972	1975	1976	1977	1978	1979	1980
Admission per 1000							
Chicago SMSA	137.9	165.5	164.5	167.3	167.5	169.3	169.8
Twin Cities SMSA	173.6	171.7	174.1	170.1	165.8	161.1	164.4
Metropolitan U.S.	145.5	159.5	159.8	161.1	156.3	157.6	160.0
Days per 1000							
Chicago SMSA	1235.7	1387.2	1396.3	1393.7	1388.4	1396.6	1413.1
Twin Cities SMSA	1469.2	1388.0	1400.2	1399.9	1354.3	1328.2	1361.5
Metropolitan U.S.	1183.3	1262.5	1262.8	1261.8	1220.1	1224.0	1242.1
Average Length of Stay							
Chicago SMSA	9.1	8.4	8.5	8.3	8.3	8.2	8.3
Twin Cities SMSA	8.6	8.1	8.0	8.2	8.2	8.2	8.3
Metropolitan U.S.	8.1	7.9	7.9	7.8	7.8	7.8	---
Occupancy							
Chicago SMSA	79.2%	80.0%	79.9%	79.5%	79.2%	79.3%	79.2%
Twin Cities SMSA	73.6%	71.7%	72.7%	71.9%	71.1%	71.7%	75.5%
Metropolitan U.S.	79.3%	77.4%	76.9%	76.1%	76.0%	76.4%	77.9%

SOURCE: 6

TABLE 1.27 HMO Hospital Utilization

	1977	1978	1979	1980
	----	----	----	----
Minneapolis-St. Paul Metropolitan Area				
Total Days for HMO Enrollees	82,833	99,904	124,369	170,654
Percent of Total Community Hospital Days	2.9%	3.6%	4.5%	5.9%
Chicago Metropolitan Area				
Total Days for HMO Enrollees	32,662	42,843	66,084	93,803
Percent of Total Community Hospital Days	0.3%	0.4%	0.7%	0.9%

SOURCE: 6, 11, 14

TABLE 1.28 Consumer Price Indices

	1970	1975	1980
	----	----	----
MEDICAL CARE C.P.I. (1967=100)			
Minneapolis St. Paul SMSA (a)	117.7	159.6	242.0
Chicago SMSA (a)	119.9	169.1	272.9
Urban U.S. Average	120.6	168.6	265.9
ALL-ITEM C.P.I. (1967=100)			
Minneapolis-St Paul SMSA	117.5	170.9	247.8
Chicago SMSA	116.3	157.6	245.5
Urban U.S. Average	116.3	161.6	246.8
RATIO OF MEDICAL CARE C.P.I. TO ALL-ITEM C.P.I.			
Minneapolis-St. Paul SMSA	1.00	0.93	0.98
Chicago SMSA	1.03	1.07	1.11
Urban U.S. Average	1.04	1.04	1.08

(a) NOTE: With 1957 as a base year, the medical care C.P.I. in 1965 was 132.5
for the Minneapolis St. Paul SMSA and 130.0 for the Chicago SMSA.

SOURCE: 32

TABLE 1.29 Estimates of Sources and Destinations of Funds for Personal Health Services (Millions)

	TOTAL EXPENDITURES (MILLIONS)			TO HOSPITALS			TO PHYSICIANS		
	1965	1970	1980	1965	1970	1980	1965	1970	1980
Minneapolis-St. Paul Metropolitan Area									
Total	$ 286.0	$ 563.2	$1,972.5	$ 112.5	$ 239.0	$ 903.8	$ 69.0	$ 125.8	$ 425.2
Private Funds	222.2	373.9	1,216.6	68.8	115.5	427.0	64.3	100.1	319.5
Direct Consumer Expenditures	146.7	228.1	653.3	19.3	24.5	85.4	42.4	57.1	162.0
Third Party Reimbursement	69.3	136.8	536.5	47.0	87.7	329.6	21.9	42.9	157.2
Direct Expenditures by Philanthropy/Industry	6.2	9.0	26.8	2.5	3.3	11.5	0.1	0.1	0.3
Public Funds (b)	63.8	189.3	755.9	43.7	123.5	476.8	4.7	25.7	105.7
Federal	30.6	120.9	537.1	19.7	78.4	356.1	1.2	18.1	78.7
State and Local	33.2	68.4	218.8	24.0	45.1	120.7	3.5	7.6	27.0
Chicago Metropolitan Area									
Total	$1,198.9	$2,199.0	$6,676.4	$474.2	$936.0	$3,071.1	$285.9	$490.2	$1,437.1
Private Funds	932.7	1,460.1	4,091.6	290.8	453.1	1,427.3	268.7	390.2	1,072.9
Direct Consumer Expenditures	615.6	890.7	2,197.2	81.4	96.1	285.5	177.1	222.4	544.0
Third Party Reimbursement	219.0	534.4	1,804.4	198.6	343.9	1,101.9	91.4	167.4	527.9
Direct Expenditures by Philanthropy/Industry	26.1	35.0	90.0	10.5	13.1	38.5	0.3	0.4	1.1
Public Funds (b)	266.2	738.9	2,584.8	183.4	482.9	1,643.8	17.2	100.0	364.2
Federal	126.9	470.8	1,846.8	82.2	305.6	1,239.3	5.0	70.3	273.8
State and Local	139.3	268.1	738.0	101.2	177.3	404.5	15.2	29.7	90.4

(a) Derived from national figures, with adjustments for population size and age distribution.
(b) Unadjusted for local differences. Compared to national figures, Minneapolis-St. Paul has a lower proportion of the population receiving public assistance but Minnesota spends more on health care per recipient. Chicago has a higher proportion of recipients but Illinois spends less per recipient.
SOURCE: 22, 23, 24, 31, 32

TABLE 1.30 Health Insurance Premiums and Benefit Payments

	1978	1980
Total and Per Capita (a) Premiums		
Minnesota	$ 833,000,000 ($ 234.98)	$ 951,000,000 ($264.39)
Illinois	3,052,000,000 ($ 304.07)	3,655,000,000 ($359.53)
U.S.	55,106,000,000 ($ 284.04)	65,285,000,000 ($324.87)
Total Per Capita (a) Benefit Payments		
Minnesota	$ 643,000,000 ($ 181.38)	$ 823,000,000 ($228.80)
Illinois	2,551,000,000 ($ 254.16)	3,211,000,000 ($315.86)
U.S.	45,604,000,000 ($ 235.07)	58,593,000,000 ($291.57)
Premium-to-Benefit Ratios		
Minnesota	1.295	1.156
Illinois	1.196	1.138
U.S.	1.208	1.114

(a) Persons under age 65.

SOURCE: 9.10

TABLE 1.31 Medicare Enrollment and Reimbursement

	1970	1975	1979
PERSONS ENROLLED			
Hospital Services (Part A)			
Minneapolis-St. Paul SMSA	158,276	182,970	210,500
Chicago SMSA	614,697	635,552	735,100
United States	20,361,000	24,640,000	26,889,400
Medical Services (Part B)			
Minneapolis-St. Paul SMSA	155,211	181,177	207,500
Chicago SMSA	595,689	624,790	722,700
United States	19,584,000	23,904,000	26,520,100
REIMBURSEMENT			
Hospital Services (Part A)			
Minneapolis-St. Paul SMSA	$ 54,502,859	$ 99,912,365	$ 173,200,000
Chicago SMSA	178,397,306	358,136,537	791,600,000
United States	4,723,800,000	11,315,000,000	11,191,500,000
Medical Services (Part B)			
Minneapolis-St. Paul SMSA	$ 15,455,013	$ 30,972,988	$ 61,600,000
Chicago SMSA	51,648,316	101,428,971	233,400,000
United States	1,824,300,000	4,273,000,000	8,400,900,000
REIMBURSEMENT PER ENROLLEE			
Hospital Services (Part A)			
Minneapolis-St. Paul SMSA	$ 344.35	$ 546.06	$ 822.80
Chicago SMSA	290.22	563.50	1,076.86
United States	232.00	459.21	713.72
Medical Services (Part B)			
Minneapolis-St. Paul SMSA	$ 99.57	$ 170.45	$ 296.87
Chicago SMSA	86.70	162.34	309.12
United States	51.06	178.76	316.77

SOURCE: 31, 32

TABLE 1.32 Public Assistance Recipients (a)

	1970	1975	1980
Minneapolis-St. Paul SMSA			
AFDC Recipients (b)	50,873 (2.8%)	86,300 (4.2%)	80,300 (3.8%)
SSI Recipients (c)	14,509 (0.8%)(d)	13,557 (0.7%)(d)	12,700 (0.6%)
Total AFDC + SSI	65,382 (3.6%)	99,857 (4.9%)	93,000 (4.4%)
Chicago SMSA			
AFDC Recipients (b)	280,079 (4.0%)	588,500 (8.4%)	509,400 (7.2%)
SSI Recipients (c)	90,726 (1.3%)(d)	85,347 (1.2%)(d)	78,400 (1.1%)
Total AFDC + SSI	370,805 (5.3%)	673,847 (9.6%)	587,800 (8.3%)
United States			
AFDC Recipients (b)	9,659,000 (4.7%)	11,401,000 (5.3%)	11,101,000 (4.9%)
SSI Recipients (c)	4,507,000 (2.2%)	4,314,000 (2.0%)	4,142,000 (1.8%)
Total AFDC + SSI	14,166,000 (6.9%)	15,715,000 (7.3%)	15,243,000 (6.7%)

(a) Total Recipients and Percentage of the Population
(b) Aid to Families with Dependent Children
(c) Supplemental Security Income
(d) Estimated values, based on actual SMSA courts for 1980 and proportional charges in national courts over 1970-1980.

SOURCE: 31,32,33

TABLE 1.33 Medicaid Expenditures Per Recipient

	1977
Minnesota	
State/Local	$ 621.19
Federal	789.59
Total	1,410.78
Illinois	
State/Local	268.10
Federal	309.58
Total	577.69
United States	
State/Local	305.73
Federal	391.33
Total	697.07

SOURCE: 12

TABLE 1.34 Total and Per Capita Local Government Expenditures on Health and Hospitals

		1962	1967	1972	1977
Minneapolis-St. Paul SMSA	$	14,416,000 (9.35)	$ 24,419,000 (14.30)	$ 66,082,000 (36.03)	$ 126,819,000 (62.07)
Chicago SMSA		67,822,000 (10.55)	73,758,000 (10.84)	166,055,000 (23.44)	276,040,000 (39.34)
United States		2,179,344,000 (11.68)	3,250,572,000 (16.36)	7,028,934,000 (33.49)	11,760,228,000 (53.41)

SOURCE: 29, 30, 31

TABLE 1.35 HMO Expenditures on Health Care

	1980

Minneapolis-St. Paul Metropolitan Area	
Total HMO Inpatient Expenditures	$ 50,808,394
Percent of Estimates Total Expenditures, All Sources	5.6%
Total HMO Medical Expenditures	$ 144,170,820
Percent of Estimated Total Health Care Expenditures, All Sources	7.0%
Total HMO Premium Income	$ 150,710,730
HMO Premium-to-Benefit Ratio	1.045
Chicago Metropolitan Area	
Total HMO Inpatient Expenditures	$ 34,226,614
Percent of Estimated Total Hospital Expenditures, All Sources	1.1%
Total HMO Medical Expenditures	$ 71,790,148
Percent of Estimated Total Health Care Expenditures, All Sources	1.1%
Total HMO Premium Income	$ 89,597,660
HMO Premium-to-Benefit Ratio	1.248

SOURCE: 11.14

TABLE 1.36 Hospital Expenses (a)

	1960	1965	1970	1975	1980
Minneapolis-St. Paul SMSA					
Total	$ 84,696,000	$ 128,667,000	$252,306,000	$463,151,000	$910,034,000
Per Capita	57.15	80.31	139.12	228.43	430.43
Chicago SMSA					
Total	276,117,000	423,454,000	878,881,000	1,798,418,000	3,514,748,000
Per Capita	44.39	63.81	125.93	275.55	494.78
United States					
Per Capita	31.32	47.27	96.99	181.02	339.89

(a) Short-term, non-federal, non-institutional (prisons, colleges, etc.) hospitals.
    Adjusted for missing values.

SOURCE: 1,2,3,4,5

TABLE 1.37 Hospital Expenses Per Inpatient Day (a)

	1978 ----	1979 ----	1980 ----
Minneapolis-St. Paul SMSA	$215.39	$240.10	$274.14
Chicago SMSA	239.37	274.56	313.23
Metropolitan U.S.	210.60	235.02	265.56

(a) Adjusted to remove outpatient expenses.

SOURCE: 6

TABLE 1.38 Hospital Discharges by Source of Payment

	1974-75 (a)	1980
Minneapolis-St. Paul Metropolitan Area	100.0%	100.0%
Commercial Insurance	39.0	39.0
Blue Cross	17.3	13.9
Medicare	19.6	24.0
Medicaid	4.2	8.7
Other Government	(b)	1.5
Self-Pay	4.5	3.7
Workers' Compensation	1.8	2.5
Unknown or Other (Includes HMOs)	13.6	6.6
Chicago Metropolitan Area		
Commercial Insurance	32.7	32.8
Blue Cross	21.8	16.0
Medicare	18.9	23.8
Medicaid	18.4	15.7
Other Government	0.5	(b)
Self-Pay	6.8	6.0
Workers' Compensation	0.9	(b)
Unknown or Other (Includes HMOs)	(c)	5.7

(a) 1974 for Minneapolis-St. Paul, 1975 for Chicago
(b) Aggregated with "Unknown or Other"
(c) Assigned to other categories

SOURCE: 8.13

SOURCES

1. American Hospital Association, Guide to the Health Care Field, 1976 Edition. Chicago: A.H.A., 1976.

2. American Hospital Association, Guide to the Health Care Field, 1981 Edition. Chicago: A.H.A., 1981.

3. American Hospital Association, Hospitals 35(15), August 1, 1961.

4. American Hospital Association, Hospitals 40(15), August 1, 1966.

5. American Hospital Association, Hospitals 45(15), August 1, 1977.

6. American Hospital Association, Hospital Statistics, 1981 Edition. Chicago: A.H.A., 1981.

7. American Medical Association, Distribution of Physicians. Chicago: A.M.A., 1965, 1970, 1975, 1980.

8. Chicago Hospital Council, Sources of Payment for Chicago Area Hospitals, 1975, 1980.

9. Health Insurance Association of America, Sourcebook of Health Insurance Data, 1981-1982. Washington, D.C.: H.I.A.A., 1981.

10. Health Insurance Association of America, Sourcebook of Health Insurance Data, 1982-1983. Washington, D.C.: H.I.A.A., 1982.

11. Illinois Department of Health, HMO Annual Reports. Springfield, IL.

12. Medicaid/Medicare Management Institute, Data on the Medicaid Program: Eligibility, Services, Expenditures. Washington, D.C.: U.S.D.H.E.W., 1979.

13. Metropolitan Health Board, Hospital Discharge Survey: 1974, 1980. Minneapolis, MN.

14. Minnesota Department of Health, HMO Annual Reports. Minneapolis, MN.

15. U.S. Bureau of the Census, Census of the Population: 1950, Vol. II, Part 1 (U.S. Summary). Washington, D.C.: U.S.G.P.O., 1952.

16. U.S. Bureau of the Census, Census of the Population: 1950, Vol. II, Part 13 (Illinois). Washington, D.C.: U.S.G.P.O., 1952.

17. U.S. Bureau of the Census, Census of the Population: 1950, Vol. II, Part 14 (Indiana). Washington, D.C.: U.S.G.P.O., 1952.

18. U.S. Bureau of the Census, Census of the Population: 1950, Vol. II, Part 23 (Minnesota). Washington, D.C.: U.S.G.P.O., 1952.

19. U.S. Bureau of the Census, Census of the Population: 1960, Vol. I, Part 1 (U.S. Summary). Washington, D.C.: U.S.G.P.O., 1964.

20. U.S. Bureau of the Census, Census of the Population: 1960, Vol. I, Part 15 (Illinois). Washington, D.C.: U.S.G.P.O., 1964.

21. U.S. Bureau of the Census, Census of the Population: 1960, Vol. I, Part 25 (Minnesota). Washington, D.C.: U.S.G.P.O., 1964.

22. U.S. Bureau of the Census, Census of the Population: 1970, Vol. I, Part 1 (U.S. Summary). Washington, D.C.: U.S.G.P.O., 1973.

23. U.S. Bureau of the Census, Census of the Population: 1970, Vol. I, Part 15 (Illinois). Washington, D.C.: U.S.G.P.O., 1973.

24. U.S. Bureau of the Census, Census of the Population: 1970, Vol. I, Part 25 (Minnesota). Washington, D.C.: U.S.G.P.O., 1973.

25. U.S. Bureau of the Census, Census of the Population: 1980, Vol. I, Chapter C, Part 15 (Illinois). Washington, D.C.: U.S.G.P.O., 1983.

26. U.S. Bureau of the Census, Census of the Population: 1980, Vol. I, Chapter C, Part 25 (Minnesota). Washington, D.C.: U.S.G.P.O., 1983.

27. U.S. Bureau of the Census, County Business Patterns. Washington, D.C.: U.S.G.P.O., Annual.

28. U.S. Bureau of the Census, County and City Data Book, 1956. Washington, D.C.: U.S.G.P.O., 1957.

29. U.S. Bureau of the Census, County and City Data Book, 1962. Washington, D.C.: U.S.G.P.O., 1962.

30. U.S. Bureau of the Census, County and City Data Book, 1967. Washington, D.C.: U.S.G.P.O., 1967.

31. U.S. Bureau of the Census, State and Metropolitan Area Data Book, 1982. Washington, D.C.: U.S.G.P.O., 1982.

32. U.S. Bureau of the Census, Statistical Abstract of the U.S.: 1982-1983. Washington, D.C.: U.S.G.P.O., 1982.

33. U.S. Department of Health and Human Services, Bureau of Health Professions, DHPA Area Resource File. December, 1980.

34. U.S. Department of Labor, Area Wage Surveys. Washington, D.C.: U.S.G.P.O., Periodic.

2

HMOs and Regulators

Regulators in Minnesota facilitated HMO development by mandating the same minimum range of benefits for all insurers, including psychiatric care and services for alcoholics and chemically dependent patients. Minnesota also introduced a mandated dual choice provision as well as standardized benefits, thus facilitating HMO competition. Minnesota regulations reveal a conscious competition strategy as expressed in hospital price disclosure, the pending abolishment of certificate-of-need regulation, and the implied change of mission for the local Health Systems Agency toward a less regulation-oriented and more competition-enhancing framework. In contrast, HMO regulation in Illinois unintentionally had a neutral to slightly inhibiting effect on HMO development. In Illinois, regulation is largely financial, limiting HMO capitalization and establishing reserve requirements. Illinois regulation, however, did not consciously promote competition.

Prior to 1970, prepaid-group-practice organizations—precursors to health maintenance organizations (HMOs)—believed that existing health care regulation established significant barriers to the formation and operation of prepaid plans. At that time, existing regulation was largely viewed by them as serving and protecting the interests of the established health care delivery and financing system. Existing medical and insurance regulations served to perpetuate the status quo. HMOs argued that specific statutes and regulations were needed for their peculiar organizational form encompassing both insurance and medical delivery

---

This chapter was written by Terry E. Herold, Project Director.

functions. HMOs contended not only that existing regulation was not relevant to their operations but also that it maintained harmful barriers. In response, HMOs sought to eliminate these barriers through legislative and legal action. Their victories during this period were primarily legal rather than legislative because the medical establishment was well entrenched in the legislative arena. The fledgling HMO industry did not possess the power or resources to have much effect on legislation.

During the first half of the 1970s, however, strides were made in removing barriers and obstacles to HMOs. Most of the HMO legislation enacted by the states occurred on the coattails of national HMO policy and legislation. In 1972, the Nixon administration launched a national health strategy that hinged on the formation and development of health maintenance organizations. Many state legislatures followed the federal lead by adopting HMO-enabling legislation. Legislation at state levels resembled federal examples and was strongly influenced by model legislation developed by the National Association of Insurance Commissioners (NAIC). State and federal legislative initiatives provided fertile soil for HMO formation.

Following the implementation of HMO-enabling legislation, the regulatory concerns of HMOs have increasingly shifted to matters of overregulation and pernicious features of the existing HMO statutes. Whereas prior to the 1970s many HMOs sought the resolution of their problems in legislation, increasingly they have become concerned about overregulation. With all the good that was accomplished for HMOs with the state and federal enabling statutes, certain features of that legislation presented the HMO with another set of obstacles that were perhaps as onerous as the ones that preceded enabling legislation.

This chapter examines regulation affecting HMO development and operation in Minneapolis-St. Paul and Chicago. It is based, in part, on information gleaned from interviews with thirty-seven respondents representing regulatory agencies and other governmental bodies at the local, state, and federal levels.

PREVIOUS RESEARCH

There was a general perception in the early 1970s that legal obstacles impeded the formation of HMOs. These issues had not been investigated systematically, so one focus of early research in this area was the relationship between specific legal conditions and the presence or absence of HMOs.

The relative importance of market, legal, and policy conditions in influencing HMO formation and growth have been studied for the period from 1970 to 1973 (McNeil and Schlenker, 1975). These researchers compared the twenty-five states with one or more HMOs in operation in August 1973, with the twenty-five states without HMOs, for laws that were usually cited as barriers to HMO development. They found some differences in the legal conditions between the state groups, but no clear conclusions could be drawn. HMOs succeeded in forming in states with every legal barrier except "strict insurance regulation," which included states with laws requiring physician control and an open physician panel. These researchers continue by reporting that a mid-1973 survey of operational HMOs by Inter-Study also indicated that legal conditions were relatively less important than other factors in limiting HMO formation and development. A legal barrier "was, in general, felt by HMOs to be only the fifth most serious formation or growth barrier they faced." Overall, these researchers concluded that the growth in the number of HMOs from 1970 to 1973 was in response to "favorable market conditions and high-level-policy encouragement by the federal government" and that legal conditions "do not appear to have greatly retarded HMO formation." Other research supports these conclusions (Goldberg and Greenberg, 1981).

In reviewing the research on HMO development, Strumpf concluded that "what may be observed about contemporary obstacles is that state legal barriers were less formidable in the early 1970s than in earlier years and state legal problems today do not seem to be much of a constraint to developing HMOs" (Strumpf, 1981). In his long experience with the federal Office of Health Maintenance Organizations, Strumpf claims that not a single federal HMO grant failed or terminated activity as a result of state legal barriers.

The latent effect of the HMO legislation, which largely eradicated legal barriers, has been to create a new set of problems which may be more detrimental than the previous barriers. The multiple, conflicting, and overlapping local, state, and federal laws and regulations are increasingly problematic for HMO operations (McNeil and Schlenker, 1975; Strumpf, 1981).

Another area of HMO research focuses on the issue of fair market competition. While early research focused on this issue, current federal interest in health care competition has added impetus to investigations in this area. Basically the fair market competition standard is that "obstacles which unfairly bar the entry of HMOs into the medical care market should be removed, but that HMOs should not receive any special advantages relative to the rest of the medical care delivery system" (McNeil and Schlenker, 1975). Several researchers stated that HMO-enabling legislation impedes the ability of HMOs to compete on an "equal footing" with insurers (McNeil and Schlenker, 1975; Luft, 1981). By attempting to protect consumers through quality safeguards, many HMO-enabling statutes slow HMO formation and growth and raise the cost of HMO care without significantly increasing consumer protection. Many of the requirements imposed on HMOs are not imposed on their competitors (insurers and providers). For example, HMOs in many areas are required to conform to insurance-type financial regulations; however, open enrollment requirements, mandated quality and utilization review, and requisite extensive financial, utilization, and quality reporting are features of HMO-enabling legislation that are often not required of insurers. HMO advertising and premiums are frequently regulated. On the other side, HMO competitors argue that HMOs have received federal subsidies through grants and loans and have received favorable federal policy consideration. In addition, many states exempt HMOs from reserve requirements required of commercial health insurers and allow HMOs to negotiate with providers for advantageous financial consideration.

POLITICAL AND REGULATORY ENVIRONMENT

The political environment is an important factor that differentiates the Twin Cities and Chicago. Examination of the political environment enables us to understand the forces that have shaped HMO legislation and regulation in the two areas. Each community has a distinctive decision-making style that is generally consistent across the entire spectrum of issues, including those related to health care and HMOs.

Minneapolis-St. Paul

Consensus is the decision-making style characteristic of the Twin Cities. The private and public sectors are closely articulated in the definition and solution of problems. The private sector tends to be interested and involved in social problems in the Twin Cities. It has taken a proactive stance by defining the problems, developing priorities, conducting research, and recommending possible solutions. Interestingly, the private sector is involved to a large extent in the implementation of the solutions it devises, either through individual or collective action. In turn, in many cases, the public sector is supportive of the private sector. Many times, the public sector assists the private sector by codifying and implementing supportive public policy initiatives.

Generally, the health care sector in Minneapolis-St. Paul is closely articulated and integrated with other interest groups. A high degree of communication exists between various interests in the Twin Cities vis-à-vis health care. This cohesiveness facilitates coordination and action on health care issues. While having different stances on particular issues, the various interests in the health care sector, i.e., physicians, hospitals, nursing homes, and health insurers, generally display a high degree of communication. An interesting aspect of the health care power structure in the Twin Cities is the prominent role that the business community has played in health care reform. The Citizens League, composed largely of corporate interests, has provided essential leadership in health care reform.

As cost containment concerns of the public and private sectors have risen over the past decade, policy makers have searched for optimal strategies to address this problem. Competitive strategies have occupied an increasingly central position in health care decision making and reform in the Twin Cities. Competition in health care was championed early on by Paul Ellwood, M.D., and Walter McClure, Ph.D., at InterStudy. Besides their role in national health policy, which came later, Ellwood and McClure educated the Twin Cities business community about its role in facilitating competition in health care. Competitive solutions to health care problems have been suggested by the Citizens League and the Minnesota Coalition on Health Care Costs, and the Minnesota legislature has incorporated competitive concepts into health care legislation. Again, the public sector serves to codify and embody in legislation many of the philosophical principles that are shared generally.

It is also important to emphasize that in the Twin Cities there seems to be a realization that competitive solutions cannot be successful without adequate planning and regulatory supports. These supports are seen by some as playing an appropriate role in fostering health care competition. It should be mentioned that there is much discussion in the health care sector and community at large about the negative consequences of competition. There is also philosophical disagreement as to whether competition in health care is necessary, appropriate, and desirable. However, competitive solutions are increasingly being incorporated into health care decisions in the Twin Cities.

The health care and community elite in the Twin Cities generally believed Minnesota's programs, policies, and legislation to be in the vanguard. A number of respondents stated that Minnesota has led the country in formulating and implementing innovative programs in social welfare. There seemed to be an attitude among political and community leaders that Minnesota can generally "do a better job" than the federal government formulating legislation relevant to their needs. There was a certain resentment of federal regulation and intervention. Respondents cited several instances in which the federal government adopted programs, policies, and legislation that was initially developed and implemented in Minnesota. Minnesotans took pride in their independence and leadership vis-à-vis federal programs, policies, and legislation.

Chicago

Politics in Chicago has long been characterized by conflicting interest groups and confrontational decision making. In general, these two elements—conflict and confrontation—permeate decision making across issues and sectors in Chicago. The public and private sectors in Chicago rarely cooperate in the definition and solution of social problems largely because of the magnitude and variety of social problems confronting Chicago and because of their intractability. As a result of diverging interests and priorities, cooperation between sectors is limited to a very narrow range of issues. Traditionally, general health care issues have not been high on the list of priorities of either the private or public sectors. The overriding issue in health care in Chicago is the provision of health care services to the very large poor population. This monumental problem has been delegated largely to the public and non-profit sectors.

The public and non-profit sectors have played a significant role in health politics in the Chicago area. They have taken the lead in problem definition and solution. In turn, the health care sector has generally been reactive to the proposals and actions of these sectors. The power of interest groups in the health care sector is highly diffuse and issue-specific. The various interests in health care do not display high levels of cohesiveness, cooperation, or communication. Power bases of the two principal interest groups—physicians and hospitals—are cross-cut in the Chicago area by city and suburban distinctions. Medicaid is the focus of much of the activity in health politics. Consequently, much of the action takes place in the state capital, yet, in contrast to the Twin Cities, the capital is 250 miles from Chicago in a rural setting. Thus, the legislators are both geographically and conceptually removed from urban problems.

Business interests have played a relatively minor role in the health care sector in Chicago. This is largely a result of the diversity, magnitude, and priorities of the employer community. The employer community is highly fractionated. More recently employer coalitions have begun to play a role in activating and organizing the employer community on health care issues. These organizations are attempting to facilitate formally the activity that occurs informally in smaller corporate communities such as Minneapolis-St. Paul (see chapter 7). Employers in Chicago are now starting to play a more active role in health politics.

Concern about rising health care costs has developed in the Chicago area during the past several years. This concern has activated both the public and private sectors. However, it is difficult to ascertain any common agenda among the relevant actors in the health care sector with respect to cost containment. First, collective decisions regarding health care issues are more difficult to achieve as a result of the confrontational characteristics of the health care sector and the community at large. Second, major health care actors in Chicago have not embraced the concept that cost containment strategies must involve broad reforms in health care finance and delivery. Most of the decision-making efforts in Chicago involve microlevel solutions. These solutions are circumscribed and thus limited in their overall impact on the health care system. Perhaps a fractionated system can act only in this manner. However, coalitions are beginning to play an important role by focusing the actions of a variety of interested parties. The agendas of these coalitions are moving toward health system reform.

The public sector in Chicago has taken a leading role in health care decision making. This has resulted from default on the part of the private sector. If anything, the private sector has taken a reactive stance. Regulatory activities in health care are guided by concerns for consumer protection, which has traditionally been provided by the Departments of Public Health and Insurance. In Chicago, with its large indigent and near poor population, this procedure has been elevated to an end in itself by many health care regulators. State regulations nearly always involve regulatory controls over supply or reimbursement. The precipitating factor for much of the state's action in health care is Medicaid expenditures.

Historically, people in Chicago looked to the public sector to define problems and propose solutions. The private sector generally reacted to these proposals. If the private sector devised a counterproposal it generally emanated from a minority of the relevant interest groups in the health care sector, e.g., the Chicago Hospital Council and the Chicago Medical Society. It seems difficult in Chicago to arrive at collective decisions in the health care sector. It is also difficult to find any common threads between proposals. In recent years the private sector has begun to take a more proactive stance on health care issues.

THE DEVELOPMENT OF STATE HMO LEGISLATION AND REGULATION

HMO legislation and regulation in Minnesota and Illinois have developed in strikingly different ways. The factors precipitating the formation of HMO legislation, as well as the parties involved, have been different in these two areas. In many ways, HMO legislation and regulation in these two areas reflect their broad political styles.

Minneapolis-St. Paul

In Minnesota, legal obstacles were encountered by the early groups interested in forming direct service prepaid-group-practice health plans. In 1937, a group of credit union leaders in the Twin Cities wanted to form a direct service prepaid health plan but were blocked by a Minnesota attorney general's opinion (Uphoff, 1980). The interpretation handed down by the attorney general stated that such a health plan would be in violation of common law, which forbade the "corporate practice of medicine." As an alternative, a mutual health insurance company was formed as a stepping-stone to a prepaid plan. The founders of the mutual were interested in activities that would change the political environment that had blocked the formation of a prepaid health plan. Since Minnesota insurance laws forbade Group Health Mutual from engaging in educational and legislative activities, a separate organization, Group Health Association, was formed. The educational and legislative activities of this organization eventually paved the way for the formation of Group Health Plan.

Beginning in 1939, Group Health Association introduced HMO-enabling statutes in every Minnesota legislative session. The statutes would have had the effect of overriding the opinions of three attorneys general holding that prepaid health plans intrinsically violated the corporate practice of medicine statutes. These early legislative efforts contended that a non-profit, member-owned plan would not violate existing law. Each time the proposed legislation went before committee, the Minnesota Medical Association argued against prepaid health plans. In addition, physicians, hospital administrators, and other members of the established health care community lobbied against the plans (Uphoff, 1980).

In addition to legal obstacles, early prepaid plans in Minnesota faced resistance from organized medicine. In 1953, when Two Harbors Community Health Association in northeastern Minnesota began an expansion program, opposition from the medical community reached a peak. The association filed suit against the St. Louis County Medical Society charging discrimination against the association's physicians, refusal of hospital privileges for the association's physicians, and general professional ostracism for denying the plan's physicians membership in the medical society (Uphoff, 1980). The suit was settled out of court in favor of the Two Harbors Association. This settlement had a profound effect upon efforts to obtain legal clearance for the formation of prepaid health plans in Minnesota.

In 1955, articles of incorporation for Group Health Plan were drafted and presented to the Minnesota Secretary of State. An opinion of the attorney general on the formation of a prepaid health plan was sought. Group Health Plan's counsel argued that a non-profit consumer-owned health plan would not violate the law since no profit would accrue to owners and that insurance laws would not apply since services would be rendered directly. With legal precedents in favor of consumer-owned prepaid health plans set by suits brought against medical societies by Group Health Cooperative of Puget Sound and the Two Harbors Association, the attorney general ruled that a prepaid health plan could form under the non-profit statute that governed hospitals. Following the attorney general's opinion, there was "no visible opposition from the State Medical Association" (Uphoff, 1980). After twenty years of legal confrontation, a legal precedent existed in Minnesota that allowed for the formation of prepaid health plans.

In the early 1970s, renewed interest was exhibited in the concept of prepaid health care. Health maintenance organizations (a newly coined term) rose to national prominence as the cornerstone of the Nixon administration's national health policy. During this period, interest in the HMO concept in the Twin Cities was also increasing. Primarily through the efforts of Ellwood, McClure, and their colleagues at InterStudy, the business community became interested in the concept. This interest took the form of the Twin Cities Health Care Development Project (TCHCDP), which played an important role in facilitating HMO development in the Twin Cities (see chapter 7). Interest in state HMO-enabling legislation grew out of the efforts of TCHCDP and InterStudy. It was felt that new HMOs would not be satisfied operating without any specific HMO-enabling legislation.

In 1971, InterStudy drafted and found sponsors for a bill that would authorize proprietary HMOs. Because the bill was introduced late in the legislative session, no action was taken on it. In 1972, the bill was reintroduced in the Senate. In addition, a state representative introduced a non-profit HMO-enabling bill in the House. There was much debate over the profit/non-profit issue. The advocates of the for-profit bill, primarily InterStudy and the TCHCDP, were concerned about capital formation for HMOs, and they argued that the ability to own an HMO and generate profits would facilitate HMO investment and development. At that point, insurance companies, providers, and business corporations were investigating the feasibility of owning and operating HMOs. The supporters of the non-profit bill, primarily Group

Health Plan but also farm, labor, and cooperative organizations, were concerned about introducing the profit motive into prepaid health care. Group Health Plan led the opposition to the proprietary bill and argued that the bill, sponsored by the "industrial-medical complex," achieved "the single purpose of authorizing profit HMOs and then attempt[ing] to regulate the mischief that is done by for-profit HMOs" (Uphoff, 1980). Group Health argued that the for-profit bill would impede the development of community non-profit HMOs by regulating the practice of an HMO without regulating fee-for-service health care providers. They posed the question, "Why should non-profit HMOs that have operated with integrity be burdened with all this regulatory gibberish?" (Uphoff, 1980). In discussing the 1973 proprietary legislation, one respondent noted that Group Health representatives argued that

> the business and professional interests [that promoted] the profit HMO concept are in most part the same as those who helped forestall authorizing legislation . . . in the past. [Because of the] success of Group Health Plan . . the forces that historically opposed the development of non-profit [HMOs] now seek to turn the application of these principles to the advantage of health care providers, insurance companies, and various other corporate business interests.

Some observers have stated that Group Health used the legislative process to its advantage by eliminating competition from proprietary HMOs. Many respondents stated that while this may have been part of their reason for opposing the proprietary HMO-enabling legislation, Group Health's opposition was primarily on ideological grounds. Their lobbying on the bill clearly identified them as a consumer interest group, thereby bringing them together with organized labor, cooperatives, and other groups interested in promoting consumer interests.

Another issue about which there was substantial debate was the regulatory intent of the bill. The crux of this debate was the balance between the financial and delivery aspects of the regulation. There was concern over the orientation of the regulators: whether it should be financial or health care delivery. Legislators ruled out the insurance department as the sole regulator quite early. They proposed, in their two bills, the Department of Health or an independent committee comprising bureaucrats from a number of departments and appointees.

The compromise legislation, the Health Maintenance Act of 1973, authorized only non-profit HMOs, contained provisions for consumer representation on the HMO's board of directors, and gave primary regulatory authority to the Minnesota Department of Health.

In drafting HMO rules and regulations, the health department staff took the NAIC model act and modified it in particular areas where the Minnesota legislation deviated. Specific features of the law and important deviations will be discussed later. In drafting the rules and regulations, a number of individuals within the Departments of Health and Insurance were consulted. After an initial draft of the regulations was completed, informal comment was solicited from existing and forming HMOs as well as from other interested parties in the health care community. Following this informal process and the incorporation of relevant comments into the regulations, formal hearings were held. Few revisions resulted from these hearings and the regulations were adopted.

Chicago

In Illinois, specific HMO-enabling legislation came later than in Minnesota. Few, if any, legal obstacles existed in Illinois for the formation and incorporation of prepaid health plans. Legislation authorizing formation of prepaid health plans had existed in Illinois since the Voluntary Health Services Act of 1951 (VHSA). This act was primarily for the formation of employer and union health plans. Many of the early employer and union health plans in Illinois were, in fact, prepaid. In addition, several of the early HMOs in Chicago, i.e., Union Health Service, Anchor, and Michael Reese Health Plan, originally served union employees. These two factors set a precedent for the formation of other HMOs in Illinois under the act.

Unions fought hard for the passage of the Voluntary Health Services Act in 1951 because it enabled them to form their own health plans. There was strong opposition to the legislation from traditional interests in the health care community. Opposition was predicated on ideological grounds, that is, that this legislation would be the first step toward socialized medicine. Underlying this ideological rhetoric was an attempt to preserve the status quo—to maintain established economic relationships. With the leadership and perserverance of organized labor, the act was passed. This legislation paved the way for the formation of Union Health Service in Chicago and laid the legal foundation for prepaid health care in Illinois.

In the early 1970s, increasing awareness and knowledge of HMOs focused legislative attention on the concept. As discussed above, early HMOs in Illinois had been organized and regulated under the Voluntary Health Services Act. The Department of Insurance was the sole regulatory agency in this act. In 1973, the Departments of Insurance and Public Health began to examine the regulatory framework for HMOs under the Voluntary Health Services Act. Their investigation found that the act was deficient and inappropriate for the regulation of HMOs. The principal deficiency was that it did not include provisions to regulate the medical delivery and quality of care aspects of HMOs. Health officials were concerned that the quality of care in HMOs must be regulated, particularly in light of what they considered to be "possible incentives for underservice present in prepayment."

Health officials also wanted the ability to monitor the accessibility of care. Also, during this period, the state was interested in the ability of HMOs to reduce Medicaid costs. The Department of Public Health felt strongly that it needed the regulatory authority to examine quality of care for Medicaid HMOs to prevent abuses that had occurred in California. As a result of these concerns, the Departments of Insurance and Public Health prepared legislation that would provide them with a specific framework to regulate HMOs in Illinois. These agencies used the model legislation proposed by the NAIC and amended it as necessary. The legislation contained provisions for the Department of Public Health to regulate the medical delivery functions of HMOs. The Department of Insurance was principally responsible for regulating the insurance and financial functions of HMOs. The departments solicited informal comment on the legislation from the HMOs in operation at the time.

In contrast to Minnesota, the public sector in Illinois was instrumental in introducing state HMO legislation. In 1974, following the formulation of the legislation, the Department of Public Health obtained sponsorship from the chairman of the Senate Committee on Public Health, Welfare, and Safety. The state legislation was passed on the heels of the federal HMO legislation.

While the state legislation was not in direct reaction to the federal legislation, several observers commented that the federal action helped make legislators aware that Illinois needed its own HMO act. The sponsor of the bill commented that since "no one understood HMOs in the Senate, there was no opposition to the bill." He stressed that there was "very little concern, either pro or con, on the bill." He also commented that there were no problems getting the bill through the House because the "concept was so new [there was] no reason to dislike it." In 1974, an HMO-enabling statute, the Health Maintenance Act, was passed in Illinois.

Separate regulations were drafted by the Departments of Insurance and Public Health. The HMO regulations from the Department of Insurance follow the NAIC guidelines and insurance principles. The Department of Public Health, while also using NAIC model regulation, convened an advisory committee to assist in drafting and reviewing their HMO regulations. The HMOs had very little input into the regulations because they had already had input into the statute.

CHARACTERISTICS OF STATE HMO LEGISLATION AND REGULATION

In evaluating the HMO statutes that were passed in Minnesota and Illinois, a number of important differences were discovered. These differences reflect different legislative and regulatory goals and intentions. Legislation may be used to facilitate and regulate HMO development and operation. The relative stress that the sponsors put on these two aspects of HMO-enabling legislation is important. A balance between facilitative provisions and regulatory provisions in the legislation is important in establishing a positive legal environment for an HMO.

Minneapolis-St. Paul

In Minnesota, as noted earlier, the principal regulatory authority for health maintenance organizations is the Department of Health. When the legislation was designed, the authors basically saw HMOs as prepaid-group-practice plans like Group Health Plan. The insurance department perceived HMOs as staff model operations, fundamentally as a group of doctors delivering health care services. It was not realized at that time that future HMOs would be organized in a variety of ways with some, such as IPA models, resembling "hybrid insurance companies." With that mind-set, regulation seemed appropriately located in the Department of Health.

This basic choice had a number of profound consequences for the regulation of HMOs in Minnesota. Some observers contended that insurance regulators tend to take a somewhat inflexible regulatory stance toward HMOs, stifling innovation. Much of insurance regulation is guided by "generally accepted insurance practices." While these principles are admittedly important and necessary, they may limit the regulators' field of vision in terms of innovation. Innovation is critically important in the development of an industry such as HMOs. However, this must be balanced with protecting the public interest. Some respondents stated that HMO regulation by the health department in Minnesota has perhaps been more permissive than it might have been in the insurance department. The health department is willing to entertain measures proposed by HMOs to ameliorate their operating problems. If a measure is effective and not proscribed by the statute, it is accepted. One example, which was cited in support of this contention, was that the HMOs are allowed copayments on preexisting conditions.

Enrollee representation on the HMO's board of directors was introduced into the legislation to provide for "consumer safeguards." Consumer interest groups and Group Health Plan were the major supporters of this provision. Forty percent enrollee representation is mandated on the board. Some of the provider-sponsored HMOs objected to this provision as a "waste of time." Some of the HMOs have turned this provision into positive public relations and have benefited from the financial, legal, and other forms of advice resulting from enrollee board members. In many cases, enrollee board members are more representative of corporate interests than the interests of consumer groups per se.

Although the Minnesota HMO statute restricts HMOs to nonprofit corporations, in recent years a number of HMOs have circumvented this issue by forming for-profit management corporations that contract with the HMOs. The HMO is essentially a "shell corporation" without employees. In another variation on this theme, a non-profit HMO can be "held" by a for-profit holding company. SHARE Health Plan is an example of both of these variations. SHARE Development Corporation, a for-profit national HMO development firm, is a holding company for SHARE and operates the plan under a management contract. Physicians Health Plan has recently negotiated a twenty-five year management contract with United HealthCare, a for-profit HMO development firm. A principal advantage of these types of arrangements is that for-profit development firms can acquire capital either through public stock offerings or through private investment, such as venture capital firms.

HMOs in Minnesota have a relatively extensive list of mandated health care services. When designing the HMO regulations in Minnesota, regulators were interested in creating incentives for the HMOs to compete in certain ways. More specifically, by mandating a relatively rich package of benefits, they would force competition in the areas of efficiency, quality, and accessibility rather than on premium price. Now, nearly all HMOs in the Twin Cities have identical benefits, including mental health, chemical dependency, and out-of-area coverage. There was some criticism that by mandating such a rich benefit package, the regulators eliminated HMOs from important markets, such as small employers.

While HMOs in Minnesota in general have more extensive benefits than conventional health insurers, there are certain areas in which HMOs do not have as extensive benefits. Conventional health insurers have to provide more extensive benefits for handicapped children, mental health, alcoholism, and drug dependency. Conventional insurers argued that HMOs have an advantage over them in the provision of the mandated levels of these benefits. Some observers argued that this omission is a result of different regulatory agencies' having separate authority over HMOs and conventional insurers. One informed observer commented that this is more a function of legislative design and claimed that the HMOs in Minnesota have effectively lobbied legislators to be excluded from certain mandated benefits. The net result is that HMOs have more comprehensive benefits than conventional insurers.

HMOs in Minnesota are not required to file their rates or obtain approval on them prior to use. Many states, such as Illinois, have this provision. Regulators in Minnesota felt that rate filings and approvals were ineffective in controlling health care costs and decided that the benefit of this provision did not warrant its inclusion.

Another area in which Minnesota HMO regulation departs from that of other states is quality assurance oversight. In many states external quality reviews of HMOs are conducted. This involves regulatory staff visiting the HMO and conducting a medical chart review. While the statute permits Minnesota regulators to conduct external chart reviews, a decision was made to emphasize the development and maintenance of internal quality assurance systems by the HMOs and to evaluate those systems rather than conducting external quality reviews.

The Minnesota HMO-enabling statute provided funds for HMO planning and technical assistance. Organizations interested in forming an HMO could apply to the state for matching funds. Several organizations took advantage of this program to assess the feasibility of establishing HMOs. This program was funded for several years.

An important feature of the Minnesota HMO regulation is the mandatory dual choice provision included in 1976. Basically, HMOs can require employers of 100 or more employees to offer an HMO, provided that 25 or more employees live in the HMO's service area. This provision allows HMOs legitimately to approach employers, and it serves an important public relations function. Respondents claimed that very few HMOs actively and forcefully use this provision.

This dual choice amendment was defeated in the legislature at least once before it was adopted. Several of the established HMOs opposed the amendment on the grounds that it was proposed at the "behest of Blue Cross-Blue Shield and segments of the state medical society as a strategy for establishing a Blue Cross HMO network." It was felt that the amendment would "solve any Blue Cross problem in marketing an HMO because they were the only health care organization that had existing relationships with providers" and that it would "give Blue Cross a great advantage not only in marketing a statewide HMO but their regular benefit package as well."

The Minnesota HMO legislation provides a minimal amount of financial oversight for the HMOs. This is mostly a result of the fact that the health department is the regulator.

Chicago

In Illinois, the primary regulatory authority for HMOs rests with the Department of Insurance, which is responsible for the review of organizational documents, provider contracts, marketing materials, rate approval, and fiscal solvency. The Department of Public Health is responsible for the administration of the public health aspects of the law. They include reviewing the quality, utilization, availability, accessibility, and continuity of services offered by the HMO. The Department of Public Health certifies to the Department of Insurance that the HMO either conforms to or deviates from the regulations and statute. The split regulatory function in Illinois works well according to representatives of the two departments. Clear definition of responsibilities aids in this smooth functioning. Some problems have been created by the HMOs "playing" the two departments against one another, but they are greatly reduced by close communication.

There are no limitations on the tax status—for-profit or nonprofit—of HMOs in Illinois, but prior approval for HMO rates is required. The Department of Insurance has forty-five days to disapprove the rates. For the majority of HMOs, the Department of Insurance stated that it does not have concerns about the rates and that the HMOs have the expertise to render justifiable rates. In reviewing rates, the Department of Insurance is not "so much looking to see that the rates are low enough but that they are high enough." They are concerned over issues of solvency. Competition, to a large extent, controls the rates, yet the Department wants to insure that the rates are not "too low."

HMO regulation in Illinois emphasizes financial safeguards and quality safeguards. Financial regulation is stressed in the statute. HMO regulation by the Department of Public Health hinges on external quality review including both site visits and chart reviews.

OTHER RELEVANT STATE LEGISLATION AND POLICY

Minneapolis-St. Paul

In 1976, the Minnesota Comprehensive Health Insurance Act (MCHIA) was passed by the legislature. This legislation has been important for HMOs in two respects. First, this legislation includes a dual option amendment that mandates qualified employers to offer HMOs. This provision directly affects HMOs. The second aspect of the legislation, which was not aimed specifically at HMOs, nevertheless had a profound impact on their growth. This provision of the Minnesota Comprehensive Health Insurance Act was designed to assist consumers and purchasers in evaluating the variety of health insurance plans available through employers in the state. Because of the large number of different plans, all with different levels of benefits and coverage, it became difficult for both employers and consumers to evaluate what they were purchasing. The act specified three levels of health insurance plans. In addition, the act mandated benefits for these plans. To deduct the cost of employee health benefits from their income taxes, employers are required by the act to offer a health insurance plan with high levels of benefits and coverage. The MCHIA effectively standardizes employee health insurance benefits and coverage. HMOs, which also are required to provide extensive benefits, are better able to be price-competitive with conventional health insurance plans.

Another piece of health care legislation passed in 1982 reflected the recent change in health care policy from an emphasis on regulation to an emphasis on competition.

> The statute reflects the desire of the Legislature to move away from regulatory control of health facility capital expenditures, and toward the promotion of price competition. Several provisions liberalize the existing Certificate-Of-Need program. . . . The statute further provides that the Certificate-Of-Need program be terminated. . . . With the intention of moving toward a more price competitive, more efficient market, the statute encourages hospitals and health professionals to undertake price reporting (Minnesota Department of Health, 1982).

This legislation cautiously approached the issue of changing from one cost containment strategy to another by providing that the Minnesota certificate-of-need law not be repealed until its effects were fully considered and alternative cost containment measures were in place and facilitating cost containment through price competition. A central part of this legislation was to encourage hospitals, physicians, and other health care providers to voluntarily disclose and disseminate price information. This provision assisted HMOs as well as insurers and consumers in identifying, and possibly in utilizing, most cost-effective providers. It may be financially advantageous for HMOs to utilize hospitals, and other health care providers, who are more efficient even though they do not offer discounts or other financial considerations. This legislation provides HMOs with more information on which to base their purchasing decisions.

Chicago

The majority of issues in health politics in Illinois focus on the Medicaid program. Policies affecting Medicaid in Illinois have a substantial impact on a large number of health care providers in Illinois. Changes regarding the Medicaid program are particularly felt by providers located in the Chicago metropolitan area. For example, a recent proposal by the Illinois Department of Public Aid to emphasize Medicaid prepayment programs as a means to contain costs created a great deal of interest and activity in prepayment programs. This has been particularly true of inner-city hospitals, which are affected most by changes in Medicaid reimbursement policies. The department requested bids from health care providers for rendering services to the Medicaid population in discrete service areas on a prepaid basis. Consequently, awareness of HMOs and prepayment has grown significantly. A number of new organizations formed in response to this solicitation of bids. These organizations are being sponsored by both hospitals and physicians.

RECENT DEVELOPMENTS IN HMO REGULATION

As a result of the fact that HMOs were new organizational forms, the legislation and regulations enacted to regulate them were also constructed anew. As HMOs matured, so have their regulators. Currently, a number of states are revising their HMO regulations in light of their experience with HMOs. HMOs in many areas are concerned that the changes being proposed in state capitals will be harmful to their growth and development. In many areas, regulators perceived that both the environment in which HMOs operate and the HMOs themselves have changed to such a degree that changes are required. Some regulators perceived that initial HMO legislation, in which HMOs received preferential treatment, was warranted for a fledgling industry operating in a hostile environment. Now, they question whether that type of treatment is warranted.

Minneapolis-St. Paul

Currently, regulators in Minnesota are proposing a number of changes in HMO legislation. Regulators are proposing changes in the area of mandated eligibility and benefits. Some of the requirements in these areas, which apply to commercial health insurance companies and Blue Cross-Blue Shield, are not currently applied to HMOs. Regulators argue that given the growth of the HMO industry in recent years, there is no valid reason for not requiring parity with other health insurers in these areas. It is argued that uniformity of eligibility and benefits is appropriate. The regulators claim that although HMOs already offer many of these features in their benefit plans, with increased competition the HMOs might eliminate them to remain price competitive. In addition, the regulators state that HMOs are "no longer the young, immature corporations" they used to be, and are now large and sophisticated enough to be fully capable of providing benefits already required of other insurers.

The regulators state that "the Health Maintenance Act of 1973 was originally drafted to oversee a young, undeveloped industry which at that time demonstrated little potential for operating harm. . . . HMOs have, in short, outgrown and, at times, outsmarted the 1973 law." The regulators propose a number of amendments to "curb" current "abuses" and minimize "risks of harm to the public." Enclosed in these amendments are provisions that will foster the "closer investigation of proprietary management contracts" and when deemed to be excessively high, provide for refunds to enrollees.

Chicago

Most of the recent changes in HMO regulation in Illinois have been a result of the maturity of the HMOs. Some of the regulations that were needed early are not needed for the mature plans. Likewise, mature plans require other regulations that are not needed by fledgling plans.

In 1982, the Department of Insurance introduced substantial amendments in reserving levels. In addition, several changes were made in the methods of financing these reserves. As HMOs grow into large corporations with substantial revenues, guidelines for HMO investments become necessary. Also as a function of HMOs' maturity and experience, the Department of Insurance is moving toward a system of "file and use" for HMO rates as opposed to the rate approval system now in operation. The majority of the HMOs are experienced in formulating rates. The need for rate filing is less for established, mature HMOs. The department will probably differentiate its procedures regarding rates according to an HMO's age.

The Department of Insurance is also addressing reporting requirements. It is working toward adopting standardized reporting to minimize problems for national HMO corporations that have plans in several states. With the variety of HMO models now in existence, the Department of Public Health has had to clarify its definition of a primary care physician as well as specifying the content of provider contracts. In addition, minimal equipment standards are needed for HMO health delivery facilities and affiliated clinics.

With the advent of other alternative delivery systems, such as PPOs, HMOs in Illinois are carefully monitoring whether legislation will regulate these entities and the extent and content of their regulation.

In Illinois, the philosophy of strong financial and medical delivery regulation embodied in the original legislation has passed the test of time. There has been no radical departure from this underlying philosophy over time, and it has been equally appropriate and effective with both fledgling and mature plans.

FEDERAL HMO LEGISLATION

The federal Health Maintenance Organization Act of 1973 was passed in recognition of the fact that HMOs needed assistance in the early stages of development. The Act provided assistance by dealing with many of the legal, financial, and enrollment barriers that plagued organizations such as HMOs in the past. The HMO act represented two innovations in national health care policy. It was the first federal act to have the explicit goal of changing the medical care system in the United States. Secondly, it represented a new approach by which change is to be accomplished—through competition (Mackie, 1981).

The HMO act specified the requirements an HMO must meet

if it chooses to become federally qualified. To receive the benefits of the act directly, HMOs must be qualified. However, some HMOs have chosen not to qualify. The principal benefits of the law are access to employers through the use of the mandated dual choice provision and the federal financial assistance available through grants and loans. A marketing advantage is the perception by some employers that federal qualification is a type of "Good Housekeeping seal." All HMOs have derived legal benefits as many states have modeled their state HMO legislation after the federal legislation. Federal qualification also has several disadvantages, two of which are in the areas of rating and benefits. HMOs in some areas might find the community rating required by the federal act too restrictive. The mandated benefit package in the federal act may be too rich for certain types of employers and for certain health insurance markets.

Over time, the importance of the federal HMO act has changed. As previously mentioned, the legal overrides have largely been adopted and incorporated into state HMO legislation. The financial assistance provided under the HMO act has been discontinued. The employer mandate and the public relations aspects of the act remain its most important features. However, in some health care markets, HMOs have gained such general acceptance among employers that they are readily accepted without the mandating provisions. This is increasingly true as premiums for conventional health insurance escalate, and employers embrace HMOs as their hope for containing their employee health benefit costs. Recently, HMOs have sought federal qualification in anticipation of Medicare capitation contracts. Federal qualification will obviate much of the documentation required of HMOs applying for Medicare capitation contracts, and will better enable qualified HMOs to enter the Medicare market than nonqualified competitors.

Minneapolis-St. Paul

At the conclusion of this study, three HMOs were federally qualified in Minneapolis-St. Paul. The supportive regulatory and market environment in which HMOs developed in the Twin Cities affected the reasons for HMOs to seek federal qualification. Largely, HMOs in the Twin Cities were developed by sponsors who provided the necessary capitalization and facilities for the HMOs to operate. A majority of HMOs in the Twin Cities were outgrowths of existing, established medical facilities and practices. In addition, HMOs entered a receptive and supportive purchaser market. Employers were familiar with the HMO concept and supported it as a result of the activities of the Twin Cities Health Care Development Project. Later Minnesota legislation provided HMOs with the ability to mandate reluctant employers. As mentioned previously, this provision is used by HMOs more as a public relations "tool" as a state endorsement of the HMO concept than as a legal instrument to force employers into offering HMOs. Finally, early on, the majority of HMOs in the Twin Cities were not interested in providing services for the Medicare and Medicaid markets for which federal qualification would have been a prerequisite. Consequently, there were few incentives for HMOs in the Twin Cities to become federally qualified.

SHARE Health Plan was the first HMO in the Twin Cities to seek federal qualification. SHARE was qualified in 1976 and remained the sole federally qualified HMO in the Twin Cities until 1981. SHARE became qualified initially to obtain financial assistance through the federal HMO grants and loans program. It was the only HMO in the Twin Cities that did not have a corporate sponsor to back it financially. It was after SHARE had obtained federal qualification that the importance of the employer mandate became apparent. SHARE began operations with one delivery site located between Minneapolis and St. Paul at a hospital that had image problems. Because of its limited accessibility and attractiveness, employers were reluctant to offer SHARE. As a result, SHARE depended on and effectively used the employer mandate to gain access to employer accounts. SHARE's use of the mandate also benefited other HMOs. Because of SHARE's limited accessibility, employers generally offered multiple HMOs to obtain the requisite geographic distribution of HMO delivery sites for their employees. SHARE also took advantage of the federal qualification to negotiate a cost contract with the Health Care Financing Administration under which Medicare beneficiaries could be enrolled. This move proved to be a harbinger of the future for the Twin Cities HMO market.

In 1981, Coordinated Health Care (CHC) received federal qualification. CHC is a relatively small HMO with limited accessibility. In addition, it is associated with Ramsey County and its public hospital. Furthermore, CHC operates largely in an area that has traditionally been unsupportive of HMOs. As a result, CHC perceived federal qualification to be useful in gaining access to the employer market. Qualification proved beneficial in this respect, but SHARE had already activated many of the employers in their area. Employers are required by the HMO act to offer only one of each of the two classes of HMOs—group-staff and IPA. Both SHARE and CHC qualified as group-staff model HMOs. CHC gained some competitive advantages in that its service area includes several counties in Wisconsin and therefore allows them to mandate Twin Cities employers who have 25 or more workers living in this area. At the conclusion of this study, SHARE's service area did not include these counties.

In 1983, Physicians Health Plan (PHP) received federal qualification. PHP sought federal qualification for competitive purposes. In the Twin Cities, federal qualification is one means used to differentiate HMOs. In addition, PHP was qualified as an IPA. Since PHP is the only IPA model federally qualified it may mandate employers regardless of whether SHARE or CHC has already mandated them. By being the first IPA in the Twin Cities to be federally qualified, PHP has in effect blocked competing IPAs from enjoying the advantages of the mandate if they decide to become qualified. Employers are required to offer only one IPA under the federal HMO law.

Chicago

Chicago HMOs faced a different set of market conditions from HMOs in the Twin Cities. The employers in Chicago were largely unfamiliar with and unsupportive of HMOs. To gain access to employers, HMOs in Chicago saw federal qualification as a necessity. In addition, by being federally qualified, HMOs were eligible for development and expansion funds.

Several HMOs in Chicago received financial assistance through the federal HMO act. NorthCare, a consumer-sponsored HMO, looked to the federal grant and loan program for its financial livelihood throughout its operation. In fact, it used the maximum amounts available under the federal HMO act. Anchor used federal money principally for its expansion. Two HMOs in Chicago, Intergroup and HMO Illinois, did not use any money under the federal program.

Chicago HMO, organized to serve the Medicaid population, was encouraged to seek federal qualification by the Illinois Department of Public Aid. After three years, HMOs serving the Medicaid population must become federally qualified for the state to obtain federal matching funds for that segment of the Medicaid population served by the HMO.

The prime reason for HMOs in Chicago to become federally qualified was to gain access to the employer market. After the HMO act was passed and before the regulations were promulgated, employers in Chicago were reluctant to offer HMOs. They took a "wait and see" attitude with respect to what they would be required to do under the act. When the regulations were established and employers understood that they would be required to offer HMOs if mandated, they reacted by offering only HMOs that were federally qualified. This created a situation that encouraged HMOs to become qualified. In addition, it gave a competitive advantage to HMOs who were qualified. Consequently, after one HMO became federally qualified, the majority of the other plans followed.

In a market as diverse and as large as Chicago, some observers claimed that early federally qualified HMOs, principally as a result of the extensive mandated benefits and the rating method, were noncompetitive with conventional health insurers on both price and services. This may have aggravated and reinforced the slow growth of HMOs, which was largely a function of the lack of employer support. In addition, since early HMO premiums in Chicago were relatively high compared to those of conventional health insurers, some adverse selection may have occurred. These problems have largely rectified themselves in recent years as a result of the rapidly escalating premiums of conventional health insurance and the ability of HMOs to contain their premium increases.

In recent years, several new HMOs in Chicago decided not to seek federal qualification. They claimed that the employer market in Chicago has grown knowledgeable and supportive of HMOs over the years to the point now that federal qualification is no longer required. In addition, these HMOs claimed that they want to preserve "maximum flexibility," which they feel federal qualification hampers.

SUMMARY

The general political environment in Minnesota supported the development of HMOs. HMO legislation in Minnesota emanated from the private sector, so the private sector had a vested interest in the success of HMOs. Essentially the public sector codified and implemented the agenda formulated by the private sector. Significant legal barriers to HMO development were perceived to exist. Minnesota HMO legislation and regulation has been supportive and has facilitated HMO development and growth. HMOs were given preferential regulatory consideration. Federal HMO legislation and federal qualification have played a relatively minor role in HMO development in the Twin Cities as a whole. State legislation provided the necessary conditions under which HMOs could develop and grow. In addition, employers were generally supportive of HMOs in this area. HMOs play a prominent role in the emerging competition philosophy influencing health care decision making in the Twin Cities. As HMOs matured, regulators called for significant changes in the regulation, which would if made erode the competitive advantages given to them as fledgling and new organizations. It is difficult to predict how this regulatory thrust will be played out and what impact any changes will have on HMO growth and development.

In Illinois, the thrust for specific HMO legislation came from regulators. Legislation existed in Illinois under which HMOs could organize and operate. Significant legal barriers to HMO formation did not exist as they did in Minnesota. Regulators were interested in specific legislation to regulate HMOs that had not been included in previous legislation. Regulators were basically interested in protecting the public interest through their regulatory activities. The HMO-enabling legislation emphasized regulation more than provisions to facilitate development and growth. This legislation was relatively neutral with respect to facilitating HMO development. Federal HMO legislation and federal qualification played a prominent role in the development of HMOs in Chicago. The federal HMO act provided HMOs with access to the employer market, which was unknowledgeable and resistant to HMOs. In addition, it provided several HMOs with a source of finances. HMOs do not occupy a prominent role in health care decision making in Chicago. This is principally a result of the fact that collective decision making in health care in Chicago is uncommon. Regulators in Illinois have not made any radical departures from the basic financial and public health regulatory philosophy existent in the original legislation.

3

HMOs and Consumers

In both metropolitan areas, consumers are the least cohesive and appeared to be the least influential of the various sectors of the health care system. Still, the community institutions and decision-making styles that they established can have a powerful influence. In the Twin Cities, consumer interests are expressed by representatives from such centralized organizations as the Citizens League (private) and the Metropolitan Council (public). In Chicago there is no central civic leadership comparable to that in the Twin Cities, but there is considerably more local and organized consumer health activism in neighborhood and special interest groups. This localized activism reflects the fragmentation of the area. Although consumers initially sponsored some HMOs, they are generally not influential in developing HMOs. The capital and organization necessary for developing health care delivery systems are too demanding for most consumer-based groups.

At the center of any health care system one finds consumers, and their perspectives and behaviors are critical to the success or failure of any organizational innovation, such as HMOs. Of course, in some sense, everyone is a consumer of health care. In much of the HMO literature, when consumers of health care are discussed, the discussion centers around "consumer satisfaction." Although satisfaction, and particularly what consumers have heard about others' satisfaction, is one element in consumers' relationships to HMOs, this study sought to gain other impor-

This chapter was written by Claire H. Kohrman, Research Project Analyst.

tant information relevant to the relationships of HMOs with consumers.

This section presents information from forty consumer informants chosen because they act as, or are seen in their community to be, skilled observers or committed participants in community or consumer activity. We sought people who were involved not only in civic activities in general, but who had been involved in, or reportedly interested in, community health issues. These informants represented churches, schools, and the press, government agencies and citizens' groups, as well as organizations serving particular interests—women, minorities, the poor, and the elderly. Some belonged to HMOs; others did not.

BACKGROUND

While there is agreement that consumers are a central part of the health care system in all communities, there is little agreement about the definition of a health care consumer. For the employer, the employee is the consumer of a health care plan, but for the HMO marketer, the employer is the consumer. Others may variously define consumers by their roles as rank and file union members, clients, patients, voters or enrollees. As Luft notes, "Definition of the consumer is open to various interpretations. Health plans may (even) solicit individuals whom they desire to have serve on the board of directors and offer them health plan memberships, thus classifying them as consumers" (Luft, 1981b). In addition to such instrumental perceptions by others, there are important distinctions among the ways that consumers define themselves.

Some consumers in both Minneapolis-St. Paul and Chicago are proactive. Their ideological perspective is associated with collectivism. Collectivism has historical roots in the settling of American farmland and was recently reawakened as a social movement in the 1960s. Collectivism is associated not only with health care but also with housing, education, and religion. These consumers choose to act out of a belief or commitment about the importance of a position or action. One Chicago consumer activist noted, "Health care is *not* like buying a refrigerator." Their conviction and tradition are characteristic of those who founded consumer-sponsored HMOs and will be discussed below.

For other consumers, though, buying health care may not

seem so different from buying a refrigerator. Their approach to health care is not ideological but simply, and often wisely, practical. It may be a reaction to a specific health care issue or a wish to correct a specific problem, e.g., high cost, poor quality, or inaccessibility. They may, in fact, not think of themselves as health care consumers until asked to serve on some committee. Federal law, as well as Minnesota law, specifies that at least one-third of the membership of the policy-making body or the board of directors of a qualified HMO shall be composed of enrollees, i.e., consumers (Luft, 1981b).

In addition to these generic variations in definitions of consumers, there are further variations in each community that reflect the nature of the communities. Consumers' perceptions and behaviors in Minneapolis-St. Paul and Chicago regarding health care, and the ways these have changed in the last fifteen to twenty years, provide an important background for understanding the different contexts in which HMOs have been initiated and developed.

It is not surprising that consumers can be informed about their community, but it is interesting to note that the very selection process of the consumers for this study (by position and recommendation) reflected and predicted the nature of the two communities from the beginning. In Minneapolis-St. Paul, which is relatively small and homogeneous and where citizens value consensus, it was not difficult to find certain consumers who were well informed about the whole community and who articulated what turned out to be a predominant view. Subsequent interviews corroborated their central perceptions and added specifics from the perspective of the particular informant.

Chicago, on the other hand, is large, fragmented, and accustomed to adversarial relationships. There it was not possible to find informants identified as representative of the general community because, unlike Minneapolis-St. Paul, Chicago has no acknowledged and centrally institutionalized consumer groups. Instead there are many capable and active representatives of specific areas, causes, and interest groups. When interviewed, Chicago informants spoke from the perspective of their own causes with little interest in issues of more general concern. Furthermore, they had little information about events outside of their neighborhood or particular concern. Thus the information on the two communities in this section not only is different, but has, by necessity, been assembled differently. Because in the

Twin Cities a number of the informants have presented quite a full synthesis of the principal community activities and attitudes, our understanding of the Twin Cities has been guided by several of their own systematic considerations. In Chicago, however, the interviews, although they often provided a great deal of information and a thorough understanding of a portion of the system, never provided an overview of the Chicago health care system. They were, instead, interesting fragments of a puzzle. These we have systematically gathered to suggest the synthetic whole.

CONCERNS AND PERCEPTIONS

In the 1960s and early 1970s, consumers across the country concerned with health care reflected the prevalent national consumer ideology. They were mostly concerned with equity in two ways. They sought an equitable distribution of good-quality care among the population—the poor and minority groups as well as secure majority groups—and they sought a more equitable distribution of power between the providers of health care (mostly perceived as doctors) and the receivers of health care (patients). Outgrowths of this latter interest are the self-help movement, the home birth movement, and the women's health movement. In the 1980s, there continues to be a significant reflection of these same concerns in Chicago consumers, but there has been a shift in a new direction in the Twin Cities.

Differences

In the Twin Cities, respondents in all sectors reflected confidence and pride in the quality of their health care. Even those at neighborhood health centers and public aid programs perceived that the Twin Cities area has excellent health care and good access to care. They also seemed warmed by the glow of the Mayo brothers' reputation, which has brought credit to the area throughout this century.

Equitable distribution of health care in the usual sense mentioned above was not a prevalent concern. For example, when a Minneapolis consumer advocate was asked, "Is there a sense in the Twin Cities that there is an underserved group?" he replied, "Yes, small business people, the self-employed, and those with problems with medical insurance." Thus it is apparent that the level and content of concern in the Twin Cities is different from those in metropolitan areas plagued by inner-city poverty and ill health.

All consumers interviewed in the Twin Cities believed the major health concern was cost containment. In the Twin Cities, the consumers voiced concerns similar to those found in other sectors of the community. In the middle 1970s, consumer groups began to give systematic attention to the problem of higher costs. Twin Cities consumers were concerned with the escalating cost of health care, and they had views on how costs should be controlled. Most consumers were aware of and approved of competition as a means of controlling costs. Many were wary of regulation. A number of consumers remembered the earlier regulatory recommendations of the Metropolitan Health Board, which almost closed some cherished hospitals in the name of cost containment, so they were willing to try competition over regulation. They were particularly opposed to federal regulation, asserting that Minnesota makes better laws and is, in fact, a model for federal legislation rather than a follower of federal action. A newspaper from the Twin Cities noted,

> ... [although] the federal government had little to do with HMO growth in Minnesota ... HEW officials point to the Twin Cities as one of the few areas in the country where the kind of HMO incentives the administration advocates actually are being demonstrated in the medical marketplace.
>
> (Minneapolis Star, 1978)

In Chicago equitable distribution of care was still perceived to be the most important health problem. Every consumer mentioned the problem of the "two-tiered system" by which quality and access to care are distributed unequally. Although excellent care is available to most of those who are working, to the affluent, and to suburban residents, equal quality care is not available to the unemployed, to the poor, and to inner-city residents (mostly non-white). A secondary but increasing concern for Chicago health care consumers was the escalation of cost. Although cost was an important focus of consumer activism, particularly in relation to Blue Cross-Blue Shield, the issue of competition as a means of lowering costs or improving care was not mentioned or was not really understood by Chicago consumers. In strong contrast to the Twin Cities, consumers in the Chicago area thought federal regulation was the best hope for improving the quality and distribution of health care.

These notable differences in health care concerns in the two communities have important implications for the development of HMOs. In the Chicago area, sophisticated consumer representatives are concerned about the ability of HMOs to serve the poor. They recognized that those on public assistance may have other needs beyond conventional medical services. Because this was a major concern for consumers in Chicago, it accounts for a major source of consumer questions about HMOs. In the Twin Cities, however, the questions regarding HMOs centered more on how they can enhance competition and on whether they can lower costs.

Although most of those interviewed in the Twin Cities did not raise the issue of maldistribution, those who represent or work with the poor did. However, the magnitude of the problem is so much smaller that it seems to make a qualitative difference in the community's perception about the broad applicability of HMOs. This is not surprising, because the Twin Cities have extensive resources for dealing with the comparatively small problem. Minnesota had the highest allotment per Medicaid recipient of any state in the nation (see chapter 1 for details). In Ramsey County, the Public Health Department arranged to supplement an HMO demonstration project for Medicaid patients with coordinated social services. SHARE opened a Thursday night free clinic for the unemployed whose benefits have run out.

Only a few of the most sophisticated consumers in the Chicago area knew about recent health care demonstration projects or about the interest of the Illinois Department of Public Aid in developing prepaid contracts for Medicaid recipients.

Similarities

Although the differences in the communities' perceptions were significant there were recurring similarities of certain perceptions and conditions among all of the health care consumers interviewed. First, consumers in both metropolitan areas had a general distrust of for-profit health care. Second, consumers were strongly influenced by the viewpoint of their physicians. Third, consumers were frequently perceived, and perceived themselves, to be ineffectual or unnecessary on boards with professionals and bureaucrats.

Although "non-profit status often reflects legal technicality rather than actual organizational goals" (Luft, 1981b), most consumers, even those who have been observing the health care system for years, have a strong aversion to for-profit health care. The Minnesota legislature, no doubt in some part responding to consumer sentiment, passed legislation requiring HMOs to be non-profit. While Illinois allowed for-profit HMOs, consumers in the Chicago area continued to express distrust of for-profit organizations in spite of evidence that non-profit organizations behave similarly to those explicitly for profit. For example, non-profit groups siphon off profits to affiliated entities such as holding companies.

Health consumers were very strongly influenced by the viewpoint of their doctor. The doctor-patient relationship, unlike other provider-consumer relationships, included elements that cannot be completely explained. For example, people believed that there was a health care crisis in America; however, they reported that they were satisfied with their own medical care (Aday, et al. 1980). In fact, high levels of satisfaction with providers were reported in almost all studies (Luft, 1981a). Consumers' concerns closely paralleled the concerns of physicians in the same community, and our interviews suggested that even the most skilled and adversarial consumer health advocates avoid conflict with physicians. When asked how they had brought their concerns about cost to the attention of physicians, the principal spokesperson for an influential health consumers' group in Chicago responded,

> (We) have stayed away from doctors . . . for political reasons. . . . They have the most powerful lobby both in Springfield and in Washington. We've tried to be very realistic about what we can do. And we have found as long as we don't antagonize the doctors we can have a field day with the hospitals and insurance companies—just as long as we leave the doctors alone.

The interviewer asked if any change in that policy was anticipated, and the informant responded that it would eventually be necessary, but we "need a complete reorganization of the system. . . . I don't see it in my lifetime."

This reluctance to confront the power of doctors coupled with admiration and close affective ties with one's own doctor has important implications for consumers' ability to advocate a health care innovation, HMOs or any other, that physicians oppose or do not actively support. Another consumer representative exemplified the abundant and perverse forgiveness consumers voiced for doctors: "Doctors are not vicious," but most "don't have time to be broad minded—that's their background." An exceptional consumer less awed by the medical profession said that there is a mystique that the health field is "highly technical and too hard to understand" and that the "doctor is well intentioned and knows best." Although this informant disagreed with that common perception, she understood that "if you go to the doctor not well, you're not going to fight with your doctor, particularly if you think he is a wonderful person."

Although one can see, particularly in Chicago, that consumers are competent and intensely active in neighborhood associations, when consumers are mixed on boards with professionals and/or others with highly technical knowledge, their effectiveness is altered. A sophisticated consumer advocate with more than ten years of experience on health committees and boards noted that although she was committed to consumers on boards, such as the HSA, she now thought it would be better if consumers had their own organization. She said that consumers "come in cold" with no experience in bureaucracies and try to work with providers and bureaucrats who have political agendas and a staff to back them up. The staff at voluntary agencies, she explained, develops paperwork to show that they are doing a lot of work and to prove that they are very much needed. The volunteers (consumers) have limited time. So, if the staff wants to run an organization, they "flood the volunteers with paperwork." Most consumers, though hopeful when they volunteer, begin to feel incompetent and withdrawn.

Some volunteers, on the other hand, are professionalized by the bureaucratic experience and lose their truly consumer viewpoint. There appears to be a paradoxical effect. Consumers who persist in their original naive or idealistic perception have little impact, and those who have impact are often drawn away from their original consumer perceptions. Thus, consumer representation among the most well-intentioned health planners continues to be a problem (Luft, 1981a).

ORGANIZATION, LEADERSHIP, AND ACTION

Questions regarding health organizations and leadership again revealed significant differences between the Twin Cities and Chicago. When asked about consumer leaders and organizations, Twin Cities health consumers named central institutions and civic leaders. They had little information about local neighborhood or special interest groups. In fact, the Minnesota informants from the consumer sector are themselves indicative of the Twin Cities consumer activity. A number of consumers or community leaders interviewed represented central community institutions, such as the Citizens League and the Metropolitan Health Board. They were extremely well known and well informed about issues throughout the community. On the other hand, those whom we interviewed from local health groups were much less well informed and active. They seemed confident that local activism was not necessary because in Minneapolis-St. Paul, the community leadership always provided leadership on important issues, such as education and transportation. Health care in the Twin Cities is seen as a matter of community and, thus, corporate responsibility. There is relatively little "grass roots" activism in health care policy.

It is not just the usual community leadership that consumers referred to. Many, but not all, of the consumers referred to a variety of other strong and broadly based sources of individual and corporate leadership in health issues. These included Paul Ellwood, Walter McClure, the University of Minnesota, and Group Health Plan. Others are mentioned more specifically in relation to HMOs and will be discussed in the next section. The consumers we interviewed in the Twin Cities took pride in these central advisors and decision-making bodies, as well as in the consensual mode in which they operate. Decision making in health in the Twin Cities is reasoned, deliberate, and focused. Consensus is developed and then voiced by institutionalized consumer or community leaders. Rarely do special interest groups or adversarial encounters get much attention. The controversial call for "bedcutting" was an exception that clarifies the general rule.

Many of the consumer respondents spoke with discomfort about the unpleasantness of the bedcutting conflict, which was reported in many newspaper articles and which sparked angry editorials. The Metropolitan Health Board, designated as the local HSA, recommended that certain hospitals be closed. It is a matter of record that the Metropolitan Health Board reconsidered its position and, motivated by the wish to avoid conflict and achieve consensus, a new report was developed. It was in that report that the recommendations for a competitive health system, with reasonable regulatory safeguards, was spelled out (Citizens League, 1981). Good leadership in the Twin Cities seems to be that which accomplishes consensus and avoids conflict.

In Chicago there is considerable leadership among health consumers, but these leaders do not avoid conflict. In health, as in other areas of community life in Chicago, activity is largely adversarial rather than consensual, and it is fragmented rather than focused. Chicago's widespread health consumer activism is based on an abundance of organizations scattered in neighborhoods throughout the city and represents special ethnicities, interests and localities. These occur in block clubs, neighborhood groups, and large umbrella organizations. One of the umbrella organizations, the Southwest Community Conference, has 130 member groups and 200,000 members.

Chicago consumers perceived the organizations and resources around them to be politicized and they themselves were very political. There are countless stories of individual successes and of the successes of some coalitions, e.g., the Association of Health Care Consumers and the Evanston Medical Consumers. However, consumers in Chicago cannot name central leaders or even major issues that unify Chicago health consumers. Despite a number of attempts to merge the metropolitan Chicago HSA and the suburban HSA, this has never been accomplished. One of the few causes that brought some of the groups together was the effort to require Blue Cross-Blue Shield to contain costs. Consumer advocates explained that this was a political move aimed at affecting the hospital through Blue Cross because hospitals could not be regulated. Blue Cross, they claimed, had 30 percent of the market and, therefore, had the leverage needed to change hospital costs.

The history of that confrontation, however, gives further evidence of not only the adversarial nature but also the specificity and fragility of many consumer groups. When Blue Cross reorganized suddenly as a private mutual company—avoiding the public hearings—the consumer group lost its cause and reported that it too would completely reorganize.

In contrast to the Twin Cities, consumers in Chicago do not consistently name certain individuals or organizations as leading or even reflecting the health concerns of the whole community. There are groups concerned with general issues of health, such as the Health and Medicine Policy Research Group founded by Quentin Young, a physician and social activist. However, the impact of such groups is reported in sectors of the community rather than throughout the metropolitan area.

Another reflection, as well as a source, of the differences in the style seen in consumers of the two metropolitan areas is the media. The press responds to, elaborates, and reinforces concensus in the Twin Cities. In Chicago, it reports, emphasizes, and helps to perpetuate the adversarial nature and fragmentation of Chicago groups.

Ironically, consumer interviews in the Twin Cities do not reflect much activism in health care, but there is consistent focused progress. On the other hand, Chicago respondents reflect high energy and activity, but they only hint at progress.

CONSUMER INTERACTION WITH HMOs

Interviews with consumers and community leaders in Minneapolis-St. Paul and Chicago provided information on the initial and subsequent responses of consumers to HMOs in each of the two communities. They further suggested the impact that consumer response has had on HMOs, as well as the impact of HMOs on consumers.

Consumers in the Twin Cities and Chicago had very different exposures to the concept and practice of HMOs, so their perceptions of and responses to HMOs are different in many ways. Despite their different exposures, they have important similarities in perception. Specifically, we spoke with community leaders and consumers about their perception of particular aspects of HMOs including access to care, quality of care, and cost of care. In addition we asked them to discuss their views on prevention, health maintenance, and education programs of HMOs. The informants were also asked to reflect on the explanation for the particular pattern of HMO development in their respective communities, and then to elaborate on both their reservations and their satisfactions with HMOs they have known and/or with the concept of HMOs.

Consumer perspectives

The two points relating to HMOs about which consumers in both communities agreed most consistently concerned their doctors and the location of their care. As has often been reported in other studies, the most important deterrent to joining an HMO is the reluctance to give up a doctor with whom one has had a long association (Lou Harris & Associates, 1980; Luft, 1981a). Often consumers said that if their physician were to retire or to join an HMO, they would join an HMO. (This may seem more likely in Minneapolis-St. Paul where 85 percent of the physicians have some relationship with an HMO, but it could also have important implications in Chicago where 12 percent of the physicians are between sixty-five and seventy-five years old.)

The second issue that seems universally important to consumers is the location of their health care facility. In the Twin Cities, where there was already widespread acceptance of HMOs, some consumers seemed to be simply waiting for some plan offered by their employer to open a facility near them. In Chicago, the absence of a facility near them was frequently mentioned as explanation for not joining an HMO—and sometimes for not even knowing about HMOs. Easy geographical access seems essential in both communities.

The most notable difference among consumers in the two communities was their level of knowledge about HMOs. In the Twin Cities everyone knows about HMOs, and most have known about them since the early 1970s. Many know the history of Group Health Plan, which began in the 1950s, and others learned about HMOs from newspaper coverage or from their employers. Every respondent in the Twin Cities knew some, if not many, members of HMOs. In Chicago, in spite of the fact that there were prepaid plans as early as in the Twin Cities, most consumers heard about HMOs only within the last two years. Even HSA members reported that they were not conscious of HMOs until 1975, when they were brought to the attention of the HSA. Although they said they may have read a newspaper article about NorthCare, or Anchor, or Michael Reese Health Plan, they thought of HMOs as localized or available only to a limited population. A staff member for the DuPage county HSA said, "HMOs are so new that people don't have any idea what they are. You have to increase the promotion." Few Chicago respondents knew anyone in an HMO, and they have only recently realized that they themselves might join.

There is not only a lack of information in Chicago but also a great deal of misinformation among people who, it seems, are otherwise informed. There is incorrect information about the number of HMOs, which are for-profit, which are non-profit, and why certain HMOs have changed management.

This notable lack of knowledge and miscommunication about HMOs in Chicago may be related in part to another important difference in the two communities, i.e., Chicagoans were not familiar with that type of medical care most like HMOs—multispecialty group practices. As is more fully discussed in chapter 5 on physicians, consumers in the Twin Cities are accustomed to the group practice setting, and they identify the idea of a "clinic" with prestigious medical establishments. In fact, one of the few reservations that consumers in Minnesota have about joining an HMO is that it does not provide coverage at the Mayo Clinic.

Chicago consumers, on the other hand, have no local experience with multispecialty group practice. Their own care has been from physicians committed to private practice or to small single-specialty group practice. Furthermore, the idea of a "clinic" in Chicago evokes the image of numerous university and county hospital clinics with poor patients, hard benches, and long waits.

In spite of these negative associations, however, consumers in Chicago did not report concern about the quality of care in HMOs. Although there were complaints among consumers about inconvenience, there were no references to poor medical care. The consumers spoke respectfully of the medical hospitals and centers associated with the best known HMOs: NorthCare, Anchor, and Michael Reese Health Plan. It seems surprising that consumers in Chicago did not even know of or remember the extensive bad press about a failed Medicaid HMO called CURE.

Satisfied, at least theoretically, with the quality of HMOs, consumers were cautious in their optimism about cost. In Chicago, where there is little information, consumers asserted that HMOs "should" lower costs. In the Twin Cities local consumer representatives made similar assertions. However, community leaders who had data from employers or hospitals and were considering HMOs in depth were puzzled about the problem of containing cost and were beginning to recognize the complexity and inequity of cost shifting within the community.

Another attribute associated with HMOs, of interest to consumers in both communities, is preventive medicine. In Chicago, consumers were enthusiastic about including prevention in a health plan. However, in Minneapolis, where they have had more experience, they were equally supportive of the idea but they were less optimistic that prevention will be a major part of HMO care. One well-placed observer reported that one-fourth of HMO patients shift from plan to plan, so HMOs are reluctant to invest in preventive care for patients who will be in another plan the following year.

Factors influencing HMO development

Given these many perceptions, we asked consumers for their understanding of the factors that enhanced or inhibited HMO development in their community. The responses were as consistent and focused in the Twin Cities as they were varied and ambiguous in Chicago. Community leaders and consumers in the Twin Cities all spoke of the strong sense of progressive community identity, Scandinavian heritage, and corporate responsibility. Most also discussed the cooperative tradition, often including the Democratic Farm-Labor Party. Some discussed the absence of urban problems that plague other metropolitan areas.

In Chicago, which is burdened by urban problems, consumers did not have a ready explanation for the slow growth of HMOs in the area. Many did not realize that they were growing significantly faster elsewhere, although those who were familiar with the Twin Cities offered the same explanation that the Minnesotans offered. Although some said "maybe because the medical societies are headquartered in Chicago," few could cite any organized opposition to HMOs. Instead, all consumers emphasized that until recently, there was a lack of interest.

There was change, however, reported by consumers in both communities. The Twin Cities consumers expected HMOs to continue growing, but they realized that growth had recently slowed. Chicago consumers were animated by the increased visibility, and they were encouraged by the increased number of facilities and the entrance of new and established names into the HMO field. Some predicted that HMOs will grow; others said they will expand exponentially.

Impact of consumers on HMOs

Luft noted that "consumer involvement in HMOs appear[s] to have little consistent effect on HMO performance" (Luft,

1981b), and as will be discussed shortly, consumers do not seem to be very active within HMOs. However, in other ways consumers have had, and continue to have, a powerful effect on HMOs. They were among the earliest and most important sponsors of HMOs, and their needs as patients and demands as activists have had impact on aspects of HMOs as general as the conceptual development of plans and as specific as their television marketing.

The impact of consumers in the two metropolitan areas studied appeared different in important ways, yet close examination demonstrated important similarities also. To analyze systematically the impact of consumer behavior on HMO development in the two cities, the first consideration will be the impact of consumers from outside of HMOs. The second consideration will be the impact of consumers within HMOs, both as board members and as enrollees.

The most notable and lasting positive impact that consumers have had is HMO sponsorship. This occurred in both communities, though at different times. Consumer-sponsored HMOs developed not only as a way to deliver health care or to contain costs but also as a form of social activism. They are statements of belief or ideology.

Although only one-third of HMOs in the U.S. were consumer-sponsored, the influence of their ideas—or at least their rhetoric—is present in all HMOs. Conceptually, the consumer-sponsored HMO is the archetype of HMOs, in that major principles embodied in the "pure" consumer HMOs became rhetorical ideals for all HMOs: care that is comprehensive, accessible, preventive, and responsive to patients.

These HMOs, their founders say, reflect collectivism, an important theme in American social and political thought—sometimes quiescent and sometimes explosive. As a historical theme, it varies in intensity and timing, and from region to region. In Minnesota private collectivism has been a dominant theme. It was as an expression of this value that Group Health Plan was first conceived in the late thirties and later developed in the 1950s by leaders who were "profoundly influenced by the philosophy . . . of the Cooperative League of the USA" (Uphoff and Uphoff, 1980).

The cooperative ideology was also at the root of NorthCare when it was founded in the early 1970s by four women in the Chicago suburb of Evanston. The women had worked together in food cooperatives and child-care cooperatives, and as part of a collectivist religious group. Their consumer-sponsored HMO was one of the first HMOs in Chicago. NorthCare was characteristic of HMOs begun by consumer activists in the early 1970s, whose founders and participants had been active in the civil rights and anti-war movements and were ready to take up a new cause. Ironically, interviews suggested that these HMOs sponsored by political activists were made feasible by funds from the Nixon administration, which was seeking ways to counter the movement toward national health insurance.

In addition to sponsoring Group Health and bringing HMOs to the metropolitan area in the fifties, consumer leaders in the Twin Cities had other positive impacts on HMOs. A number of examples follow. The Citizens League supported HMOs both for their health care virtues and because they "provide incentives" to cost-effective medical care. The league's public deliberations and reports were said by those consumers, who were simply reactive, to have caught their attention and made them favorable toward HMOs. A second way that the community helped HMOs to gain momentum was through the press. There were not only factual reports of the development of HMOs and extensive educational articles but also frequent editorials and letters about the virtues of HMOs. It was clear from the interviews that once HMOs gained momentum, they were supported as a matter not only of improved health care but also of community pride and identity. The third example describes not so much a positive impact as a powerful competitive impact in the Twin Cities. It was noted earlier that both employees and employers are consumers for HMOs. Because employers in the Twin Cities assume a paternalistic role toward their employees, consumers reported that when their employer chose to offer HMOs, it gave HMOs credibility in their eyes. After consumers were offered more than one HMO, their sophistication and the competitive environment caused service differentiation among HMOs.

Although HMOs in Chicago are less developed, consumers in the community have had an impact. Interviews in Evanston suggested that in 1970 Evanston Hospital was drawn into its important role in NorthCare's development because of demands from consumers for more community spirit and activity. Consumers who participated in Blue Cross cost containment hearings reported that pressure from health consumers in the Association for Health Care Consumers against Blue Cross's rate increases caused Blue Cross to return to the second set of hearings with a proposal for the HMO network. In Chicago, unlike in the Twin Cities, there has also been some apathy or negative impact among consumer groups as well. Some groups reported that they did not support HMOs even as members on the HSA boards. In addition, a number of health consumer groups decided not to coordinate support for HMOs because, with the costs already escalating, they "could not justify supporting more health organizations."

Although consumer impact on HMOs from outside was evident in both metropolitan areas, consumer impact from within HMOs is more ambiguous. Research on effects of consumer participation within HMOs is scanty, but one study noted that one difficulty was a lack of broad-based interest and that only a small, select group of consumers served as council members (Harrelsomn and Donovan, 1975). Our research gave further evidence of this problem. Luft asserted, "The potential for consumer influence is the greatest in the consumer cooperative plans" (Luft, 1981a). In fact, in Group Health Plan, consumers' impact was crucial. Consumers actually made financial contributions to bail it out of financial difficulty in its early days. In most ways, though, consumers as members of HMOs show little interest in the running of the HMO. As one consumer activist in Chicago said, they "do not carry the candle." At NorthCare, all the founders emphasized their initial commitment to consumer participation. They chronicled their commitment in their first public document, which they took to Evanston Hospital. In retrospect, however, they noted that without their having realized it at the time, a small self-selected elite became deeply involved, but the larger membership hardly participated. Most members interacted with their HMO just as they had with their previous provider. This was consistent with Mercer's finding that less than 1 percent of the Group Health Cooperative membership actively participated in its operation (Mercer, 1973).

Reciprocal impacts

The impacts of consumers on HMOs and of HMOs on consumers are often inextricably interwoven. First, the phenomenon of consumer professionalization will be discussed, followed by further discussion of reciprocal impacts including the effects of competition.

For the self-selected elite consumers mentioned above, a complex reciprocal interaction was taking place. As they became more involved and sophisticated about the complexities of running a medical delivery system, they reported that they themselves became "professionalized." For example, in NorthCare, eight consumers were intimately involved. Four participated in the initiation stage and four more joined in the "second generation." Although each had at least a bachelor's degree, none of the eight had any background in health care delivery. Of the seven who continued working until NorthCare opened its doors to patients, all are now professionals in some field of health administration. All, we found, were conscious of their changed perspective. Although they remembered vividly their earlier viewpoints, commitments, and hopes, they were acutely aware that their experience making the HMO viable, caused them to make compromises continually. It is interesting that founders of NorthCare were so conscious of the tension between some of their initial goals and the realities that they institutionalized the dichotomy by creating two separate organizations: Consumers Health Group and NorthCare. Consumers Health Group continued the ideological activities, and NorthCare became increasingly practical and viable.

Not always, however, are these tensions so clearly dealt with. Consumer members on HMO boards are reported to frequently have a negative impact. To physicians considering joining an HMO the presence of board members who are outside of medicine in general turns them away, and, furthermore, as was the case with Group Health Plan, weakens the group reputation as a quality medical care system. Consumer board members have another effect that might have a negative financial impact on the HMO. They often support open individual enrollment, which is an integral part of their ideological commitment but which has been a serious financial hazard to beginning HMOs. This issue, founders say, almost prevented NorthCare from opening. Consumers' boards are considered so problematic that a community leader in the Twin Cities said that he thought St. Louis Park's MedCenter Health Plan would not have started if the present legislation requiring one-third consumer representation had been in place then.

Even though consumers as official representatives within HMOs have little positive impact, administrators of the prepaid plans noted that when consumers, as enrollees, became more sophisticated, the plan must attend to their interests because they can have a powerful impact. An administrator of a medical center with both fee-for-service and prepaid patients emphasized the potential power of consumers. He explained that the plan must be very careful:

> A fee-for-service (FFS) patient who has been coming here for years and years on FFS may come tomorrow on a prepaid basis, and if you start treating them differently it will be immediately obvious to them and (pause) they will disappear the next time they get the chance, so I think that keeps us where we need to be, that is providing the same level of service for all of our patients irrespective of their financing.

As consumers become sophisticated about the delivery of their health care there is a strong reciprocal effect on them. The informed consumer must take more responsibility and make more choices. In the competitive health market the consumer will need more information about cost and about care. The historically paternalistic system in which patients turned themselves over to the all-knowing practitioner is beginning to change.

SUMMARY

In this comparison of two metropolitan areas, consideration of consumers in the two communities is particularly interesting because one can conclude that they are simultaneously the most influential and the least influential. Because the nature of the communities—that is, their social history and their decision-making style—is seen to be among the most significant explanatory differences in this comparative study and because consumers, as citizens, are responsible for their communities, consumers can be viewed as the single most important influence on the development of HMOs (or any social innovation) in their communities. On the other hand, if one looks for direct influence of consumer groups or consumer activism on the direction of health care in either community, one finds little impact. Although consumer-sponsored HMOs are symbolically important and although certain groups do make sporadic efforts in reaction to specific problems (such as increased premiums or decreased access), consumers as a whole do not form a self-conscious or unified constituency. Rather than acting in concert, they fragment into subgroups in which some other identity or role is salient. For example, they act primarily as employees, labor union members, or often as patients of certain doctors or medical groups. This overall absence of a group consciousness as health care consumers, as well as their lack of professional experience, reduces consumers' effectiveness and allows them little more than token participation in the development of health care policies or plans, including HMOs.

4

HMOs and Hospitals

In the Twin Cities, low hospital occupancy rates, active price competition prompted by regulatory action and third-party payers, and effective communication between hospital administrators have provided an atmosphere conducive to HMO development and growth. The combined effect of low occupancy, and financial as well as managerial resources, is that most hospitals have both the ability and the incentive to respond to HMO initiatives. Chicago hospitals are much more diverse in occupancy rates and available resources, resulting in a tendency to respond negatively to HMO initiatives. Active service competition and limited communication between hospital administrators have also provided a neutral to poor environment for HMO development and growth in Chicago.

In this century, hospitals became a central focus of virtually all health care delivery because of their ability to concentrate financial, technological, and human resources and because of the favorable climate of third-party reimbursement for inpatient care. During the past few years, however, a troubled economy and escalating hospital costs have led third-party payers to seek alternatives to traditional health care financing and delivery. HMOs, as one alternative, offer hospitals both challenges and opportunities.

This chapter presents information from interviews with forty-eight influential people in the hospital communities of

---

This chapter was written by Ellen M. Morrison, Research Project Analyst.

Minneapolis-St. Paul and Chicago. The respondents were selected from state and local hospital associations, hospital consulting
firms, multi-hospital systems, and free-standing hospitals. Hospital administrators represented community hospitals, teaching
and research medical centers, and inner-city and suburban hospitals. These included both hospitals with and those without HMO
affiliations.

HOSPITAL MARKET CHARACTERISTICS

Previous studies explored existing HMO-hospital relationships (Luft, 1978; Fink and Trimmer, 1981; Kralewski, et al.,
1982). One of the objectives of this current study was to explore
why hospitals do or do not enter and maintain relationships with
HMOs.

Some general characteristics of a hospital community that
affect market receptiveness to HMOs are capacity, utilization, occupancy, and cost. An examination of hospital system indicators
over the period from 1970 to 1980 reveals important differences
between the hospital communities of Minneapolis-St. Paul and
Chicago on those three characteristics.

In the early 1970s, high capacity, high utilization, and low
occupancy rates were characteristic of the Twin Cities hospitals,
while low capacity, low utilization, and high occupancy rates
were characteristic in Chicago. From 1970 to 1980, significant
changes occurred (see figure that follows).

Capacity decreased in Minneapolis-St. Paul and increased in
Chicago during the 1970s, resulting in both metropolitan areas
having 4.9 beds per 1000 population in 1980. Admissions per
1000 population, inpatient days per 1000 population, and average length of stay decreased in the Twin Cities. Although average
length of stay decreased in Chicago, admissions and inpatient
days increased. In 1970, admissions and inpatient days were substantially higher in Minneapolis-St. Paul than in Chicago, and
average length of stay was lower in the Twin Cities. By 1980,
admissions and inpatient days were lower in Minneapolis-St.
Paul than in Chicago, and the two metropolitan areas were equal
at 8.3 days for average length of stay. Hospital occupancy rates,
while still lower in Minneapolis-St. Paul than in Chicago, have
increased in the Twin Cities and decreased in Chicago. Cost,

Hospital Market Characteristics

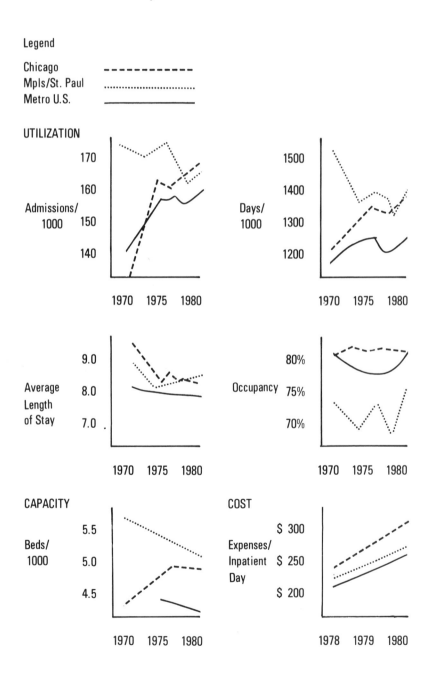

Legend

Chicago   - - - - - - - - - - -
Mpls/St. Paul   ....
Metro U.S.   _____

UTILIZATION

Admissions/1000

Days/1000

Average Length of Stay

Occupancy

CAPACITY

Beds/1000

COST

Expenses/Inpatient Day

indicated by expenses per inpatient day, has increased in both communities, but less so in the Twin Cities than in Chicago. High capacity and low occupancy are danger signs for the inpatient-centered hospital. Hospitals in Minneapolis-St. Paul have faced these danger signs for several years and have developed innovative approaches to cope with changing market demands. Chicago hospitals appear to be fast approaching a state of high capacity and low occupancy. The head start that Twin Cities hospitals had on Chicago in dealing with these dangers is reflected in the advanced state of competition between hospitals there.

HOSPITAL COMPETITION

Hospital representatives discussed two forms of competition —service and price. Service competition was described as competition for physicians who in turn bring in paying patients and add prestige to the institution. Price competition was described as competition for price-sensitive buyers of health care. To the extent that insured patients pay deductibles and copayments, they are price-sensitive buyers. However, given that employers, insurers, and the government pay the lion's share of hospital expenses, they are the primary targets of price competition.

Service competition is a long-standing tradition according to hospital administrators. Price competition is in different stages of development in Minneapolis-St. Paul and Chicago. A critical point is that the market is different in these two forms of competition: in service competition, the "customer" is the physician; and in price competition, the "customer" is the buyer of hospitalization. A successful hospital administrator can determine from the environment which form of competition, or which combination of the two forms, is best suited to increasing patient volume at any given time.

To complicate the issue, the hospital, as an institution, is held accountable, to some degree, for serving the public good. Hospitals will not be allowed to compete without restraint if that competition results in underserving the poor or elderly. Dorman reported concern that a truly competitive system would threaten inner-city hospitals that are the only source of care for the poor and elderly (Dorman, 1982). Also, a competitive model jeopardizes costly teaching institutions and consequently the funding of medical education. Even in the Twin Cities, where hospital competition is heralded by many as the answer to escalating health care costs, competition is monitored to protect the public good.

Questions regarding hospital competition received a broad range of responses. A common response to a question on competition was "First tell me what you mean by 'competition'." In the Twin Cities, respondents appeared to have thought at length about HMOs, cost containment, and health care planning. Their responses, however, differed as greatly from one another as did responses in Chicago, where it often appeared that respondents were thinking about the issues for the very first time. A possible explanation for such a variety of responses is the complex nature of competition.

Responses from the interviews reflected two important competitive differences between Minneapolis-St. Paul and Chicago hospitals: first, their ability to compete, and second, the competitive initiatives in which they are involved.

Ability to compete

Minneapolis-St. Paul

Although Twin Cities respondents were quick to point out the important differences between Minneapolis and St. Paul, they also acknowledged several factors that allow hospitals there to compete equally with one another. Geographic concentration of the population was mentioned frequently as a factor facilitating competition. Travel times within the metropolitan area are short, so most hospital administrators considered all other metropolitan hospitals to be their competitors, at least those that offered similar services. Ventures such as industrial medicine arrangements and preferred provider organizations are common between hospitals and corporations located very near one another. However, hospital administrators were not concerned about potential difficulties marketing health care when employees work far from where they live, a concern frequently voiced in Chicago.

The ethnic and economic homogeneity was also credited for facilitating equal competition. The predominance of Scandinavian descendants, discussed in earlier chapters, promotes a perception of shared culture and values between hospital personnel and potential patients. Consumer prejudice against hospitals because of the ethnic or racial composition of the hospital's personnel or the surrounding neighborhood was not an issue there. Economically, the Twin Cities are more affluent and homogeneous than most metropolitan areas. Few hospitals in the Twin Cities could be described as "inner-city" hospitals, with the high percentages of poor and minorities, Medicaid recipients, and charity cases that the term implies. A Chicago respondent with experience in the Twin Cities claimed that, for a normal medical or surgical problem, he would put any member of his family into any hospital in Minneapolis or St. Paul, an endorsement he would not make for Chicago. Twin Cities respondents sometimes characterized the population of Minneapolis as white-collar Lutherans and that of St. Paul as blue-collar Catholics, but hospital competition is not reported to reflect these differences. Even administrators of hospitals with conspicuous religious affiliations did not specify their target patient population in terms of religion or neighborhood.

Another factor in any hospital's ability to compete is the level of administrative sophistication. In the Twin Cities hospital administrators sense the disintegration of their formerly collegial network and the development of a new genre of administration, characterized by competitive management practices. The University of Minnesota has traditionally been the main source of Twin Cities hospital administrators. Until recently, those administrators, often former classmates, have maintained a cooperative environment within the hospital community. One respondent said that older hospital administrators viewed their profession as a calling, similar to the church or social services. Joint ventures, shared services, and multihospital arrangements were facilitated by this mission-oriented collegial network. As the market becomes more competitive, many of the past cooperative efforts are no longer appropriate given current economic conditions. Administrators of long tenure describe the painful process of learning to "hold their cards closer to the chest," and new administrators are being trained within this competitive environment. The respondent cited above described this new group as approaching hospitals as a business, albeit a business with a "social tint."

A final factor regarding ability to compete concerns a "competitive environment" (Christianson, 1981). Twin Cities respondents in all sectors overwhelmingly support competitive rather than regulative approaches to problem solving in the health care field. The 1981 Citizens League report is an example of this support. Another respondent stated the support in terms of voluntarism: "[Minnesotans feel strongly] that regulation can guide policies and monitoring, but implementation should be voluntary." Given the nature of the regulatory environment of Minnesota, support for competition is not surprising. However, respondents described an unusually adversarial incident which may have catalyzed acceptance of the competitive approach.

In 1981, the Metropolitan Health Board, the local HSA, compiled a report on hospital overbedding. The recommendations of the report included closing several hospitals. One of the hospitals targeted for closure was the only Jewish hospital in the Twin Cities. The HSA's recommendation awakened old responses to anti-Semitism, and public sentiment supported protecting this hospital from closure. During this uncharacteristic turmoil, the hospitals and their supporters argued that the battle for survival should be fought in the marketplace. Support grew for the argument that competition, not a regulatory body, should determine "who will live or die." By the time public hearings were held on the report, the HSA had retracted its recommendations.

Hospital administrators perceive that competition, on service and price, is positively sanctioned by the community. This sanction frees administrators to compete overtly. Many administrators find this aggressive atmosphere a challenge as well as a refreshing change in health care management.

Chicago

The environment in which Chicago hospitals operate can be described appropriately as heterogeneous. Whereas analysis of the Twin Cities hospital community was largely a result of summarizing consistent, supporting data, the Chicago analysis has been a greater challenge of synthesis. In Chicago, responses are unique to each institution. Chicago hospitals are to some extent islands unto themselves, reflecting the social, political, economic, and ethnic diversity of the metropolitan area. Chicago hospitals' ability to compete with one another on price and service is influenced by this diversity.

Chicago hospital administrators did not consider all other Chicago hospitals their competitors. Chicago hospitals do not compete equally with one another. Analysis of individual hospital statistics and administrators' perceptions revealed important differences in location, ethnicity, and economics.

The dispersion of seven million people over 3724 square miles is one reason why all Chicago hospitals do not compete directly. Inner-city hospitals do not emphasize attracting suburban patients, or vice versa. Although the city's medical centers draw patients from all over, their attraction is limited to specific sophisticated talents and equipment.

The interaction of economic, ethnic, and racial factors increases the city–suburban distinction. Chicago has a much larger nonwhite and indigent population than the Twin Cities. Similar to other large cities, Chicago's inner city decayed over its long history. Flight to the suburbs by middle-class and upwardly mobile whites has divided the urban and suburban sections of the metropolitan area.

Chicago has been known traditionally as a city of neighborhoods. Ethnically and racially segregated groups are often separated by only a park or city street. These groups have their own markets, restaurants, recreation areas, and hospitals. Consumer preferences regarding the racial or ethnic composition of a hospital's personnel or the surrounding neighborhood play an important role in Chicago. Furthermore, racial and ethnic characteristics are frequently linked with economics. Neighborhoods may be described as "poor blacks" or "working-class Poles."

Most community hospital administrators respond to questions regarding their patient populations in terms of the demographics of the surrounding neighborhood, and that neighborhood may change over time. Local community hospitals are vulnerable to the economic conditions of their surrounding neighborhoods. Variation in resource availability makes hospitals unequal competitors.

Hospitals' ability to compete is also inhibited by the heterogeneity of management styles and business acumen. Although some graduates of the University of Chicago and Northwestern University's hospital administration programs remain in Chicago, these graduates do not consider themselves part of a network of locally trained administrators. Bearing in mind that respondents were not chosen randomly, Chicago hospital administrators differed from one another more often than Twin Cities administrators in type and place of education. This diversity in training is reflected in the diversity of management styles and business acumen. Some Chicago administrators are already actively assessing environmental changes and taking aggressive competitive measures, while others appear overwhelmed. One respondent stated that many "can't decide whether [hospitals] are businesses or charitable enterprises". He described Chicago hospitals as "a backward, sleepy market with some dazzling exceptions."

There is an important interaction between management acumen and resource availability. Resource availability is critical to an administrator's ability to take competitive risks. Management acumen is critical to determining the range of strategies from which an administrator can choose. One inner-city administrator with a degree from a prestigious university and twenty years of experience reported that during his tenure, his hospital had changed from predominantly private patients to approximately 60 percent Medicaid and Medicare. He reported that the conflict between what the state pays for medical care and what it demands in terms of stricter building codes leads to a no-win situation for older inner-city hospitals. Although his knowledge and experience might yield innovative strategies, battling for survival in a resource-scarce environment left this administrator "firefighting" with reactive strategies.

The environmental factors discussed above affect the ability of Chicago hospitals to compete with one another equally. However, the form of competition—price or service—is determined both by environmental factors and by the developmental phase of the hospital industry in a community. Interviews with hospital representatives support the claim that Chicago hospitals are, as a whole, still in the initial expansion phase of their evolution.

Institutions that serve a public interest, such as hospitals, are subject to public adjustments during their initial expansion. The Twin Cities hospital industry has experienced expansion, overexpansion, and retrenchment through public intervention as well as changing economic and market conditions. Until recently, the Chicago hospital industry had not experienced retrenchment. Administrators reported relative ease receiving or circumventing certificate-of-need requests for expansion. Circumvention has been facilitated by confusion in the HSA regarding grandfather clauses or specific implementation. Certificate-of-need requests for equipment also received favorable HSA judgments. One administrator implied that certificate-of-need equipment requests were just a slowing down process. He represented a common philosophy in Chicago by implying that the government cannot deny an organization the right to buy a piece of equipment.

The lack of effective public sanctions to reduce capacity and cost has enhanced service competition. Hospital administrators reported knowing about duplicative services and equipment in neighboring hospitals, but they point to the disincentives of sharing, particularly losing patients to the other institution. One administrator described a failed attempt to share a linear accelerator with a nearby hospital. Both administrators negotiated without conceding anything. Negotiations broke off when the initiating institution decided that it could not afford to share the cost of a separate site and would therefore locate the accelerator on its own grounds.

Without sufficient sanctions against new construction or equipment, regulatory agencies have been unable to enforce price competition. Perhaps more important, Chicago hospitals receive no support for competing on price. Insurers and employers in Chicago are just now beginning to look seriously at hospital costs, and their attempts at cost containment have primarily targeted waste, e.g., billing for services not received, unnecessary lab tests. These efforts place the responsibility of waste detection and prevention on the patient or the physician, not on the hospital. For example, a few companies in Chicago have offered their employees rewards for finding errors in their hospital bills.

Hospitals have had few incentives to lower room rates or per case cost. Insurers and employers have not been sensitive to those changes, at least not sensitive enough to restrict their beneficiaries' access to costly hospitals. The government also plays an important role in Chicago because of the large number of state and federal beneficiaries. Hospital administrators claimed that Medicaid and Medicare reimbursements are so low that hospital charges must be high to compensate. Discussing productivity one respondent claimed, "There's no incentive to [look at productivity] given the present cost reimbursement system. You get no brownie points for keeping charges low."

Direct public intervention and private and public reimbursement mechanisms have enhanced expansion and overexpansion in the Chicago hospital industry. Retrenchment has occurred within the past few years because of the economy. Hospital administrators report that, although they have the right to expand and to buy equipment, they cannot afford it. Census is dropping, and with it, revenues. Medicaid and Medicare reimbursements are becoming more restrictive and private third-party payers are beginning to verbalize anger about cost shifting.

In Chicago, then, retrenchment has been the result of economic necessity rather than public intervention. Two separate incidents were described in interviews of hospitals banding together to prevent certificate-of-need approval for expansion by another hospital. One incident involved legal action to prevent the construction of a new hospital, and one involved administrative pressure to dissuade one hospital from a "greedy" request—the hospital wanted to expand by 200 beds, the exact number of beds that the HSA had determined the entire area was lacking. In both cases, rare consortiums of hospitals acting in self-interest achieved the same results as a strict regulatory agency.

The recent retrenchment of Chicago's hospital industry is not the result of intentional public intervention. Further expansion may still be in the industry's future, particularly if the economy takes a favorable turn. Greater evidence lies in the rarity of competitive efforts. In contrast to the Twin Cities, multihospital arrangements, vertical integration, and diversification efforts in Chicago are the "dazzling exceptions," not the norm.

Competitive initiatives

Minneapolis-St. Paul

The competitive environment enhances the development of numerous initiatives by hospital administrators. Each institution's competitive efforts are unique in their combination. Examples are discussed here as efforts to increase census, multihospital arrangements, or changes of mission.

Although Twin Cities administrators recognize that inpatient care is not the only role of the hospital, they still operate within certain boundaries of physical plant capacity and overhead. Administrators described several competitive options to increase census. These included seeking HMO contracts, increasing marketing efforts, and either expanding specialty services or abandoning low-volume specialty services.

Many hospital administrators discussed seeking HMO contracts as a strategy to increase patient volume. The administrator of one tertiary care hospital explained that the primary objective of an HMO contract is to lock in a group of patients who previously visited other institutions. After meeting that objective, fi-

nancial incentives are provided to the HMO to deliver more patients, such as giving volume discounts. A crucial part of his
decision to pursue a given HMO is the number of patients the
HMO controls, given the probability that HMO members will use
fewer hospital services.

A related consideration is the number of other hospitals affiliated with the HMO. Fink and Trimmer demonstrated that in a
community where the prepaid plan's market share is 25 percent,
as the percent of areawide hospitals affiliated with a prepaid plan
increases, the control of the plan over any one of the affiliated
hospital's utilization decreases (Fink and Trimmer, 1981). Therefore, when the HMO market share is high, as it is in the Twin
Cities, the distribution of HMO business is an important variable.
A hospital with an exclusive or a near-exclusive HMO contract
may reap the highest rewards, in terms of increasing volume,
through HMO business. One respondent described substantial
HMO contracts as windows that open only for a short time. When
an HMO allows bidding on a contract for all or most of its area
members, administrators must act quickly or lose the opportunity.

The marketing of hospital services has historically been
limited by professional norms and standards similar to those of
physicians. Particularly during the initial expansion phase of the
hospital industry when service competition was predominant,
hospital administrators perceived a superior product as the best
marketing tool. Currently in the Twin Cities, administrators respond primarily to a price-sensitive market. While a good reputation can be communicated to the physician market through professional networks, it is quite difficult for a cost-efficient hospital
to communicate this quality informally to the buyer market.

Hospital administrators in the Twin Cities reported recently
"beefing up" their marketing strategies. Advertising, through the
media and by direct mailings, is one strategy. Another is to approach employers directly to market employee assistance programs, health promotion classes, industrial medicine services,
and preferred provider arrangements. An administrator of a multihospital system that has a preferred provider arrangement
stated, "If hospitals are smart, they'll be in touch with all of the
businesses around them. . . . Hospitals have got to know who
their business people are; who their market is."

Specialization is one last indication of efforts to increase
census. Rather than attempting to do a little bit of everything,

most hospital administrators in the Twin Cities described the specialty services that they provide or that they refer to another institution. Specialties frequently mentioned as referral services are cardiac surgery, high-risk obstetrics, psychiatry, and chemical dependency.

Psychiatry and chemical dependency services have experienced substantial growth recently. A knowledgeable respondent reported that approximately 25 percent of the chemical dependency beds in the country are located in the Twin Cities area. This has been explained as an entrepreneurial response to the Minnesota Comprehensive Insurance Act of 1976, which mandates a broader package of insurance benefits. According to the 1981 Citizens League Report, Minnesota has more mandated benefits than any other state.

Multihospital arrangements range from formal multihospital systems owned by a parent corporation to informal agreements between hospitals to share laundry services or a CT-scanner. The key ingredient in multihospital arrangements is consolidation of resources and risks. Increasing buying power and decreasing individual hospital risk allow hospitals within a system more freedom to compete, both on price and on service.

Multihospital arrangements have flourished in the past fifteen years. Formal multihospital systems, virtually nonexistent fifteen years ago, included 30 percent of the nation's hospitals in 1981 (Goldsmith, 1981). Hospitals in the Twin Cities participate in a wide variety of arrangements.

In 1979, Mason and Melum described four non-profit multihospital systems operating in the Twin Cities: Fairview Community Hospitals; Minneapolis Medical Center, Inc.; Health Central, Inc.; and United Hospitals, Inc. (Mason and Melum, 1979). These systems were primarily the result of mergers and acquisitions of operating free-standing hospitals, and some of the systems have expanded by constructing new hospitals in underserved areas.

In 1982, the Minneapolis Medical Center, Inc. corporately reorganized, developing a holding company, Lifespan. In 1983, United Hospitals merged with Metropolitan Medical Center, which is itself the product of a complex history of mergers and public-private shared space and services. In May 1983, the first for-profit hospital chain entered Minneapolis when the Hospital Corporation of America signed a three-year management contract with Mount Sinai Hospital.

The four non-profit systems mentioned above are all based in the Twin Cities, and each owns at least two hospitals in the Minneapolis-St. Paul area. In addition, they all have management contracts and shared service affiliations with numerous other institutions in the Twin Cities area, in rural Minnesota, and in other states. The degree of centralization of decision making, resources, and risk varies between and within organizations. Twin Cities area hospitals are very active in multihospital arrangements outside the realm of ownership and management contract. In 1979, Mason and Melum described three nonincorporated joint ventures: one single-function shared service corporation, and two condominium arrangements (joint construction of buildings) (Mason and Melum, 1979). As mentioned earlier, these cooperative efforts may have been facilitated by the presence of a network of University of Minnesota graduates in hospital administration. By consolidating resources in informal multihospital arrangements, hospitals became better prepared to compete with nonaffiliated hospitals. Ironically, affiliated hospitals also became better prepared to compete on price with one another.

Hospital administrators appear skeptical of the recent public embrace of competition. Bitter competition between institutions could reduce or eliminate hospital involvement in cooperative arrangements such as shared space and services. However, the loss of group purchasing power and other economies of scale may force up the price of hospital services, in turn threatening their ability to compete.

Perhaps the most aggressively competitive strategy a hospital can take is to redefine its mission as an organization. Given that price-sensitive buyers, including HMOs, want to reduce hospitalization, many hospitals are looking outside inpatient care for revenues. One respondent reported that he warns hospital administrators, "If you have more than half of your total financial or dollar volume in the inpatient side by the end of this decade, you're probably in real serious trouble." In an American Hospital Association publication on the changing role of the hospital, inpatient options are discussed as only one of many options for hospitals adjusting to changes in the health care market (Melum, 1980). Respondents discussed high participation in activities traditionally considered outside the realm of a hospital.

Hospital administrators described a recent transformation in their hospitals from providers of inpatient services to providers of health care services. This transformation is principally the result of two management strategies: vertical integration and diversification. While diversification, in its broad sense, includes all of the activities of vertical integration, the two strategies differ in purpose. Vertical integration enhances a hospital's control over its inpatient business, while diversification enhances a hospital's financial stability whether related to its inpatient business or not.

Vertical integration is defined as "acquisitions and development of new forms of delivery of health care to capture and control more of the inputs which lead to inpatient hospitalization" (Goldsmith, 1981). According to Goldsmith, the "inputs" to the health care systems are the patients and the health professionals who serve them. He discusses backward integration in terms of gaining control over a flow of health professionals and forward integration in terms of gaining control over a flow of patients. If, however, the focus of vertical integration is, as Goldsmith states, inpatient hospitalization, it can be argued that the crucial input is the patient. Personnel, physical plant, and equipment are all necessary for the hospital's survival, but patients are the purpose for which those resources are gathered. Therefore, an alternative definition of vertical integration is suggested: backward integration as diversification into ambulatory care in order to draw referrals into the hospital, and forward integration as diversification into long-term, chronic, and home health care in order to maintain "control" over patients after acute hospital episodes.

Hospital administrators in the Twin Cities discussed several backward integration strategies. Investing in an HMO or a PPO links a hospital into ambulatory care with potential for inpatient referrals. A public hospital, St. Paul Ramsey Medical Center, sponsored an HMO in response to the loss of public aid patients who had, after the passage of Medicaid legislation, a free choice of provider. Employee assistance programs and wellness clinics are also examples of backward integration.

Backward integration into ambulatory care is potentially threatening to physicians. One hospital administrator offered a very clear and colorful explanation of this development:

> Traditionally, we have sort of kept out of each others' sandboxes. If it was in the hospital—and that was where most of the technology and everything was—then it was in the hospital's arena, and the outpatient care was more or less the physician's arena. Now you're seeing physicians starting to buy major pieces of technology, setting up ambulatory

surgery centers, etc. Hospitals, in order to survive, are going to have to do some of that too, and physicians will say, "Hey, wait a minute. You're getting into my sandbox!" and that's going to cause some stresses and strains. I see more joint venturing going on between doctors and hospitals, in order to minimize that strain.

Forward integration into chronic care, home care, and hospice programs is in the early developmental stages. Restrictive Medicare reimbursement policies for extended and alternative care are named most frequently as the sources of this slow growth. Given the increasing age of the population, programs and services for the aged have high potential for growth in the near future.

Diversification into new lines of business can take several forms. As discussed above, hospitals may diversify by vertical integration. They may also diversify into related businesses, such as hospital supplies, consulting, and health insurance. Last, they may diversify into businesses completely unrelated to health care, such as gas stations or supermarkets. The overriding benefit of diversification, as described by respondents, is the income received from "unregulated" business, which in turn supports the hospital's main business—inpatient care.

Administrators voiced concern about their hospitals' ability to survive in a market of decreasing census, increasing restriction, and cutbacks from the private and public sectors. One response to these problems is to restructure corporately, designating some portion of the new corporation to be for-profit. Thus, earnings from for-profit ventures can subsidize losses from nonprofit business.

Chicago

In Chicago, the importance of service competition results in strained cooperative efforts and capital-intensive competition, e.g., buying new equipment and developing specialty care units. Hospital administrators in Chicago reported a heavy dependence on inpatient business and concerns about dropping census. As with all issues, though, there is a wide range of actions in response to those concerns. Some administrators actively seek new opportunities to reduce dependence on inpatient care or to enhance census, while others continue using tried-and-true methods to attract inpatients.

In Chicago, HMOs are unattractive alternatives for increasing census because the potential increase in census is small and the potential for difficulty with medical staff is great. The potential increase in census resulting from HMO contracts is small primarily because the HMO market share in Chicago is so small. However, the geographic dispersion of current and potential HMO members is also important. HMOs commonly use more than one hospital, to enhance convenience or to purchase specific services at lower cost. HMOs affiliated with only one hospital limit their ability to attract new members. HMOs with numerous hospital affiliations risk losing members if they reduce hospital affiliations. One suburban respondent reported that hospital-sponsored HMOs in the inner city had attempted to market in his area, but they were unsuccessful because of their hospitals' location.

The areawide HMO market share is low. In addition, the probability of an HMO contract's funneling all HMO members into one hospital is low. Finally, HMO members use hospitals less; therefore, HMO members represent less potential business. These factors in combination provide little incentive for a hospital administrator to seek out any HMO arrangement, especially one involving a discount.

Some Chicago hospital administrators reported that the potential census gain from a HMO would need to be high before they would consider it because they anticipated difficulty with their medical staffs. Given the importance of service competition, hospital administrators often discussed the importance of congenial relationships with their admitting physicians. Chapter 5 presents a discussion of physicians' resistance to and suspicion of HMOs and of the limited kinds of HMO affiliations that physicians may be willing to consider.

Although HMO affiliation is not favored to increase census, Chicago administrators showed speculative interest in PPOs. One administrator stated that HMOs are just a transition to PPOs or other forms of health care delivery yet to be developed. This administrator is studying several PPO arrangements amid a flurry of feasibility studies financed by hospitals. To date, there are no PPOs in Chicago. Several administrators reported having completed HMO feasibility studies in the past and decided not to pursue HMO sponsorship. The next few years will reveal whether the difficulties hospitals face in working with one another and in challenging traditional medicine will result in a similar fate for PPOs.

One option to increase census is to maintain current capacity while the population increases. Hospital administrators are faced with potentially conflicting demands in this regard. Certificate-of-need approval and the construction of new facilities are so time-consuming that hospitals must project demand years in advance. In recent years the economy has negatively influenced health care demand overall, but immigration to some suburbs has increased demand in those areas. Administrators want to see census high, but the hospitals best suited to compete for physicians are those with ample space and services. Another conflict involves self-interest. As described earlier, some hospital administrators are banding together to prevent expansion by other institutions. While institutions attempt to expand individually, each hopes to prevent others from expanding.

The difficulties of cooperation in Chicago are reflected in the structure of multihospital activities. When asked about shared services, group purchasing, or other multihospital activities, administrators referred almost unanimously to the Chicago Hospital Council and the Illinois Hospital Association. Both these organizations offer their services as facilitators to group action by hospitals. Small consortia of hospitals exist, but most of these have no professional staff and very limited functions. One such group dissuaded one of its members from petitioning for the "greedy" certificate-of-need proposal mentioned earlier. One consortium, an outstanding exception, hired staff and developed several shared service projects for member hospitals, including a blood bank. The blood bank has become the primary activity of the consortium; its other activities, such as group purchasing and long-range planning, have now been combined into a subsidiary of the Illinois Hospital Association.

A recent development in multihospital activity was initiated by the Chicago Hospital Council. It has since formed a separate organization called Metro-Care. Metro-Care is a consortium of twenty-nine Chicago-area hospitals that has responded to an Illinois Department of Public Aid request for proposal for a Medicaid prepayment plan. The state is seeking providers who will deliver health care services to Medicaid beneficiaries for a predetermined fee per person. Hospitals risk losing Medicaid business if they are not chosen by the state. The significance of that risk varies from the percentage of a hospital's revenues coming from Medicaid patients. Furthermore, many respondents claimed that the risks are almost as high for hospitals with large Medicaid populations that are selected as providers. That is, even though the current Medicaid reimbursement is reported to be inadequate, the proposed prospective payment system would call for more services at prices bid competitively. Many claim that the state is asking for more but paying less. Hospitals serving many Medicaid beneficiaries risk substantial losses whether or not they become providers of prepaid care.

Metro-Care holds two advantages for member hospitals. First, the risk of losing Medicaid revenues as a result of not being selected as a provider is reduced. The organization is more able to offer a comprehensive competitive bid than most individual hospitals because it can select from a wide range of services and prices at member hospitals. Second, all member hospitals share the risk of losing Medicaid revenue as a result of being chosen as a provider.

Whether or not Metro-Care is selected as a provider for the Medicaid prepayment program, leaders of the organization reported that Metro-Care will become a preferred provider organization for private payers. Given Chicago's historical lack of involvement in shared services and multihospital arrangements, it will be interesting to observe the progress of this organization over time.

Although more than one-third of Chicago hospitals are members of multihospital systems, approximately 45 percent of those hospitals are affiliated with systems outside Chicago (AHA, 1981). Twelve multihospital systems are based in Chicago with twenty-two Chicago-area hospitals. However, eight of these are long-standing systems affiliated with the Roman Catholic church, and one is affiliated with another church. The three systems developed recently appear to be competitive initiatives. All three are non-profit; each owns and operates at least two hospitals in the Chicago area; and none has ownership or management affiliations with hospitals outside the Chicago area. Evangelical Hospital System differs from the other two systems by acquiring operating hospitals. The hospitals in the Evangelical Hospital System range from troubled inner-city to profitable suburban institutions. The pooling of resources helps inner-city hospitals to survive public aid cuts, bad debts, and costly physical plant repair.

It is interesting that administrators of all three organizations were nominated by informants and/or other respondents as influential. One administrator of a Catholic church system was nominated also. However, of the hospitals that are affiliated with multihospital systems based outside Chicago, no administrators were considered influential in the Chicago hospital community. The affiliated hospitals are not unusually small or overrepresented in the inner city or outlying areas. It could be argued that administrators of hospitals affiliated with non-Chicago-based multihospital systems are not as invested in the Chicago hospital community as are administrators for free-standing hospitals or Chicago-based systems. These administrators may seek to gain influence within their hospital systems rather than within their immediate environment.

Whether Chicago hospitals are members of long-standing religious systems, newly incorporated religious systems, or investor-owned chains, it is significant that the systems were not conceived in Chicago. If the systems were developed as competitive initiatives, they were conceived by administrators and benefit parent organizations in other cities. Of course, many organizational strategies benefit member hospitals in Chicago, e.g., group purchasing, long-range planning, and insurance coverage. However, the ultimate decision makers for many hospitals are not located in Chicago. In both the business and hospital communities of Chicago, the locally based, locally invested, elite group of decision makers appears to be absent. This may partially explain the absence of strong cooperative or competitive hospital movements in Chicago.

Efforts by Chicago's hospital administrators to increase census and their involvement in multihospital institutions differ from efforts in the Twin Cities in quality and quantity. This difference also applies to vertical integration and diversification. According to one respondent, only "a handful of organizations in this city have reorganized corporately." Some are aggressively involved in integration and diversification, and others are either still in the planninng stages or moving more slowly.

One suburban hospital, the "dazzling exception" referred to earlier, has taken giant strides. The parent organization and its subsidiaries have diversified into wellness clinics, preventive sports medicine, industrial medicine, substance abuse programs, and numerous other activities. Consulting and management contracts with local hospitals are clearing the way for mergers and acquisitions.

Some similar innovative efforts are underway at a large inner-city hospital. However, these strategies are exceptional in Chicago. One respondent explained, "It's hard to innovate when you're drowning." The financial crises faced by many free-standing hospitals make it difficult to consider corporate reorganization. Lesser efforts to diversify are inhibited by requirements for initial capital investment.

HMO-HOSPITAL RELATIONSHIPS

Because they offer ambulatory and inpatient care, HMOs must associate with hospitals. HMO-hospital relationships range from HMO ownership of a hospital to a limited service agreement between a hospital and an HMO. The common types of HMO-hospital relationships fall between these two extremes.

In any HMO-hospital affiliation, the HMO and the hospital are in a "resource dependent relationship"; that is, each organization provides some resource to the other. A symmetrical relationship exists when this exchange is equally important to both organizations. The symmetry or asymmetry of the relationship is determined, in part, by the scarcity and significance of the resources exchanged (Pfeffer and Salancik, 1978). An HMO provides a hospital with patients and receives hospital access for its members. The type of relationship that develops is influenced by the significance and scarcity of inpatient business to the hospital and by the significance and scarcity of hospital access (or discounted hospital access) to the HMO.

Each type of relationship has different levels of resource dependence. The potential for a symmetrical relationship increases from very low in HMO-hospital ownership to very high in HMO-hospital service and financial agreements.

Only two HMOs in the United States are built on the model of hospital ownership: Kaiser-Permanente Medical Care Program and the Group Health Cooperative of Puget Sound (Seermon, 1981). Only Group Health Cooperative also owns the medical group that serves its members. Kaiser's medical group is a separate legal entity that contracts exclusively with Kaiser.

Zelten identifies five advantages of a hospital-based HMO: 1) continuity of care; 2) composite medical record; 3) financial advantages, such as elimination of duplication and matching of service demand with supply; 4) predictability of allocating inpatient services; and 5) elimination of contract stipulations (Zelten, 1979). Still, some major barriers to HMO-hospital ownership make this strategy rare. First, a membership of approximately

125,000 is needed to support a 200-bed hospital (using Kaiser planning figures of from 1.6 to 1.8 beds per 1,000 members at 85 percent occupancy and 500 inpatient days per 1,000 members). Currently only eighteen HMOs in the country have over 100,000 members (InterStudy, 1983). Requiring 125,000 HMO members to be within reasonable distance of one 200-bed hospital poses a major strategic problem.

Second, hospital construction and acquisition are problematic. Hospital construction by HMOs involves certificate-of-need regulations, and in many areas it is very difficult to receive permission to construct new facilities. Acquiring an existing hospital involves the financial and managerial problems that made the acquisition candidate available and a medical staff that may oppose HMOs.

In the few cases of HMOs' owning hospitals, the resource-dependent relationship is asymmetrical. The hospital is completely dependent on the HMO for all resources. A complete reversal of that relationship exists in the case of hospitals' owning HMOs. No HMOs are fully owned by hospitals (Seermon, 1981). A national census of HMOs in 1977 identifies nine hospital-sponsored HMOs out of 165 HMOs existing at that time (Office of Health Maintenance Organizations, 1977). "Sponsorship," however, was not defined; but it implied that a single hospital had been solely responsible for the development and financing of the HMO, although from inception the HMO was a separate legal entity. "Hospital-affiliated HMOs," as the term is used by InterStudy, includes HMOs solely sponsored by hospitals, and those jointly sponsored by hospitals and other organizations (e.g., insurers and physicians' groups). "Hospital affiliation" can also mean that a hospital was instrumental in the HMO's development, providing loans, personnel, facilities, or other means of support. InterStudy identified thirty-seven hospital-affiliated HMOs in January 1981, not including HMOs affiliated with academic medical centers.

The advantages to a hospital of sponsoring or affiliating with an HMO vary with external environmental conditions. Primarily an entrepreneurial strategy, HMO sponsorship helps maintain or increase a hospital's market share or provides more comprehensive health care to hospital employees at lower cost than otherwise possible. Specific strategies will be discussed below in the context of the two metropolitan areas.

Four types of organizations were ranked by Johnson on their

capacity for HMO sponsorship or affiliation (Johnson, 1981). Prepayment carriers (i.e., insurance companies) were judged most capable of entering the HMO market based on the following factors. These factors are critical to successful HMO development:

- organizational structure;
- actuarial know-how;
- marketing know-how;
- information processing experience;
- utilization control experience;
- understanding of physicians;
- capitalization strength.

Hospitals ranked second, well below prepayment carriers but ahead of medical groups. Commercial corporations were ranked last. Johnson judged hospitals particularly weak in organizational structure, actuarial know-how, marketing know-how, and capitalization strength.

The potential conflict of objectives between HMOs and their sponsoring hospitals also hampers cooperation. While hospitals want to increase census and utilization, HMOs want to reduce hospitalization and overutilization of ancillary services.

The resource-dependent relationship in HMO sponsorship and affiliation is more symmetrical than in HMO hospital ownership. Although the organizations may be bound by a common parent organization and interlocking boards of directors, the HMO and the hospital are legally differentiated. Each may freely seek resources from and provide resources to other organizations. Many hospital-sponsored or hospital-affiliated HMOs eventually use hospital services from other sources, and sponsoring hospitals frequently have agreements with other HMOs. Each becomes less critical to the other when resources are readily available elsewhere. Of course, the relationship could become symmetrical if the organizations gained rather than lost importance to one another by each monopolizing the resources exchanged. However, given antitrust laws and the huge public demand for health services, monopoly over hospital services or health care coverage is problematic legally and financially.

As explained, formal relationships of ownership and sponsorship between hospitals and HMOs are relatively rare. A variety of service and financial arrangements are more common.

Hospital service arrangements may be formal contracts, providing all available services to HMO members or providing special services offered by that hospital. The first example is a "full service contract," and the second is a "limited service contract." Informal arrangements are mediated by admitting physicians who are HMO providers; the hospital provides full services to such a physician's patients and bills the HMO as it would an insurance company.

When a hospital and an HMO have only a service relationship, by contract or through admitting physicians, the HMO pays the hospital billed charges for services received by members. Examples of payment mechanisms other than billed charges are these:

- discounts (as a percentage of full charges or as cost-plus);
- current Blue Cross reimbursement rates;
- retrospective formulae;
- capitation;
- all-inclusive-rates preadmission;
- all-inclusive per diem rates;
- leased beds;
- charges to maximum total reimbursements;
- billed charges with hold-back provisions;
- year-end settlements with risk-sharing;
- advance payment deposits and guarantees of maximum HMO dollars and patient-day volumes (Seermon, 1981).

Financial arrangements between HMOs and hospitals are almost always formalized by written contract. The relationship may be initiated by either organization, and many factors influence their decisions to participate. Factors that influence an HMO's decision include preexisting ties to the hospital or its medical staff, cost per inpatient day, willingness to negotiate reimbursement, hospital reputation, and hospital location. Factors influencing a hospital's decision include preexisting ties to the HMO, the potential increase in census to be gained through a financial agreement, and the potential loss in census if an agreement is not established and the HMO terminates the relationship.

Service and financial arrangements have greater potential for symmetry than hospital ownership or hospital sponsorship or affiliation. When two previously independent organizations exchange resources, exchange theorists argue, the resources exchanged are likely to be of equal importance to both organizations (Blau, 1964; Downs, 1967). It is important to understand that resources, in this case, are not exclusively measured in dollars. Hospitals with convenient locations or strong community reputations hold resources that are valuable to HMOs. In turn, HMOs with prestigious physicians or physicians with established admitting privileges hold valuable resources for hospitals.

INTERACTIONS OF HMOs AND HOSPITALS

The mutual impact of hospitals and HMOs is a complex issue. Hospitals and HMOs differ in their impact on one another from organization to organization and from market to market. Multiple factors influence their mutual impact. For example, the HMO market share, a measure of success, determines the extent of HMO impact on hospitals. Primary and secondary data from this study support the contention that both internal and external factors determine the HMO market share. The fact that hospitals, together with other actors in the HMOs' environment, have impact on the HMO market share, which in turn has impact on hospitals, is the key to the complexity of hospital-HMO mutual impact. To address the full range of issues gleaned from this research, the following sections focus on generic topics, then on topics of particular relevance in Minneapolis-St. Paul and Chicago.

Hospital impact on HMOs

Organizational

The most direct organizational impact a hospital can have on an HMO is by sponsoring an HMO. HMO sponsorship entails the provision of finances, management, personnel, and facilities. A sponsoring hospital can further influence its HMO by successfully marketing the HMO to hospital employees, arranging for staff privileges for HMO physicians, and accepting preadmission lab tests performed in the HMO. Sponsorship by a prestigious teaching hospital can enhance an HMO's credibility to potential members and to potential physician providers. However, the traditionally high cost of care in teaching hospitals can adversely affect an HMO's savings ability. Initially, hospital sponsorship has great impact on the sponsored HMO. Over time, if the HMO stabilizes financially and markets effectively to other employee groups, the hospital's influence will decrease.

Hospital impact on HMOs is also evident in HMO joint sponsorship and HMO affiliation. Joint sponsorship by a hospital and another organization (e.g., a physician group, a union, another hospital) results in the same amount of support to the HMO as in full sponsorship but less total impact from the hospital. Affiliation also has positive impact on the HMO, by means of instrumental loans of capital, personnel, or other means of support. Both joint sponsorship and affiliation with a prestigious hospital can enhance the plan's marketability to consumers and providers.

Hospitals have organizational impact on HMOs through service and financial agreements. Researchers found convenience, physician preference, and reputation to be important variables in HMO selection of hospitals (Appel and Aquilina, 1982). A service agreement can enhance the HMO's marketability by increasing the HMO's prestige, credibility, and convenience to members for inpatient care. A financial agreement that stipulates some discount or risk-sharing has all of the positive impact of a service agreement, in addition to the benefit of paying less than billed charges.

At some time the HMO may wish to renegotiate a service or financial agreement. At this point, physician and patient preferences may make it difficult for the HMO to change hospitals if it is unable to negotiate successfully. Even in a market area where HMOs are very active buyers, such as Minneapolis-St. Paul, HMOs do not "shop" for low-cost hospitals. "HMOs can only be as selective and price sensitive in their choice of hospitals as their physicians and members will allow" (Appel and Aquilina, 1982).

Two factors influence a hospital's willingness to cooperate with an HMO: the hospital's capacity to respond to HMO initiatives and its incentive to do so (Kralewski, et al., 1982). Adequate financial and managerial resources are required for a hospital to sponsor or affiliate with an HMO. Furthermore, the incentives a hospital must have range from anticipation of gain from HMO involvement to the anticipation of loss if involvement is rejected.

Extensive capital is not required for a hospital to enter a service or financial agreement with an HMO, but hospital location and reputation are important variables. A hospital that lacks the resources to maintain its physical plant and to attract qualified health care professionals will not attract HMOs seeking service or financial arrangements. If an HMO did pursue an arrangement with a financially troubled institution, the hospital would probably deny the HMO a discount or risk-sharing contract. Conversely, financially healthy hospitals that have the capacity to respond to HMO initiatives often lack incentives to do so. If census and revenue are high, the potential negative impact of an HMO arrangement may outweigh the potential positive impact.

Environmental

Hospitals have environmental impact on HMOs through their collective receptiveness to HMOs. The receptiveness of a hospital market to alternative health care delivery systems appears to depend on two conditions: the competitive state of the market and the political state of the hospital community.

Hospital competition has been discussed extensively. The relevant variables that influence the impact of hospitals on HMOs are areawide occupancy rates and the type of competition —service or price—prevalent in the market. When occupancy rates are low, hospital administrators report more receptiveness to alternatives that might increase census. On a larger scale, low areawide census enhances hospitals' receptiveness to HMOs and increases the likelihood of competition for HMO business. This competition has positive impact on HMOs. When areawide occupancy rates are high, the impact on HMOs is likely to be negative. Variability in occupancy rates presents a complex challenge to HMOs. When occupancy rates vary greatly between hospitals or between residential areas, it may be that other variables intervene, such as location, available resources, and management sophistication.

The prevalence of service competition or price competition in a hospital market influences hospital impact on HMOs. The interactions with and impact of price-competitive hospitals differ substantially from those of service-competitive hospitals.

In a service-competitive environment, whether hospitals are healthy or troubled financially, HMO utilization control mechanisms will meet more resistance from physicians and hospital administrators, because neither buyers nor users of health care services are price-sensitive. HMOs will also have difficulty marketing their services to employers and employees in a service-competitive environment. Firms are likely to offer generous health coverage with low deductibles and copayments if management is not price-sensitive in its health insurance buying (see chapter 6).

No market exists in which hospitals compete solely on price. Both "service-competitive" and "price-competitive" designations should be considered ideal types, used only for explanatory purposes. However, in a market where hospitals compete on price, in addition to service, patients are attracted through the buyers of health care as well as through physicians. Price-competitive hospitals, therefore, have incentives to compete for buyers, including HMOs. In a market where all hospitals compete, many will satisfy the convenience and reputation requirements of HMO members, and many will have the financial capacity to offer HMOs discounts and risk-sharing agreements.

Two aspects of the political state of the hospital community influence hospital impact on HMOs: the ability of local hospitals to communicate and unite on issues, and the ability of state and local hospital associations to influence legislation regarding HMOs. Interview data suggested that if hospital administrators in a market area have well-established communication patterns and are able to confer on events and issues relevant to the hospital community, they are likely to be proactive. Whether this communication and unity have a positive or a negative impact on HMOs depends on the position administrators take. HMOs will feel positive impact if hospital administrators philosophically support the HMO concept or agree that HMO involvement is an appropriate financial or political strategy. Conversely, if administrators collectively reject HMO initiatives, HMO development will be impaired.

If communication and unity are low in a market area, administrators are likely to be reactive. New health care options may be poorly approached, or understanding may vary individually. When approached by an HMO, the administrator may have little information on which to base a decision. The administrator will also have less information concerning community and other provider response to such a decision. The impact on HMO development of poor communication and disunity is likely to be negative because of inertia.

State and local hospital associations may be powerful forces to enhance or inhibit HMO development. Depending on the strength of the organization, lobbying at the state level can influence the timing and provisions of HMO-enabling legislation and other relevant regulations. A local association can act as a unifying agent for normally uncooperative administrators by disseminating information regarding pending legislation. The impact on HMOs will be positive or negative depending on the stance of these organizations toward HMOs.

Minneapolis-St. Paul

The hospital community of Minneapolis-St. Paul is distinguished by its homogeneity, its cooperative history, and its current level of price competition. Community input and leadership in the hospital community are also unusual. These factors have resulted in positive impact on HMOs.

Three hospitals in Minneapolis-St. Paul have been directly or indirectly involved in HMO sponsorship. Given the small number of hospital-sponsored and hospital-affiliated HMOs nationwide, this level of sponsorship activity in one community is unusual. Beyond providing start-up financial and technical resources, the sponsoring hospitals have benefited their HMOs by marketing the HMO to hospital employees, absorbing tension from fee-for-service medical staffs, and entering discount and risk-sharing agreements.

Service and financial agreements with hospitals have also had positive impact on HMOs. Many factors contributed to the homogeneity of high-quality institutions and to hospital accessibility in Minneapolis-St. Paul. Most Twin Cities hospitals have some financial agreement with at least one HMO. Service agreements are most often limited agreements in the Twin Cities, and allow HMO members access to the specialized techniques and equipment of teaching hospitals. One interesting disadvantage is the proximity of the world-famous Mayo Clinic. For a long time, Minnesota residents have thought of the Mayo Clinic as a medical panacea, but no HMO has a service or a financial agreement with the clinic. Some respondents in each sector considered the inability to seek treatment at the Mayo Clinic a deterrent to joining an HMO.

The environmental conditions that influence hospital impact on HMOs have enhanced HMO growth in the Twin Cities. Occupancy rates are low, leaving many hospitals "desperate for patients" (Kuntz, 1983). HMOs and other third-party payers are negotiating successfully for discounts to the disadvantage of some hospitals.

A price-competitive strategy exists amid service competition. This helps HMOs by increasing the universe of hospitals that are attractive to HMO members and that have the capacity and the incentive to pursue HMO initiatives.

Political conditions have also supported HMO growth. Information regarding new health care initiatives, such as HMOs and PPOs, spreads quickly. The early support for the HMO concept by business leaders, legislators, and community groups in the Twin Cities would have made rejection by hospitals politically and financially unwise. Therefore, many Twin Cities hospitals gave active or passive support to HMO development.

High consumer and business activity in hospital policy in Minneapolis-St. Paul influences hospital impact on HMOs. Both the Citizens League and the Twin Cities Health Care Development Project are examples of organized local influence on health care delivery. Minneapolis and St. Paul also have hospital trustee councils that allow hospital board members to have policy input beyond their individual hospitals. The West Metro Trustee Council, of Minneapolis, is reported to have a collaborative relationship with the local HSA and to be proactive on most issues. The East Metro Trustee Council, of St. Paul, is reported to be more reactive and to have an adversarial relationship with the HSA, especially regarding bed-cutting and hospital closure policies. Trustees have been supportive of HMO growth, although more so in Minneapolis than in St. Paul.

Organized activity by laypeople in hospital policy and the history of consumer action in cooperatives and community organizations have inhibited the lobbying effect of state and local hospital associations. Given the strength of the consumer's voice in hospital activities, consumer support of the HMO concept has aided HMO growth and development.

Chicago

Organizational impact of hospitals on HMOs in Chicago has been primarily the result of hospital sponsorship. The two major medical centers that sponsored HMOs offered considerable start-up financial and technical resources to their HMOs. These HMOs were conceived, in part, as a result of labor demand for comprehensive health services, and hospital employee participation in the plans has remained high. The medical centers enhance their HMOs' credibility by the technical and academic prestige of their institutions. To date, this credibility has outweighed the high cost of care in teaching hospitals. Convenience has been the primary reason for use of other hospitals by the HMOs.

Another example of hospital and medical staff support for an HMO during its early stages does not involve formal sponsorship or affiliation. The one consumer-sponsored HMO in the Chicago area was aided informally by a prestigious hospital located in the same suburb. The founders of the HMO used established social networks to procure participation and advice from members of the medical staff of this hospital. The prestige of these physician providers was described by one founder as a chief marketing tool. Physicians who became especially involved in the HMO's development helped obtain hospital space and cooperation. It may be that the HMO would not have survived its developmental stage without the assistance of these providers.

Hospitals have had little impact on HMOs through service arrangements. Since group, network, and IPA physicians do not change admitting privileges as a result of becoming HMO providers, the issues of hospital convenience, reputation, and physician preference are moot.

Hospitals in Chicago differ significantly from one another in financial resources. Many respondents reported that inner-city hospitals have low censuses and revenues, whereas suburban hospitals are generally strong. Inner-city hospitals may have the incentive to respond to HMO initiatives as a means to increase census, but they do not have the resources to offer discounts or to attract HMO members. Suburban hospitals have the capacity to respond to HMO initiatives but no incentive. Indeed, there is almost an inverse relationship between capacity and incentive in the Chicago area. An administrator of a hospital in a very wealthy suburb stated simply that residents of his community could "afford to buy their own health care"; they have no reason to sacrifice choice and convenience for cost-savings.

The environmental impact of hospitals on HMOs in Chicago has been negative, in terms of both the competitive state of the market and the political state of the hospital community. Occupancy rates in Chicago differ between the suburbs and the inner city, but overall they have been high. Variability in occupancy rates among residential areas presents marketing problems to HMOs. Hospitals with low occupancy rates are frequently located in economically troubled areas and present barriers to HMO relationships because of physical plant, personnel, and location. The prevalence of service competition inhibits hospital incentive to pursue or accept HMO relationship. Some administrators claimed that the potential for losing actively admitting physicians because of conflict over HMO involvement was sufficient reason to avoid the issue.

The lack of communication and unity among hospital administrators has resulted in a great range of understanding about HMOs. Some administrators have made well-informed decisions to pursue or reject HMO involvement, but others rely on hearsay. One administrator reported that he had heard that HMOs pay each of their physicians "$200 for every day the physician knocks off a patient's hospital stay" compared to the hospital's average length of stay. Poor communication among hospital administrators allows such rumors to linger.

Administrators' disunity is evidenced by the paucity of successful cooperative efforts in Chicago. The lack of neighborhood hospital leagues has made the local hospital association the sole catalyst of community hospital efforts.

The state hospital association is a very powerful lobbying organization. Unhindered by organized consumer input at the state or community level (although in Illinois, such input would not necessarily be pro-HMO), the hospital association is reported to rival the state medical society in political clout on health care issues. As stated earlier, hospitals and HMOs have inherently conflicting interests regarding hospital utilization. This conflict and the power of the state hospital association have gummed the path of HMO development. Although both the hospital association and the state medical society officially claim a neutral position on HMOs, organized provider promotion of the HMO concept is neither politically nor financially strategic in Illinois.

HMO impact on hospitals

Organizational

An HMO may have organizational impact on a hospital whether or not it has a relationship with that hospital. HMOs may reduce the hospital's market share by enrolling individuals who previously used the hospital. The volume of the loss depends on the number of HMOs in the hospital's market area and their enrollment success. Physicians who become providers for IPA models may, for convenience, place their IPA and fee-for-service patients in one hospital. As one hospital administrator pointed out, "If those physicians who bring a couple percent of their patients here weren't allowed to do so, they'd be encouraged to go elsewhere—not only with their HMO patients, but with their non-HMO patients." A hospital without an IPA relationship, therefore, risks losing fee-for-service patients who previously used the hospital. The volume of this loss depends on how many of the hospital's admitting physicians become IPA providers and whether those physicians were active admitters.

The potential positive impacts of HMOs are described by Motzer in terms of offering reasons for hospital involvement with HMOs (Group Health Association of America, 1981):

1. referrals to institutional and/or physician subspecialties within the hospital;
2. opportunity to develop organized ambulatory care programs or upgrade existing ones;
3. new settings for hospital educational programs;
4. increased probability of positive reactions from local health systems agencies in securing approval for other projects planned by the hospital;
5. less dependence on solo practice physicians for admissions;
6. increased prospect of additional revenue from ancillary services (e.g., clinical lab testing, radiology, emergency room);
7. fewer collection problems (e.g., bad debts, late payments, paperwork);
8. vehicle for stimulating interest in preventive care and health promotion;
9. opportunity to expand expertise in collection and use of patient, provider, and facility statistics; and
10. increased hospital market share.

If a hospital insures its own employees through an indemnity insurer, and employees use other hospitals, the hospital pays premiums to the insurer while "subsidizing a competitor's bottom line" (Goldsmith, 1983). If the hospitals that employees use are more expensive than their employer, the hospital's benefit costs could increase. Hospital HMO sponsorship, although potentially increasing premium costs, owing to first-dollar coverage and ambulatory care benefits, increases the probability of the hospital's use by its own personnel.

Interviews with health care respondents and data from secondary sources reveal potential negative impacts of an HMO on a hospital. The primary impact is that HMOs decrease hospital utilization. Administrators reported that HMO members use fewer hospital days for all services and procedures. Speculation about reasons for this falls into two categories: "selection effect" and "HMO effect." The selection effect argues that individuals who enroll in HMOs, gainfully employed and younger than the general population, require less inpatient care. Difficulty in collecting accurate data about HMO enrollees' pre-HMO health care has prevented confirmation of this claim. However, as discussed in chapter 7, when HMO premiums were higher than indemnity insurance premiums, respondents suspected that individuals willing to pay the premium differential were those who expected to use many services. This might counteract the selection effect from younger, healthier enrollees.

The HMO effect argues that HMOs reduce hospitalization by means of numerous management techniques. The claim that HMOs reduce the need for hospitalization by providing preventive care has not been proven empirically (Luft, 1978). However, HMOs do require ambulatory rather than inpatient care for some surgical and medical procedures, and often HMOs negotiate with hospitals to perform preadmission testing in the HMO rather than the hospital. HMOs often require a preadmission certification process and do not reimburse for weekend nonemergency admissions. Ongoing utilization review programs in HMOs provide data for control policy decisions, such as negative sanctioning of high-use providers. Finally, it has been suggested, though not documented, that utilization awareness learned by HMO physicians spills over into the physicians' fee-for-service practice. As larger numbers enroll in the different types of HMOs, more data will become available concerning the differential presence of these effects in group, staff, network, and IPA models.

While decreased utilization is the primary concern of hospital administrators, there are times when increased utilization is also problematic. Some hospital administrators reported that because HMOs treat the less major medical problems on an outpatient basis, HMO members who are hospitalized require a greater intensity of care and support services. The average cost per case, consequently, is perceived to be higher for HMO members than for fee-for-service patients.

Another utilization issue is that HMO business is not uniformly distributed across hospital departments. Because young, employed individuals are overrepresented in HMOs, their members use fewer patient days in cardiac surgery and renal dialysis but considerably more days in obstetrics. Soper reported that while a 25,000-member HMO may have an average daily hospital census of only twenty-five patients, a high delivery rate could increase the hospital's deliveries by fifty per month (Group Heatlh Association of America, 1981). Uneven distribution could place unanticipated strain on particular hospital services and departments.

The final issue relates to the total volume of HMO business. If one HMO maintains a high patient volume in a hospital, administrators report concern about the HMO's potential to dominate the hospital's destiny, particularly the types of services offered and the emphasis on primary care. If two or more HMOs together maintain a high patient volume in a hospital, these HMOs may negotiate discounts on risk-sharing. The hospital is in a poor bargaining position, even though discounts or risk-sharing may require the shifting of costs to the decreasing numbers of fee-for-service patients.

Environmental

Interviews and data from secondary sources revealed that HMO impact on hospitals changes as HMO market share increases. When HMO market share is low areawide, HMO impact is limited. Individually, an HMO with a low market share cannot have positive impact on a hospital by noticeably increasing the hospital's market share or its revenue from ancillary services. Conversely, that HMO can have little negative impact on a hospital in terms of decreasing utilization or differentially influencing specific hospital departments. Even when market share is low, however, resistance from fee-for-service medical staff can strain relations with the hospital administration. There are also some negative effects on hospitals that are a function of low HMO market share. When HMOs are just starting and have small enrollee populations, hospital administrators are concerned that HMOs might fail, leaving the hospital with bad debts. Also, when HMOs are developing, numerous problems occur regarding reimbursement guidelines and member education. Administrators report incidents of conflict because an HMO member used hospital services incorrectly and/or hospital personnel were unfamiliar with HMO reimbursement policies. These incidents are especially common in connection with emergency room services.

When HMO market share is high, HMOs have great impact—positive and negative—on hospitals. HMOs bring sufficiently many patients into hospitals to influence revenues. Strong IPAs can negotiate discounts for the IPA and fee-for-service patients brought in by IPA physicians. When market share is high, HMOs also affect the demand for hospital services. Gary Appel, president of the Council of Community Hospitals in the Twin Cities, reported that from 1977 to 1981 HMO enrollment increased by 15 percent of the population in Minneapolis-St. Paul. In that time period, HMO patient days decreased by 13 percent. This simultaneous increase in HMO membership and decrease in patient days threatens hospital survival. An interesting side effect of increased areawide impact, however, is decreased impact by individual HMOs. Two key variables influence the effect of an HMO on a hospital: the percent of areawide beds affiliated with prepaid plans, and the percent of areawide enrollment market share in prepaid plans (Fink and Trimmer, 1981). As HMO-affiliated beds and enrollment increase, the individual impact of each area HMO decreases.

Minneapolis-St. Paul

With approximately 25 percent of the market, HMOs have had substantial organizational and environmental impact on hospitals in Minneapolis-St. Paul. Approximately two-thirds of the hospitals in Minneapolis-St. Paul have contracts with HMOs calling for reimbursement on a basis other than billed charges (Kralewski, 1982).

Reports from administrators regarding initial acceptance of HMO involvement confirmed the checklist of potential positive impacts of HMOs. Some hospitals initiated or accepted HMO relationships recently—within the past four or five years. Among these hospitals, the most common reason given for HMO involvement was maintenance of the hospital's market share. Administrators were quick to point out that they did not anticipate an increased market share as a result. Administrators perceived HMO involvement as one of many strategies to combat further decline in their market share. Hospitals having HMO relationships older than ten years were less likely to report market protection or enhancement as a reason for their initial involvement. Their reasons included support of the HMO concept and previous ties to a physician group that sought HMO involvement.

Although most Twin Cities hospitals have some type of HMO relationship, only a handful of hospitals receive a significant percentage of their admissions from HMOs. Because of HMO utilization controls and selection effects, an HMO market share of 25 percent translates to 8 percent of total patient days (Appel, 1982). Therefore, most administrators can offer favorable contracts to HMOs without seriously affecting their bottom lines. However, in a price-competitive market, such as Minneapolis-St. Paul, other buyers of health care demand hospital discounts. The combined impact is potentially serious. In the Twin Cities, third-party payers, including HMOs and PPOs, are "pushing hospitals to the wall for price discounts, and industry observers fear that many hospitals, desperate for patients, are making bad deals" (Kuntz, 1983).

The few hospitals with significant percentages of admissions from one HMO voiced concern about the HMO's ability to dominate their destinies. One hospital that receives 57 percent of its admissions from HMOs, primarily from one HMO, is building up its private medical staff. The administrator of another hospital, with 60 percent of its admissions from HMOs, also primarily from one HMO, reported concern that the hospital's fee-for-service primary care physicians must compete with the HMO physicians. It is interesting that most Twin Cities administrators reported that the initial negative response of fee-for-service physicians to HMOs has subsided over time. This is due, they said, to a growing familiarity with the HMO concept, the allaying of fears that HMO care is inferior, the success of physician-sponsored IPAs, and acceptance of the inevitable.

The estimates cited earlier regarding decreasing individual HMO impact as areawide HMO impact decreases do not necessarily hold true in Minneapolis-St. Paul. Important differences exist in the size, age, and concentration of hospital penetration among HMOs there. The oldest and largest HMO in the area concentrates a significant number of its members in one hospital, so its individual impact is high. Other HMOs, however, particularly network and IPA models, do not concentrate patients, so their impact is diluted.

Chicago

A city as diverse in its interests as in its population, Chicago is probably more representative of other large American cities than is Minneapolis-St. Paul. In Chicago's hospital community, both organizational and environmental factors have contributed to inhibit HMO development and growth. In turn, HMOs have had negligible organizational and environmental impact on the hospital community.

In Chicago, HMOs have an areawide market penetration of approximately 3.5 percent. Thus, HMOs do not have enough membership strength, individually or collectively, to have significant impact on area hospitals. Only very recently did HMOs in Chicago negotiate sucessfully for reimbursement on a basis other than billed charges. Service arrangements with hospitals have not brought enough HMO members into hospitals to influence hospital revenues or utilization. However, the presence of HMOs and the potential for HMO-hospital relationships has been sufficient to motivate hospital medical staffs to communicate concern to administrators.

Some interesting side effects of low HMO market share were revealed in interviews. Physicians for group, network, and IPA models continue to use those hospitals they had before becoming HMO providers. Few discounts have been negotiated, and service contracts do not require high-level hospital input. HMOs are billed like any other third-party payer. The presence of HMO patients in the hospital, then, is not due to a decision by the hospital administrator that could be influenced by board members, the medical staff, or other hospital personnel. The presence of HMO patients is the collective result of individual physicians' decisions to become HMO providers and to admit those patients to the hospital. In Chicago, therefore, physicians are mediating the relationship of HMOs and hospitals.

The other effects of low HMO market share described earlier are also evident here. Chicago administrators voiced concern about HMOs going "belly up," leaving the hospital with bad debts. Respondents also discussed billing problems with HMOs. One administrator said the lack of understanding by patients is "one of the real flies in the ointment with HMOs." He explained further, "Marketing and education differ. HMOs are quick to compete in price but don't educate the patient about losing his or her physician, and I think it's done out of design sometimes because if they told the people, they wouldn't sign up."

SUMMARY

In both Minneapolis-St. Paul and Chicago, certain characteristics of the hospital community have been discussed as important to the understanding of interactions between hospitals and HMOs. Hospital market characteristics influence the degree and type of hospital competition. Both market characteristics and competition are influenced by historical, economic, and social variables. All of these variables influence HMO market share and the mutual impact of HMOs and hospitals.

In addition to directly influencing HMO development, hospital market characteristics influence the degree and type of hospital competition. In Minneapolis-St. Paul, administrators reported that hospital price competition increased in the 1970s. The financial interests of each individual institution advocate maintaining current facilities while maintaining or increasing utilization. Given that capacity and utilization were decreasing areawide, this institutional goal became a "zero-sum game." One institution must lose if another gains. Price competition for buyers of inpatient services, including HMOs, increased along with an already active service competition as a means of maintaining and increasing census. Because of the ethnically and economically homogeneous population, the accessibility of hospitals, and the similarity of resource availability to hospitals in the Twin Cities, hospitals are able to compete with one another on a relatively equal footing, both on service and on price. Minneapolis-St. Paul hospitals possess both the ability and the incentive to respond to HMO initiatives.

The competitive and political climate of the hospital market in the Twin Cities has enhanced HMO development and growth, and the high HMO market penetration has resulted in great interaction and impact between HMOs and hospitals. Individual organizational interdependence and impact vary greatly between institutions, but looking at the market area as the unit of analysis, one can see that HMOs and hospitals exchange measurable quantities of vital resources and therefore have impact on one another's success and survival.

In Chicago, hospital respondents reported that service competition is very strong. Spurred by rising admissions, inpatient days, and beds, in addition to ethnically and economically differentiated service areas, hospitals have sought to expand facilities, buy equipment, and increase the convenience and attractiveness of their services. In a growing industry, the "zero-sum game" is not in play. That is, it is possible for one institution to gain without another one losing. In fact, with such distinct service areas and distinct differences in resource availability, one hospital's success may be irrelevant to another's. HMOs, as price-sensitive buyers of inpatient services, face difficulties in negotiating service and financial agreements unless they have the ability to bring in significant numbers of patients. HMOs in Chicago are not yet large or geographically concentrated enough to have that ability. The differences in service areas and resource availability result in a negative correlation between ability and incentive to respond to HMO initiatives. The competitive and political climate of the hospital market in Chicago has inhibited HMO development and growth. Low HMO market share results in low HMO-hospital interaction and little impact between organizations.

5

HMOs and Physicians

Certain responses of physicians to HMOs were similar in both metropolitan areas, but their behaviors differed. Physicians in both areas feared erosion of the physician-patient relationship. They also feared increased bureaucratization of medical practice. In the Twin Cities, the physician community is a homogeneous group with a recognized leadership. In Chicago, physicians have no cohesive professional identity or leadership. In both areas, physicians worried about the potential for poor quality of care or "undertreatment" resulting from excessive concern about containing costs. The medical practice patterns and the health care concerns are very different in the two communities. The Twin Cities and Minnesota have the highest proportion of physicians in private group practice in the country, serving a homogeneous, healthy population. This, it would seem, made shifting to HMOs easier. In Chicago, physicians are much less likely to have the background or inclination to enter such arrangements, and they are not convinced that HMOs can solve the major problem of providing health care to the poor.

In an increasingly complex health care delivery system, physicians continue to be central actors. While their fees account for only 15 to 20 percent of health care dollars spent (Fuchs, 1974), it is clear that, as a Chicago representative of organized medicine noted, "Physicians are responsible for another 60 cents on every dollar." Furthermore, much of the lay public perceives

---

This chapter was written by Claire H. Kohrman, Research Project Analyst.

"health care" and "physicians" to be synonymous. The physician is "captain of the team"; "it is impossible to make significant changes in the medical field without changing physician behavior" (Fuchs, 1974). It became clear from our study that physicians' behavior and the structure of health care are tightly interwoven. Thus, physicians' perceptions and behavior have an important impact on their communities' attitudes about health care, as well as on the development of any change in the health care delivery system. Furthermore, physicians do not reflect solely their local area; they form a "community within community" (Goode, 1957); their attitudes and behavior reflect the norms not only of their geographic community but also of their professional community.

We interviewed sixty-three informants to understand the perspectives of each of the medical communities. Most were physicians selected from the medical sector. Others were physicians working primarily in other sectors. These included a selection of administrators of medical groups or agencies, and physicians with varying responsibilities and forms of practice. The practitioners we interviewed represented solo practice and different forms of group practice, fee-for-service, and various forms of prepayment. In addition to practitioners, we spoke to physicians in universities; in state, county, and city agencies; and in national, state, county, and city medical societies.

PHYSICIANS' VALUES AND THEIR CHANGING ROLE

To understand physicians' roles in the development of HMOs, it is useful to consider first the historical development of the physician's role and patterns of practice in America in the twentieth century. Those behaviors that have inhibited or enhanced HMO development are rooted not only in particular conditions of the individual communities, but also in the historical norms and practices of the profession as a whole.

In the 1980s, when the 360,000 physicians in America enjoy a relatively secure and autonomous role, "competition" is seen as a new mode for, and challenge to, the medical profession. Before the twentieth century, however, the predecessors of modern medicine competed with naturopaths, homoeopaths, assorted patent medicine men, and faith healers, as well as with each other, for the privilege of healing late nineteenth century ills.

Considering both the history and the structure of medicine, Starr notes,

> In the nineteenth century the medical profession was generally weak, divided, insecure in its status and its income, unable to control entry into practice or to raise the standards of medical education. In the twentieth century, not only did physicians become a powerful, prestigious, and wealthy profession, but they succeeded in shaping the basic organization and financial structure of American medicine (Starr, 1982).

In other countries physicians also constitute a powerful and prestigious profession, but it is particularly in the United States that the profession has always had freedom not only in the "art and science of medicine" but also "in methods of organization, delivery, and payment for their services" (Anderson, 1968). Official organizations representing the medical community through this century developed an increasingly specific set of policies and official statements to reflect and to shape the norms of practicing physicians. The twentieth century saw a dramatic rise in both technology and bureaucracy, and, in the name of professionalism, the medical profession allied itself ideologically with technology but claimed to oppose bureaucracy.

Although bureaucracy was becoming an inevitable part of physicians' daily lives (Starr, 1982), the profession battled both its public and its private forms, opposing not only federal controls but also private group practice and private health insurance. After the challenging report of Flexner in 1910, physicians were rigorously educated and credentialed, and they "claimed specialized, technical knowledge, validated by communities of their peers." They invited the otherwise repugnant touch of the state only for medical licensure. During that time physicians practiced their science independently and were "uneasy with organizations that potentially threatened their autonomy" (Starr, 1982). Protecting the autonomy of physicians was one of the medical profession's central concerns. Private fee-for-service practitioners did not want any mediators interfering in their role with their patients. When physicians found themselves free to design their own practices they were almost never cooperative. For example, although there were twenty-three specialty fields in 1923, "there was very little coordination and cross reference of such skills. In the course of a year a patient might [need to] call on ... five specialists ... with little coordination of treatment" (Stevens, 1971).

During that same period, however, companies with many employees, particularly in remote areas, had an interest in providing medical care to their employees and in controlling the providers. Contracts for industrial practice were developed especially in the mining and lumbering industries as well as in the railroads. By 1930 these programs covered more than one million employees and an undetermined number of dependents in the mountains and mill towns of America (Starr, 1982).

Although medical societies recognized the necessity of contract practices for remote areas, they "regarded it [in other areas] as a form of exploitation because it enabled companies to get doctors to bid against each other and drive down the price of their labor" (Stevens, 1971). They fought it. For example, in 1908 the physician who had been the company doctor at Sears, Roebuck felt forced to resign from the company because the Chicago Medical Society had excluded him from membership on the grounds that his service to employees' families constituted "an unethical invasion of private practice" (Starr, 1982). In addition to censuring these disapproved forms of practice, medical societies in such areas as the Pacific Northwest, where contract medicine was especially prevalent, competed by forming their own prepaid plans. Known as "medical bureaus," these plans offered care by any member of a local medical society in exchange for a fixed prepayment to the bureau. However, in these plans, individual physicians were paid on a fee-for-service basis and not on a salary, and patients could choose their own doctors. Thus, organized medicine could simultaneously perpetuate its ethics and protect its professional interests (Fitzmaurice, 1959). It is notable, however, that these isolated efforts to establish contract practices and medical bureaus had little impact and were able to set no precedent for mainstream medicine.

Early in the century, before World War I, another form of medical association, private group practice by specialists, was developing. The most notable prototype was the Mayo Clinic of Rochester, MN, begun in the 1880s (Starr, 1982). After World War I there was an intense growth of private group practice. By 1930 there were from 1500 to 2000 physicians involved in 150 physician-owned and physician-managed group practices. "In Minnesota, it was claimed that there were few towns of 10,000 or more inhabitants without one or more private group clinics" (Stevens, 1971; Starr, 1982).

However, this surge was temporary. Although a number of those specialist group practices survived, they threatened the viability and legitimacy of general practice; they competed with solo practitioners in specialty practice. As a result, the "initial enthusiasm [for specialty group practice] within organized medicine was replaced by a spirit of caution, followed by hostility" (Stevens, 1971).

Since that time, form of practice has continued to be one of the major political issues of the American Medical Association (AMA), and the AMA has strongly supported solo, fee-for-service practice. As Freidson notes, "the term 'solo-practice' is as often ideological as it is descriptive" (Freeman et al., 1979). Because AMA membership is rooted at the local county society level, "admission is entirely at the county society's discretion" (Freidson, 1970). Thus, county medical societies have been able to deny membership to physicians "who worked on an economic base repugnant to local members." For example, physicians who practiced in the Elk City Cooperatives, the Puget Sound Cooperatives, and the Health Insurance Plan for Greater New York were at one time denied membership (Freidson, 1970). Even today, "under the watchful eye of the AMA Judicial Council, multispecialist group practice has remained . . . in the background rather than in the vanguard of health services, a possibility rather than the model for organizational reform" (Stevens, 1971).

The AMA's effort to control the form of medical practice has been asserted in many ways, ranging from peer pressure to extended anti-trust law (Goldberg and Greenberg, 1977). Furthermore, "this policy is rationalized more on 'ethical' than on technical grounds" (Freidson, 1970). It is interesting to observe that political issues of power and resources, i.e., who treats which patients and how much they are paid, are considered by organized medicine (and were discussed by most physicians in interviews) as moral issues of good and evil. Again, Freidson writes, "Much of what has been called 'ethics' and certainly the common rules of etiquette [right and wrong] is designed to prevent 'unfair' internal competition and preserve comparative equality of opportunity in the medical marketplace at the same time as it preserves an impeccable front of silence to the outside world" (Freidson, 1975).

In addition to concerns about group practice, there are other political issues, perceived as issues of medical ethics, with which the medical profession has perpetually struggled. Some issues are with those outside of the profession and others are within the profession. These issues are of particular interest in this report because HMOs raise or aggravate each of these issues, and they have appeared throughout the interviews with physicians. There are a number of areas in which physicians worked to establish professional authority or sovereignty (Starr, 1982). Organized medicine has stated clearly as a first principle that no third party should come between doctor and patient. Thus they oppose working for laypersons or hospitals. They are also opposed to government regulation of medical practice, and they contend that paraprofessionals cannot operate independently of a physician (AMA, 1981).

First, the medical profession asserts that it is unethical for physicians to work for laypersons; only physicians can supervise physicians. This has created a continuing argument against salaried physicians and is to this day an unresolved problem in HMOs with lay board members. Interviews with physicians and administrators of even the consumer-sponsored HMOs demonstrated that lay "interference" is still perceived as a problem, and these interviewees commented without hesitation that only an exclusively medical board can deal with professional issues of medical colleagues.

Second, there has been a historic, tenuous balance of power between medical staff and hospital administration. The interviews suggested that actions by both physicians and hospitals regarding HMOs were in reaction to real or anticipated behavior on the part of the other.

Third, the historic attitudes of organized medicine toward government regulation of medical care included the major, successful campaign against national health insurance and the opposition to federal grants to HMOs. Much of the explicit as well as the subtle opposition to HMOs was based on the perception that HMOs were "like socialized medicine" or "a step toward socialized medicine."

Fourth, physicians have worked since the 1930s to secure a position free from the competition of paraprofessionals. In the

1930s "non-physician specialists were subordinated to the doc-tor's authority" (Starr, 1982), and "their work [now] is given legitimacy in relation to physicians' work" (Freidson, 1970). But HMOs raised again the specter of paraprofessionals gaining more status. In official statements from its 1981 conference, the AMA opposed federal programs to train physician assistants, sup-ported certification rather than licensure, preferred that physi-cian assistants be hired by physicians, and supported a require-ment that physician assistants be supervised by physicians.

The development of HMOs not only awakened controversy with those outside of the profession but also aggravated historic problems within the profession. Issues of specialization, and the differing—sometimes conflicting—interests of specialists and primary care practitioners are closely connected with the histori-cally volatile issue of referral patterns. The development of HMOs brought out old arguments against "closed panels," "con-tract medicine," and "fee splitting." It also intensified another aspect of specialist versus primary care physicians' tension, that is, the differing interests of teaching hospitals and nonteaching hospitals (Starr, 1982). The interdiction against advertising was also a symbol of professionalism as well as a way of controlling competition. The importance of these concerns within the profes-sion will be discussed in later sections.

COMPARISON OF TWO MEDICAL COMMUNITIES

This section considers more specifically the two medical communities of this study. It compares their general character-istics and the relevant historic patterns of practice and leadership in each metropolitan area. Note that although this study com-pares two areas, each of the metropolitan areas has two notable subcommunities, of which the residents are particularly con-scious. In the Twin Cities, residents perceived important distinc-tions between Minneapolis and St. Paul. Likewise, Chicago resi-dents drew distinctions between the suburbs and the city. Although differences do not seem always as salient to the outside observer as they do to residents, certain distinctions do seem relevant and will be noted in the discussion of medical practice and leadership.

Patterns of practice

In the history of American medical practice, Minnesota has been a leader in the development and acceptance of group practice. Multispecialty group practice was introduced early by the Mayo brothers, and it is widely accepted throughout the state. While across the United States 26.2 percent of physicians practice in groups, in Minnesota 67.3 percent, and in Illinois 23.3 percent, practice in groups (AMA, 1982). Furthermore, the sizes and kinds of the groups are different in Minnesota and Illinois. In Minnesota there are more physicians practicing in many fewer groups; i.e., 5,481 MDs practice in 350 groups, but in Illinois 5,066 MDs practice in 518 groups. Among Illinois' groups there is a prevalence of small, single-specialty groups, whereas in Minnesota, on the model of the Mayo Clinic, the groups are larger and more frequently multispecialty (AMA, 1982).

However, with the exception of their response to group practice, the range of physician behavior in the Twin Cities was very similar to that in Chicago. The Minnesota medical community did not historically initiate forms of practice different from those initiated in the Chicago area. In both areas interviews with physicians suggested a similar history of conservatism mixed with innovative efforts. In the Twin Cities, however, the environment seemed at least to tolerate, and sometimes to support, a minimal level of innovative efforts. For example, in Minnesota, Group Health Cooperative was begun in 1957, and although its beginnings were very slow, it kept the idea of prepaid health care alive and later flourished (187,000 members in 1982). During the same period, in Chicago, Civic Medical Center was begun in the downtown area to offer prepaid health care, and though it stayed open until the early 1960s, interviews suggested that it drew little interest or support and had no impact on the shape of health care in the Chicago area.

In both communities, a number of physicians reported that after their experience in World War II they felt committed to continuing cooperative practice; but the results in the two communities differed. In Minneapolis, a group with that commitment formed St. Louis Park Medical Center, the prestigious multispecialty group that was later very influential in building acceptance for HMOs in the Twin Cities; but in Chicago physicians making similar efforts to develop multispecialty clinics reported that they were unable to spread the idea or to develop a reputation that would draw sufficient support to have citywide impact. Thus, Chicago is still a community largely of neighborhood-based solo practitioners and some small specialty group practices. Multispecialty group practice is very infrequent.

The distribution of types of practice is varied in Minneapolis. Minneapolis has both large fee-for-service, multi-specialty group practices and prepaid group practices. One physician explained, "Here it's hard to find a solo practitioner, . . . [group practice] has been the pattern for ever and ever."

It is interesting to note that the Twin Cities of St. Paul and Minneapolis, although similar, are not identical. In fact, St. Paul resembles the Chicago medical community in some ways: most of its physicians practice in solo practices, or in small, single-specialty group practices, often distributed, as in Chicago, in ethnic neighborhoods. The implications of these different patterns of practice will be discussed in the section on the reciprocal impact of physicians and HMOs.

Leadership and participation

It was noted earlier in this chapter that in the American medical community there is an interesting tension between a strong tendency to avoid change in organizational forms and practice and a commitment to change that is associated with therapeutic or technological progress in medical care (Coleman, et al., 1966). Also, there is strong resistance to any participation or "interference" from laypersons. These characteristics suggest that meaningful leadership for physicians must come from professional peers and that innovations are more likely to be accepted if they are sponsored or directed by physicians. Physician peer leadership is important for the development of HMOs—leadership not only within the community but also within the HMOs themselves (Meier and Tillotson, 1978).

Interviews in the two communities showed that while there are committed leaders in both metropolitan areas, in the Twin Cities there is a focus of leadership and a commitment to responsible participation; throughout the community, respondents mentioned certain names repeatedly. Furthermore, the medical societies have widespread participation, as reflected by their relatively high membership numbers; 69 percent of the physicians in Hennepin County belong to the Hennepin County Medical Society, and 84 percent of the physicians in Ramsey County belong to the Ramsey County Medical Society. Perhaps more important, medical community leaders in the Twin Cities do not work only within medicine; they cooperate and participate actively in major community forums of all kinds. For example, in the early 1970s, influential physicians from both St. Louis Park Medical Center and the Nicollet Clinic were serving in the Citizens League when plans were developed for their physician-sponsored prepaid plans. Thus they were benefiting from the advice and developing the cooperation of other sectors in the community influential in the success of the plans.

Twin Cities medical leaders also worked cooperatively with leaders in other areas, particularly business, to confront problems of cost. In the early 1970s physicians in Minneapolis voluntarily decided to develop their own peer review. Although they developed the Foundation for Health Care Evaluation on the premise that physicians must review themselves, they nonetheless turned to industry, the health department, etc., for participation on their board, and thus elicited the cooperation and support of industry in the development of the Foundation.

Another important element in the Twin Cities medical community is the sense that this medical community is distinctive and "way ahead." This is stated clearly by those who have had experience outside of the Twin Cities amd can make comparisons. This sense of pride seemed to be self-perpetuating and self-motivating. Physicians' success in influencing the results among themselves—in "keeping destiny in [their] own hands"—caused the Twin Cities physicians to be, in turn, even more progressive and to stay ahead of regulations. The following observation characterized their pride in independence from regulation. After discussing the rapid growth of the major Twin Cities HMOs, a physician explained, "Someone had to show that private practice could probably do a job better and cheaper than national health insurance or federal bureaucracy." It is significant that this physician identified HMOs—when run by physicians—as "private practice." In another interview the exchange went like this:

> Physician: When the government came with their regulation we were usually 'way ahead in terms of understanding ... I think that we feel a sense of responsibility as far as the Feds are concerned, realizing that they're a bunch of people who are as hu-

man as we are, and looking for leadership in these
areas, so we've always had a sense of providing the
leadership. That sounds arrogant, I guess, but that
really is the underlying sense in our private practice
community in the Twin Cities. . . .
Interviewer: And when federal regulation comes?
Physician: . . . We've anticipated it and have our
own system in place so it causes little ripple . . . The
practices of utilization review and supervision have
taken place by our own private efforts so government regulations are not so odious, when all things
are being done by peers.

Physicians in the Twin Cities reflected the larger community
in another way. The medical leadership was very conscious of
the importance of consensus and avoided confrontation. Descriptions by physicians of the early stages of both Physicians Health
Plan and the group-model HMOs demonstrated this consciousness. A founder of a Twin Cities HMO said that the decision to
start the HMO was preceded by months of discussion but was
never put to a vote because a vote creates "polarization" rather
than "consensus."

In Chicago, the process is different. Consensus is infrequent
even within physician groups, and the medical community as a
whole is fragmented, with no recognized focus of leadership. Although Chicagoans interviewed in other sectors commented
about Chicago being the headquarters of organized medicine,
physicians themselves did not mention the AMA or its local affiliates as being important. Of the 13,659 physicians in Cook
County, only 49 percent belong to the Chicago Medical Society
(Chicago Medical Society, 1982). Furthermore, interviews suggested that only a small, dedicated group—perhaps 300 physicians—is truly active.

Historically, the suburban medical societies and the Cook
County Medical Society have not worked together. Attempts to
merge the suburban and urban HSAs failed, and a politically active Chicago physician reported that one suburban medical society would not cooperate at all with HSAs. Reflecting the Chicago
Medical Society's slightly different view, he said, "We don't
really approve of [HSAs] but [they're] going to be making some
important decisions and we'd at least like to get our two cents in;
and if we don't agree we can express our concerns."

Interviews also showed that physicians in Chicago moved

toward peer review reluctantly. The local professional standards review organization, the Chicago Foundation for Medical Care, experienced "considerable antagonism" from practicing physicians. In contrast to the Twin Cities, the Chicago review organization was encumbered by resistance from within the profession, and it did not seek or develop cooperative relationships outside of the medical community. Furthermore, although Chicago has five major medical centers, community physicians did not mention these centers as sources of leadership. Physicians acknowledged the idealism, skill, success, or power of certain physicians within the centers, but they did not see the centers as having citywide implications.

Chicago physicians are neither risk-takers nor progressive actors. In a speech to the Chicago Medical Society in 1970, Dr. W. C. Bornemeier, then president-elect of the AMA, made a statement that described, to the extent it is possible to do so, the Chicago medical community:

> The physician has been trained in medical school and in his practice to accept change slowly. Until material and methods have been proved to be safe and effective, we consider it dangerous to move too rapidly. If we as doctors grasped each new suggestion before adequate study, we would kill more people than we cure. We have earned the label of conservative and we must continue to wear it wisely and well (Chicago Medical Society, 1970).

It appears that the difference in leadership between the Twin Cities and Chicago is more than simply quantitative or incremental. In the Twin Cities, focused and proactive leadership and medical community participation make it possible for physicians to keep ahead of federal and local regulatory efforts. It is possible for physicians to feel that they are keeping their destiny in the hands of the profession. Thus, there is little cause for reactive behavior, which in other communities is often triggered by interference from individuals or bureaucracies outside of the profession. Because of this complex interactional process, Twin Cities physicians often initiate change themselves. Chicago physicians, however, who are more characteristic of the overall American medical community, find that "it [is] dangerous to move too rapidly" and, as a community, they do not participate voluntarily in change.

HEALTH CARE CONCERNS

The significant differences between the medical communities of the Twin Cities and Chicago were most apparent in the nature of their fundamental concerns about health care. Their diverging concerns may have an important impact on their perceptions of and responses to HMOs.

In Minneapolis-St. Paul the concern most frequently expressed by physicians was for containing cost in the delivery of effective health care. The respondents there also often raised the issue of competition among physicians, and between physicians and hospitals, as an increasingly frequent and inevitable characteristic of their practices. They were aware that competition is a mechanism for containing costs. Furthermore, as noted earlier in this chapter, physicians expressed overall pride in both the excellence of the medical profession and the health of the community in the Twin Cities.

In Chicago, questions regarding quality of care and the overall health problems of the community received notably different answers, and physicians there did not spontaneously raise the issues of cost and competition. Regarding quality, there was considerable variation in response, reflecting the heterogeneity of the medical community. More important, however, the health problems of the community elicited a *unanimous* response. Virtually all physicians interviewed in Chicago talked about the "two-tiered system." They mentioned, usually early in their interview, their awareness of and concern about inequality of care between affluent, suburban residents and the poor, inner-city population, many of whom, they said, are on public aid or are without aid. In contrast to Minneapolis-St. Paul, the cost of health care in Chicago was mentioned only as a secondary issue and usually only in the context of problems of public aid reimbursement. When probed, Chicago physicians acknowledged that cost is important, but it is not the most important issue. Furthermore, physicians who were interviewed in early and middle 1984 never spontaneously raised the issue of competition within the medical profession, and even when probed, they asserted that although they have heard about it, they had not yet perceived increased competition among physicians.

Physicians' concerns in both communities reflected local conditions. The demography of physicians and patients and the economic and health status of the patient populations in each area are vastly different. In Chicago there are relatively fewer physicians and more patients; the patients are poorer and twice as likely to depend on public assistance; there is relatively less money available from public assistance; and the health status of the population, suggested by the sensitive indicator of infant mortality, is not a source of pride. The numbers of physicians, the relative dependence on public aid, and the comparative infant mortality rates are shown in the figure below.

Levels of Public Aid, Health Status, and Physician Resources

	Chicago SMSA	Cook County	Minneapolis-St. Paul SMSA	Hennepin County	Ramsey County
Population	7,103,624	5,253,655	2,113,533	941,411	459,784
Aid to Families with Dependent Children (AFDC)					
Families	157,000	146,200	29,500	14,500	7,900
Families/1,000 Pop	22	28	14	15	17
Individuals	509,000	475,900	80,300	39,800	21,800
Individuals/1,000 Pop	72	91	38	42	47
Children	359,000	335,700	53,400	26,300	14,400
Children/1,000 Pop	51	64	25	28	31
$/month in 1000s	$ 46,209	$ 43,15	$ 9,461	$ 4,645	$ 2,529
Supplementary Security Income (SSI)					
$1000/month	$ 11,107	$ 10,340	$ 1,526	$ 832	$ 445
SSI/1,000 Pop	$ 1,564	$ 1,968	$ 722	$ 884	$ 968
Infant Mortality (1978) (Deaths under 1 yr./1,000 births)	16.9	18.4	11.9	11.8	13.2
Physicians/100,000 Pop	192	210	192	283	223

The problems of the communities differed not only in content but also in the way they were dealt with and in their effects. Paradoxically, the major issues of cost containment and competition in Minneapolis-St. Paul have been dealt with as elements or symbols of consolidation rather than dissension, even for the medical community. Instead of focusing only on the divisive aspects of competition and escalating costs, the community also emphasized the opportunity for innovation and leadership in a new phase of health care delivery. HMOs provided, and were supported as, an important source of cost containment through competition, without excessive regulation. Thus, they became another source of medical community pride.

In Chicago, however, physicians approached HMOs cautiously. Dr. Dolkert of the Chicago Medical Society, in 1970, reflected the characteristic attitudes of Chicago physicians as they considered HMOs in light of their most pressing health problems:

> As far as group practice is concerned, prepaid health insurance programs, or closed panel types of practices, models of which are portrayed by the Kaiser Permanente plan, . . . all are propounded on the basis of reduction of total health care costs. . . . These are important considerations, but do not provide any basic contribution to the major health care problems for the deprived segments of our population. The plans described are largely applicable to the employed population, whereas our major and most immediate concern should be for the indigent. . . . For the 30 percent of the population without any third party payment plan, which is composed of the indigent ghetto populations of Chicago, and in some areas this number approaches 50 percent, there are no funds available for medical care. If we are to avoid a two standard system of medical care, . . . it is essential that some means be provided for these persons to have access to the same health care system as everybody else (Chicago Medical Society, 1970).

Data from 1980 (see page 177) reconfirmed Dr. Dolkert's remarks from 1970. In the Twin Cities, where a population with well-above-average economic resources and considerably better-than-average health is being cared for by more than the average number of doctors, physicians realistically saw issues of cost to the payer and competition among providers as their most salient problems. HMOs in that context have been, and continue to be, acutely relevant. But in Chicago, where the economic resources of the population are well below average, and the physician numbers are relatively low, it was equitable distribution of health care itself and not its cost or competition among providers that seemed most salient to physicians. Thus, because HMOs are generally perceived as an alternative form of health care for a population that is middle-class, stable, and employed, HMOs have not appealed to Chicago physicians as an important solution for their most pressing concern.

PHYSICIANS' RESPONSES TO HMOs

Analysis of physician responses to HMOs in the two metropolitan areas reveals not only the dynamics of the two communities in response to HMOs but also the nature of physicians as a profession. We found that since the 1950s, each community has had physicians who have been committed and creative advocates of HMOs as well as those who have been persistent opponents. Still, most physicians in both communities responded to the norms of their profession as well as reflecting the modes of practice and decision making in their community.

In both communities, the range of responses to HMOs among physicians was the same, that is, no responses were unique to one area; however, the distribution of responses was very different. Those responses that are consistently different among physicians in both communities are considered before those responses that are consistently similar.

Differences

This section examines contrasts in 1) physicians' level of awareness and communication about HMOs, 2) physicians' level of understanding of the organizational forms of HMOs, and 3) physicians' expectations of HMOs.

The first prepaid group practices emerged at about the same time in Minneapolis-St. Paul and Chicago. The initial responses of physicians were similar in both cities. However, in 1982 and 1983, all the physicians interviewed in the Twin Cities were aware of the history of HMOs in their community, whereas in Chicago few physicians were aware of the history of HMOs.

Physicians in the Twin Cities knew of HMOs early because of efforts by Group Health to open a prepaid group plan. At first, it remained small and was not respected by most of the physicians, but it was known in the medical community. Physicians inside and outside of Group Health Plan reported that in its early days the plan won little regard from the medical community largely because it was not begun by physicians. It was thought to be "out of the mainstream," "an experiment," and "socialistic, with mostly part-time physicians." One physician, now a leader in HMO development, said, "[Group Health] was looked on from the professional side as a cut-rate way of doing business." Group Health persisted, but it was so far outside the mainstream of medicine that when physicians from St. Louis Park Medical Center and community leaders from the Citizens League began looking for models of prepaid group practice, they looked to Kaiser Permanente in California. Throughout the 1960s and early 1970s, the medical community continued to be aware of, but benignly to neglect, Group Health, which was supported then by a small loyal following drawn largely from labor and the University of Minnesota community.

That early awareness of Group Health was insufficient to interest practicing physicians in HMOs. When St. Louis Park Medical Center, a highly respected multispecialty group practice run by physicians, entered the HMO market in 1972, however, it changed the image of HMOs for physicians as it did for others in the community. St. Louis Park was convincing, respondents said, not only because it was run by physicians but also because the physicians who ran it (colleagues known personally or by reputation) clearly provided "good medicine."

At St. Louis Park, the physicians chose to call the prepaid plan "an experiment," and they started it slowly within the larger multispecialty group practice, gathering cooperation and acceptance as they went. They were not overtly threatening. The patterns of cooperation and communication in the Twin Cities medical community muted opposition because respected physicians took leadership roles. The intense commitment to communication and cooperation was expressed in the interviews as a distaste for, and even fear of, disunity in the medical community. One administrator said,

> There was the fear that this could actually make our Twin Cities into little feudal states in which hospitals would be the castles and they would have their little area around them that would be theirs. . . . This would really fragment the medical community.

In Chicago, on the other hand, the medical community was fragmented already, and although the development of prepaid plans in many ways paralleled their development in the Twin Cities, it did not elicit the same perceptions and responses from physicians. For example, Civic Medical Center, the prepaid downtown Chicago group mentioned earlier, began no later than Group Health and continued into the 1960s, but it had no conceptual importance to physicians. Those who did remember it said that although it had "responded to a need" during the Depression and had continued for many years, it never thrived. After almost thirty years, Civic Medical Center finally closed. One respondent said, "It was ahead of its time. . . . I think they were too isolated."

Because the Chicago medical community is fragmented, isolation is a recurring theme. Developments in one part of Chicago can remain a mystery to those in other parts. When the Union Health Service was begun in the mid-1950s, it caused little interest in the medical community. More strikingly, when Anchor and the Michael Reese Health Plan were developed by physicians in the early 1970s—even earlier than St. Louis Park Medical Center—they remained unknown to all but a few physicians.

Physicians who were aware of Michael Reese Health Plan or Anchor did not disregard them or regard them poorly. Like St. Louis Park Medical Center in Minneapolis, Michael Reese Hospital and Rush-Presbyterian-St. Luke's were respected, major medical centers. However, Chicago physicians believed the innovations were geographically localized and/or related only to certain interest groups.

Communication is so minimal in Chicago that even the negative history of HMO efforts was not communicated. In 1975 and 1976, there was sensational coverage in all the major news media regarding a now-defunct Medicaid HMO, alleged to be giving poor service and misusing funds, yet few physicians in Chicago—including those opposed to HMOs—mentioned it in interviews.

The interviews with physicians in the two metropolitan areas also revealed a different level of understanding of the structures and organizational forms of HMOs. All the physicians interviewed in the Twin Cities had similar knowledge about HMOs. They knew of the different HMOs in their community; they understood the general operation of prepaid group practice; and most of them clearly understood the differences among the three types of organization—staff, group, and IPA. The many sources of their rather complete information offer insight into the dynamics of the community. They had learned from personal participation (85 percent of physicians are now associated with HMOs in some way); from their colleagues in the profession, whom they knew from training and from working together; from medical society bulletins and meetings; and from other physician cooperative organizations, such as the Physicians Metro Task Force.

In contrast, the wide range of physicians interviewed in Chicago demonstrated an equally wide range of understanding of HMOs. All physicians knew of prepaid group practice, but few knew anyone who practiced in or with an HMO. Few could name more than one or two HMOs in the area, incorrectly recalling their location, affiliation, sponsorship, or other details. Only those Chicago physicians in leadership roles in the development of HMOs understood the differences between the forms. Others who declared an interest in becoming affiliated or starting an HMO rarely knew the implications such affiliation would have on their practice. They perceived rather that the HMO would change hospital behavior. Although informative articles and reports of meetings about HMOs had appeared in the Chicago medical society newsletter, most physicians had not read or heard of the information either at meetings or from their colleagues.

The third way the physician communities differed may be the most abstract, yet one of the most consequential. There is a significant difference between the Twin Cities and Chicago in the physicians' expectations of an HMO. The early forms of HMOs were staff and group models, which can be understood best in comparison to the well-respected multispecialty group practices or multispecialty clinics, such as the Mayo Clinic and St. Louis Park Medical Center. In the Twin Cities, many of the physicians had some part of their training in such settings.

Physicians had not always respected multispecialty group practices. In "the early days . . . thirty some years ago [St. Louis Park Medical Center] was looked on as being socialist—group practice was pretty pink," said an early participant. Once multispecialty groups gained esteem for their high-quality practice, private practitioners reported that they found the groups problematic and competitive because once a solo practitioner referred a patient to the multispecialty group, the group could exclude the physician from the referral patterns. Thus, some physicians in the Twin Cities claimed that the large multispecialty group practice was the chief competitive departure and that the HMO, with prepayment, was simply a refinement. It is appropriate to note here that the response among Twin Cities physicians was not uniform. Generally, physicians in St. Paul, largely solo practitioners in a comparatively heterogeneous community, responded more slowly and reluctantly to HMO development than did Minneapolis physicians. Although there was an effort in 1970 to start a primary care HMO in St. Paul, respondents reported that an "articulate," "persuasive" private practitioner "blew it out of the water." He convinced the board that such health care delivery was immoral and would interfere with the doctor-patient relationship. When interviewed, the practitioner himself said that he had been able to "dig the moat around St. Paul for a few years." When St. Paul's Ramsey County Medical Society was invited to join the Hennepin County Medical Society in the formation of Physicians Health Plan in 1973, the physicians in Ramsey County rejected the plan and excluded themselves from the independent practice association that covered the other six metropolitan counties. In all cases, when one considers both the resources and the burdens of the Twin Cities, St. Paul seemed more like Chicago than did Minneapolis, and so were the perceptions and responses of its physicians to HMOs.

In Chicago, physicians' perceptions and expectations of group and clinic practice contrasted sharply. The scarcity of multispecialty group practices in Chicago was reflected in the perspective of physicians interviewed. Although some individual physicians in Chicago spoke eloquently in favor of group practice, few had any experience with prestigious multispecialty groups. Often their experience was not with the Mayo Clinic, St. Louis Park Medical Center, Marshfield Clinic, or the Cleveland Clinic, but with outpatient clinics in sprawling medical centers, in city and county hospitals and in military and Veteran's Administration hospitals where most Chicago physicians did much of their training. Thus, the mental association for these physicians was of impersonal institutions with ugly halls, long waits and too many bleak patients. Rarely knowing HMO physicians, Chicago physicians were most likely to believe that less competent physicians are associated with HMOs—foreign medical graduates and inexperienced physicians who cannot get a practice started or who "want an easy life." They often predicted that as soon as HMO physicians got practices started, they would leave the HMO.

Also, Chicago private practitioners were concerned about disrupting the system of medical staff privileges. In the Twin Cities, physicians commonly have privileges in several hospitals throughout the city, but in Chicago, where the community is large, fragmented, and heterogeneous, physicians' practices are localized, and they maintain tight control on hospital privileges. One physician summarized the concerns reflected in many interviews:

> This is a mainly one hospital per doctor town. Although [in other cities where I've practiced] you were expected to be on staff of every hospital in town . . . here, by and large, most people admit to a single hospital and are on a single hospital staff. So, its a lot different. When you have an [HMO] office, the whole office has to get on one hospital staff in order to function. Then that is threatening to the staff—they think the guys are going to take it over!

The other concern noted above, and felt sharply by most physicians in Chicago, was that HMOs serve those who are basically healthy and employed, ignoring the acute health care problems of the poor. The Chicago Medical Society assigned a Blue Ribbon Committee to the task of creating an alternative proposal —the Chicago Plan—for distributing health care to the poor of Chicago with private practitioners rather than HMOs. Luft has examined HMO programs for the poor in demonstration projects and in "real world situations" and he reports both problems and possibilities (Luft, 1981a). The complexity of poverty, the structural requirements of HMOs, and the lack of experience make it impossible to say yet whether HMOs for the poor will be a "viable combination." However, there are more demonstration projects being tried, and in March 1983, Illinois was inviting proposals for prepaid plans to provide health care for those on public aid in the state.

Similarities

The similarity of responses among physicians in both communities can be discussed as distinct perceptions or convictions that were closely related. They were related in that they reflected intrinsic parts of the physicians' professional role. First, physicians characteristically emphasized the doctor-patient relationship as the center of high-quality medical care. Second, physicians stressed the importance of personal and professional independence, emphasizing autonomy from government. Third, physicians in and out of HMOs shared similar perceptions regarding physicians who practice in HMOs. Fourth, physicians raised a number of miscellaneous recurring concerns associated with their profession that do not appear in other sector interviews.

All but one of the sixty-three physicians interviewed subscribed to that belief system or "service ideology" (Luft, 1981a) that identifies the doctor-patient relationship as the key to good service for the patient. For physicians, good-quality health care was symbolized by the doctor-patient relationship. Physicians' mode of responding in interviews suggested the centrality of their personal role in medical care. In contrast to those in other sectors, physicians did not distinguish between their personal and professional identities. For example, hospital administrators and insurance executives always distinguished between their personal opinion and the view that came from their role as representative of an organization. Physicians did not differentiate. Furthermore, they implied that elements not related to patients, such as income or administrative responsibilities, were of comparatively little interest or importance.

This focus was widely held by physicians and has persisted over time. As far back as 1933 during the development of group practice the central concern was "to preserve the relationship between the patient and the physician ..." (Shouldice and Shouldice, 1978). Fifty years later, when physicians talked about prepaid group practice, they voiced the same concern. Data from this study were consistent with those gathered by other researchers with other methodologies who report similar categories of physician perception and conviction. These convictions are evident both in their specific attitudes about HMOs (Luft, 1981a; Lou Harris & Associates, 1982) and in their attitudes toward the practice of medicine more generally (Becker, et al., 1961; Bosk, 1979; Freidson, 1970).

The one physician interviewed who did not share this belief system was an important and informative one. Dr. Bruce Flashner, the founder of "emergicenters" in Chicago and one of the leaders of a dramatically growing movement developing short-term free-standing ambulatory care clinics, disputed the "service ideology." He asserted that patients are often more interested in getting efficient, immediate care for minor but acute problems than they are in establishing long-term doctor-patient relationships. The powerful negative response of organized medicine to the concept and ideology of the free-standing emergency center is evidence of the exceptional and threatening nature of Flashner's point of view.

As evidence of the importance to patients of the doctor-patient relationship, private practitioners in both Minneapolis-St. Paul and Chicago told several anecdotes of HMO members who pay to come to them as well. Furthermore, even those physicians seeking ways to deliver public health care to the poor in Chicago still emphasized the right of every patient to establish a relationship with a physician of his or her own choice. A Chicago inner-city practitioner worried that if Medicaid paid for HMO enrollment, the patients would lose that right.

Woven into the physicians' understanding of the doctor-patient relationship was also their serious concern for the quality of health care. Yet it was so woven into their ideology that there seemed no adequate objective measure of quality. "In fact, the value the profession attaches to medical care quality seems inversely related to our ability to measure quality" (Luft, 1981a).

Thus, it seemed that the ambiguous nature of quality made it all the more intense an issue. This issue elicited strikingly similar responses among physicians in the Twin Cities and Chicago. Physicians, in and out of HMOs, reported that they are always concerned not about what does happen, but about what might happen to the quality of patient care under the changed incentives of HMOs.

Physicians in our study reported that in "the early days of HMOs" they sometimes thought the care was "not mainstream," but none said that they feel that way now. Physicians worried, however, that the potential for poor quality is there because of "undertreatment." This concern is not new with HMOs. Observers have noted a characteristic worry among physicians in all practice settings about "undertreating" at the level of diagnosis (too few tests) or of therapy (insufficient hospitalization, drugs, or outpatient visits). Physicians reported that because of pressure from peers and the malpractice climate they use a lot of tests and treatment. Some health observers have argued that with different incentives physicians will change their behavior to reduce tests. These physician interviews suggested, however, that to reduce testing and procedures is a qualitatively and ideologically different process than to increase testing and procedures (also Foldes, 1983). As discussion later in this chapter demonstrates, reductions can be made satisfactorily, but the process is slow and complex.

A similar concern for physicians in both areas was that the turnover of physicians in HMOs might reduce quality. They said that high turnover in HMOs will interfere with the development of lasting doctor-patient relationships and will, consequently, diminish the quality of care.

As another aspect of quality, physicians deemphasized or rejected some issues as unimportant. Most notable among these are economic issues. Although external evidence does not always seem consistent with self-perceptions, physicians in both communities denied any interest in their fees or billing. They also asserted that fees are not what is important to patients. This has two important consequences for physicians in their interaction with HMOs in both communities; the first concerns their response, and the second, their experience and competencies.

In both communities, physicians who *supported* HMOs saw the HMO organizational characteristics as a way of protecting the physician from concerns about cost to the patient. They said that although the physician may be required to explain costs to the management, cost concern is absent from the doctor-patient relationship. In contrast, those who *opposed* HMOs objected to the explicit concern by a medical organization with financial issues. They asserted that the cost containment objectives inherent in an organization that provides both care and health insurance are likely to be "harmful" to the patient. They preferred the system of third-party payers as a way of removing the issue of cost from the doctor-patient relationship. In some cases neither the doctor nor the patient may ever know what the treatment actually costs. A few physicians, particularly in Chicago, said that patients overuse physicians' services, and they asserted that some copayment would help contain costs. This, however, was an occasional rather than a frequent observation.

A second consequence of the intentional exclusion of business matters from the professional role is a pervasive lack of experience and competence in matters of management. There has been a notable absence of economic training in medical education. Not until the late 1970s were there any courses in medical schools about costs or cost containment, and those courses were in only some medical schools and were characteristically not part of the core curricula. In both communities, physicians, and those who work with them, regretted this lacuna in their capabilities.

Physicians in Minneapolis-St. Paul and Chicago reported that they have been idealistic about running HMOs—both staff and IPA models. They acknowledged that more is needed than "happy patients" and "good doctor-patient relationships." Their lack of preparation in business matters is a consequence of education and socialization that physicians generally share.

The second major similarity of physicians we interviewed concerned independence and autonomy. This is complex, and like the doctor-patient relationship, it is central to physicians' perceptions of themselves. Recent studies of physicians offer seemingly conflicting results. One study notes that "the major group of medical concerns that physicians have about the future of medical practice relates to the loss of autonomy mainly as a result of regulatory interference and external intervention" (Lou Harris & Associates, 1982), yet the same study shows physicians moving increasingly "away from office-based solo practice" and "toward salaried employment and toward hospital- and group-based practice". Furthermore, one study evaluating physicians' support for HMOs asserts that "the autonomy issue is largely a nonproblem" (Luft, 1981a).

Physicians interviewed in both Minneapolis-St. Paul and Chicago consistently discussed the importance of independence. One practitioner typified the attitude as he discussed historical objections to closed panel HMOs:

> One of the major principles of medical ethics is that physicians should control medical practice; that lay people, lay boards, and administrators should not control medical practice ... There was a lot of bad feeling—feeling that [the closed panel] was unethical, if not downright illegal.

The same respondent went on to explain that Physicians Health Plan, the IPA in Minneapolis, had overcome many of the problems of closed panel HMOs but that he is "not sure it's going the way physicians would like it to go" ... because "by Minnesota statute it must have a large consumer representation ..." and thus "very minimal physician control."

Even in Group Health Plan, in which cooperation and consumer participation are a mainstay of the organization, physicians asserted their independence from nonphysician administrators and sought progressive changes in the structure of the committees in order to have more independence and direct access to the board. Furthermore, they formed a separate association because they continued to be dissatisfied with the representation of physicians' interests. In addition, there is a medical advisory board which, one physician reported, "is used as backup in difficult disciplinary problems—to keep confidentiality." The physician continued, "It was not appropriate to take [matters of discipline of physicians] to the lay board. The judgment of physicians' competence had to be made by other physicians. That was important."

Still, change is occurring. Older physicians are coming to accept decreased autonomy and younger physicians are developing more modest expectations of autonomy. Autonomy nonetheless remained significant in physicians' discussion of HMOs. Interestingly, they cited the importance of autonomy both in support of, and in opposition to, practice in HMOs. Those who opposed HMOs saw them as additional interference with their practice mode; those who supported HMO practice gave a more complex explanation. They noted the pressures on health care and perceived that the public is demanding change. Thus, they preferred to develop something physician-controlled—and physician-owned, if possible—to avoid working in a bureaucracy imposed and controlled by nonphysicians. A private physician, when asked if he had practiced with an HMO, replied, "No, I prefer not to; I like independence." However, he supported HMOs because "society and medicine are becoming so complex that we have to have some kind of organization," and he preferred HMOs to national health insurance.

This response was characteristic of the dilemma that Enthoven observes physicians are feeling now. Although physicians have opposed competition in health care and have been committed to a "free choice of doctors," the resulting costs have been so high that the system is drawing unwanted regulation and bureaucracy. Most doctors dislike the prospect of such detailed bureaucratic controls even more than the prospect of economic competition (Enthoven, 1980).

The third similarity among physicians in the two communities is their perception of those physicians who practice in

HMOs. Doctors in both communities perceived correctly that physicians who choose to practice in HMOs are likely to be younger than those who don't. They also perceived that physicians who are in transition—just out of training or new to an area—are more likely to practice in HMOs. Thus, they believed *incorrectly* that there is an exceptionally high turnover rate among HMO physicians. In fact, turnover rates for physicians, once they have been with a plan for more than two or three years, appear to be very low (2 to 3 percent) (Shouldice and Shouldice, 1978). This compares favorably with turnover at Veteran's Administration hospitals or in the military. Most turnover occurs during the 2 to 3 year probationary period (Luft, 1981a). One more perception was notably similar among physicians who had been involved with HMOs from the early days. They perceived that physicians who join HMOs are changing. Whereas in "their day" physicians who worked in HMOs were informed about and politically committed to HMO practice, the physicians now join for other reasons and "know nothing of ideology—or the cooperative movement." Often, they reported, there is more interest in "life style, e.g., regular hours, fewer on-call evenings, and free weekends."

There was a final group of miscellaneous concerns unique to the physician sector and expressed similarly in both communities. Many of these concerns were related to aspects of medicine that physicians perceived as their communal responsibility but are not cost-effective. Medical education and clinical training have been a large hidden cost of university and related hospital medicine. If medical care must be cost-effective, physicians asked, who will pick up the cost of the extra hours and tests for medical students to learn their profession? These same physicians also noted that HMO setting provides an excellent base for teaching primary and outpatient care. These forms of care are the dominant portion of a nonacademic physician's practice, but they have been neglected in the usual university settings. Physician educators in Minneapolis-St. Paul and Chicago saw HMOs as an excellent opportunity to improve physician training, but at the same time they saw no way to pay for it.

Similarly, psychosocial disorders and other chronic illnesses cannot be made cost-effective. Physicians asked where the costs will be shifted in a system that must be cost-effective. Physicians also feared that a cost-oriented system will discourage clinical research, stifling innovation and medical advances. For example, there was a rumor in the Twin Cities that one patient with a bone marrow transplant absorbed half of the Group Health Plan's profits for one year. In addition, some physicians in both communities asked, who will care and pay for those who are too sick to qualify for an HMO?

Finally, another finding reflects an interesting element of the physician communities' history. In both Minneapolis-St. Paul and Chicago, physicians who served in World War II spontaneously referred to their experience in the military as an important factor in their decision about their practice. A significant number of physicians in leadership positions in both communities said that group military practice provided professional freedom to focus on the medical problems of patients in a supportive atmosphere with peers readily available for consultation. In fact, St. Louis Park Medical Center was begun by physicians returning from World War II; and in Chicago, a number of physicians practicing in the few multispecialty groups or HMOs began their practices right after the war. On the other hand, another significant group of physicians in both communities said that inefficiencies in the military bureaucracy persuaded them to practice independently. A third group of military alumni supported HMOs. Seen by themselves and their colleagues as politically active and astute, they preferred private HMOs to government programs.

INTERACTIONS OF HMOs AND PHYSICIANS

To accomplish a comparison of the communities it is useful to consider separately the impact of physicians on HMOs and the impact of HMOs on physicians. This is an artificial distinction, but it is useful heuristically. In fact, the impacts seem largely reciprocal. Physicians sometimes create HMOs, and where there is a greater penetration of HMOs, the impact on physicians is greater. It has been reported that the most common effect of local prepaid groups is that physicians consider joining or starting an IPA or a closed panel HMO (Lou Harris & Associates, 1982). Thus, cause and consequence become intermingled in the reality of everyday events. Also, a number of contextual factors discussed in other chapters—for instance, corporate leadership, hospital overbedding, and particularly the decision-making style of the community—can create an environment that draws physicians along as integral members of the community. Thus, impact is the product of both actions and the environment. In the Twin Cities, physicians' early negative impact was not lasting, and their positive impact was multifaceted and prevalent. In Chicago, the negative impact has persisted since HMOs were first known, and the positive impact, though clearly present, has been isolated and less significant.

PHYSICIAN IMPACT ON HMOs

Minneapolis-St. Paul

Negative impact

In addition to the early negative response to Group Health Plan from most physicians in Minneapolis and St. Paul, Ramsey County physicians continued to resist HMOs and are partly responsible for the considerably slower growth of HMOs in St. Paul than in Minneapolis. Ramsey County physicians, who are generally resistant to federal involvement, were particularly opposed to SHARE, which was federally qualified and located in St. Paul.

Certain physicians had a more negative impact than others; specialists were generally less cooperative than general physicians both inside and outside HMOs. Tension between specialties is reported to have been a problem in staff model HMOs, also. The impact of uncooperative physicians was felt acutely. In 1982, the potential for negative impact on new health care systems in the Twin Cities was demonstrated further by a controversy about a PPO. It was reported that a major hospital system with many affiliates planned a PPO to be based in the hospital and had a feasibility study prepared by the consulting arm of the hospital corporation. Physicians felt that they were not consulted, so they did not cooperate. They claimed that they had "forestalled the development of PPOs in the area for 10 years."

Another source of negative impact from physicians in the Twin Cities is their relative weakness in administration and management. Their lack of understanding of business and management is said to have caused a difficult beginning for the Physicians Health Plan. However, the response of physicians to this weakness may, in fact, be considered as part of the positive impact of physicians in Minneapolis-St. Paul.

Positive impact

In spite of—or perhaps because of—physicians' lack of preparation in management, they have developed close associations with medical managers. The Medical Group Management Association reported that Minnesota has developed a mature management association (founded in 1951) that represents 45 percent of the state's physicians and is closely integrated with the Minnesota Medical Association. As a result, the management association acts only through the medical association. Physicians in this cooperative effort have had a positive impact on the development of HMOs with good medical managers. Furthermore, having learned to participate effectively in management, physicians have not developed the characteristic adversary relationships with nonmedical administrators.

The most important positive impact in Minneapolis-St. Paul has been the development of strong, respected multispecialty group practices. These have been a source of strength in the development of HMOs for a number of reasons: multispecialty group practices socialize physicians to practice cooperatively in collegial networks, accumulate capital, and, most important in the Twin Cities, provide a simultaneous source of leadership and competition.

It was noted earlier that multispecialty group practices are the model of medical practice on which HMOs are built. Physicians with opportunities to train in such settings, as they have had in the Twin Cities since the late 1940s, are more likely to understand the administrative necessities and to appreciate the cooperative setting. In addition, established multispecialty group practices have management patterns and a financial base from which to try innovation. Such was the case when St. Louis Park Medical Center decided to "experiment" in 1971 with a prepaid comprehensive component. The attention of physicians was drawn to the fact that St. Louis Park's MedCenter, and also the Nicollet-Eitel HMO, were run by physicians. This was a crucial step in their subsequent participation.

Another source of positive physician impact was the presence of Dr. Paul Ellwood, who developed a base for HMO advocacy in the Twin Cities. Physicians reported that they knew of his efforts, but many believed that his focus was national rather than local. Other individual physicians had impact through their leadership in county and state medical societies. They were particularly important in the development of Physicians Health Plan, which is largely responsible for raising physician HMO participation in Minneapolis to 95 percent.

In sum, while Minneapolis-St. Paul physicians have reflected the conservative nature of their socialization to the profession of medicine, they have at the same time responded primarily as integral members of their resourceful and progressive community. They have had a positive impact on the development of HMOs.

Chicago

Negative impact

In Chicago, the qualities of cautiousness and traditionalism characteristic of the medical profession are intensified by the conservative, fragmented, and adversarial nature of the metropolitan area. Despite localized positive and negative effects, the overall result of physicians' HMO-related activities is a virtual absence of impact on the development of HMOs.

Physician respondents noted that from the beginning of prepaid health care in Chicago, there were "frank reprisals" from physicians against their "wayward colleagues." This response was common among "fee-for-service peers who tend to take umbrage at a mode of practice that cordons off the members from the general flow of referrals within the medical community" (Brown, 1983). Chicago physicians, who were staff members in only one or two Chicago hospitals, often barred HMO physicians from staff privileges and made it impossible for their hospital to form agreements with HMOs. Primary care physicians, including those in the Academy of Family Practice, openly opposed HMOs. They claimed to the public in general and to their patients in particular that HMO competition was unfairly (federally) subsidized. Less explicit, but frequently mentioned as having local impact, were pressures brought by physicians through their social networks. Physicians discouraged their friends in business from offering HMOs to their employees.

Finally, and perhaps most important, few physicians in Chicago have experience with group practice. Solo, fee-for-service, neighborhood practice predominates in Chicago, and inexperience with group practice greatly inhibits HMOs. Positive influences from HMOs are neutralized by physicians who fear the unknown. At one time, physicians in Chicago opposed any form of group practice. Later, when fee-for-service group practice, principally of small, single specialty groups, was accepted as a concept, there was strong opposition by organized medicine to prepaid group practice (Boehm, 1976). Chicago physicians suggested that there continues to be skepticism, disrespect, and hostility toward HMOs by individual physicians.

However, Chicago physicians have not ignored HMOs. In the late 1960s and throughout the 1970s, alternative forms of delivery were discussed methodically by the Chicago Medical Society, just as they were in the Twin Cities. In early 1971, the Chicago Medical Society approved "a not-for-profit corporation of physicians sponsored and owned by the society to design and administer prepaid medical care programs . . . without a dissenting vote" (Chicago Medical Society, 1971). Yet, only the portion of the original program that related to quality assurance through peer review survived. That professional standards review organization, which was started in Cook County in 1976, is reported to have always been unpopular with practicing physicians in the Chicago area. In 1976, it was the nation's largest review organization—and perhaps the most unwieldly. Later, on the subject of an association-sponsored IPA, there was official ambivalence. In May 1980, the Chicago Medical Society concluded that "the subject of HMO/IPAs [was] complex . . ., important and urgent . . . and should receive further study . . . [therefore] CMS should not either ally itself with, or indicate, more support of any HMO/IPA" (Chicago Medical Society, 1980). The ambivalence was created by and has contributed to inertia among physicians. By 1983, Chicago physicians reported that although they are still unsupportive of HMOs, "they are stopping peer pressure against them."

Positive impact

Although inertia in the medical community as a whole opposes HMOs, certain physicians in Chicago have had a positive impact on the success of individual HMOs. Anchor, Michael Reese Health Plan, and Intergroup had founding physicians. At NorthCare, the medical director was recruited by the consumer sponsors at its earliest stages, and that person has guided the medical activities of the plan since its opening.

HMO IMPACT ON PHYSICIANS

Minneapolis-St. Paul

While the development of Group Health Plan had little effect on physicians, the beginning of MedCenter Health Plan and, in 1972, of Nicollet-Eitel Health Plan drew their attention. Some physicians considered HMOs closely, but most physicians reported that they were not yet concerned about competition. One knowledgeable physician from the Hennepin County Medical Society explained that they started a feasibility study in 1973 motivated by the establishment of MedCenter and Nicollet-Eitel;

> ... the greatest impetus [toward Physicians Health Plan] was the fact that the hospitals were really looking seriously at starting their own hospital-based HMOs in our community. I think that was the most scary thing to the rank and file physicians who at that time felt really no threat at all from Group Health or [any other plan that was just getting started] ... But the physicians do have a great deal of respect for how hospitals can get things done. [Physicians] also have a fear that hospital administrators, when they do something, don't really include physicians in their thinking process.

Thus it appears that at first HMOs were not viewed as direct competitors, but rather as ways that the physician's traditional competitor, the hospital, might become more powerful. The physician continued,

> Even though the threat and fear of losing one's practice wasn't there yet, there is a lot written about fear as a motivator; but speaking for the practicing physician, I really think that when Physicians Health Plan started that was not the greatest thing. There was the fear of hospitals doing this, and that was a great big unknown. We certainly weren't afraid of the other HMOs which were so young. Today is certainly different.

The bulletin of the Hennepin County Medical Society confirms this report. In a "Prepaid Group Practice Committee Update" it was reported that a "discussion followed regarding the concerns of those present over the development of a multiplicity of HMO plans by our local hospitals and the Blues." Further-more, HMO physicians and organizers arranged to get admitting privileges. One Twin cities physician reported that "the heads of the medical board invited heads of county medical societies to dinner and told them what was developing and asked that they make a statement of acceptance. This paved the way and there was never any barring." A sense of the momentum and the com-petitive impact that HMOs were developing is evident from an-other physician's account of resistance from some fee-for-service medical staff.

> Yes, there was some hostility but it was handled by the administrators—the realists in the situation. We were invited by (the hospital) administrators and they told it to their staff—not underhanded—a friendly way. It was a matter of survival for the hos-pital; the administrator appealed to a self-interest of the medical staff—if they wanted to continue to exist. Now we've become pretty close to being dominant—also a problem.

Physicians sense that there was then a rapid growth of HMOs. As more physicians joined HMOs, the HMOs became more competitive and again more physicians joined.

With the addition of competitive forces in the health care market, physicians both inside and outside HMOs reported greater intraprofessional tension among primary care physicians, specialists and subspecialists. HMOs affected the different groups differently. Not only do specialties command different salaries (Meier and Tillotson, 1978), but primary care physicians felt almost irresistible pressure to join an HMO. Certain special-ists were vulnerable, but others, who were more scarce, resisted joining because they knew their services would be needed whether they were HMO participants or not. While many pri-mary care physicians felt powerless, certain specialists were re-sentful of the power of primary care physicians in a competitive market to act as "gatekeepers," altering the established referral networks. Several excerpts from a letter to the editor in Min-nesota Medicine exemplify the palpable frustration and recall historical arguments.

> The term "cost containment" has assumed a propa-ganda mystique.... Trendy terms from "think

tanks" propose new programs under the buzz word
of "competitive model" . . . In this environment, it is
essential that physicians observe and buttress the
ethics of precise medical practice which place the
patient's interest paramount. Some of the newly
proposed prepaid plans have features that appear to
run contrary to the ethical standards of our Minnesota Surgical Community [such as] . . . specific
features designed to discourage specialists' referral
and to induce referral to a specialist care on an economic basis (lowest bidder). To quote from the
American College of Surgeons statement on principles, "any form of inducement to refer a patient to
another physician other than for superior care to be
secured, is unethical." Lowest bid is not a basis for
referral under such a principle. . . If (the primary
care physician) can find a more compliant specialist
who will provide the service cheaper, he will retain
more money for himself . . . a sanctioned method of
"indirect fee splitting." The American College of
Surgeons and our own Minnesota Surgical groups
have given decades of diligent effort to stamp out
the pernicious harm of fee splitting. . . . We owe it to
ourselves to see that the voice for patients' rights
and medical ethics is not dragged down in the hard
sell patois of the used car lot (Minnesota Medical
Association, 1981).

Dermatologists were also distressed. The chairman of the
American Academy of Dermatology claimed, "Denial of self-referral flies in the face of competitive medicine; it also creates
friction between primary care physicians and specialists because
one group—the specialists—becomes dependent on the other for
business."

Some specialties are difficult to retain in a system emphasizing cost-effectiveness. Mental health services have presented
problems for HMOs and their physicians. Risk-sharing arrangement with psychiatric groups have had a troubled history. However, in response to HMOs, a mental health group, the Metropolitan Clinic of Counseling, was developed in 1975 to serve HMOs.
The clinic provides mental health and chemical dependency services and is itself much like an HMO. It contracts with the
HMOs, and both share the financial risk. The clinic has more

than fifty professional employees. All are salaried, except the psychiatrists, who have contracts.

Intraprofessional problems are present not only in the network HMOs but also in the staff models. Distribution of extensive and predominantly routine primary and simple trauma care among physicians who prefer to practice their specialty is problematic. Group Health Plan hired family practice physicians to cover primary care, then found dissension within the organization because of historical resentment among medical school departments about subsidized family practice programs. Although there was resistance to non-board qualified physicians, "their unequal status finally became untenable," and they were recognized as a department.

The University of Minnesota Medical Center, the source of alumni throughout the Twin Cities, has been strongly affected by the competitive environment. Several adaptations at the center are important. Respondents explained that university physicians believed that their beds were more expensive than comparable community beds, and that they worried about the census. As a result, they tried two new programs: 1) a nonacute medical surgical ward, where the costs aren't any higher than other hospitals in the community; and 2) an ear, nose, and throat station from which patients could go home on the weekends. But as further evidence of the intense competition, "it didn't take off" because the same-day surgery section was expanded and became very popular as an alternative. In addition, Group Health Plan negotiated contracts with the university for obstetrics service, and the department is now very dependent on that population for their training programs.

Though St. Paul has responded more conservatively to HMOs than Minneapolis, the effects of competition are felt. By 1981 it was claimed that competition would create alternative delivery systems and that doctors would be forced to compete with hospitals (Ellwood and Ellwein, 1981). In May 1983, twenty of twenty-eight community hospitals were participating in the AWARE program, a PPO sponsored by Blue Cross-Blue Shield. Conflict developed regarding participation. According to Dr. Roy, president of the Ramsey County Medical Society,

> The carrot for a participating physician is of course that you will see more patients yet you will [be required] to accept the payor's version of the reason-

> able charge as payment in full and you cannot bill
> the patient for the additional amount . . . whether
> these charges represent the real costs of providing
> care or not (Ramsey County Medical Society, 1983).

Furthermore, Dr. Roy noted that although increasing numbers of physicians are electing not to accept Medicare assign-
ments, ". . . there are very definite legislative gestures to mandate
assignment and perhaps not at the 75th percentile of '79 figures."
He continued the lament, "It seems everywhere we turn we en-
counter pressures to participate in health care programs, and fewer and fewer occasions arise for the physician to work directly
with patients on the issue of medical costs. . . . If you do not elect
to participate, there may be more waiting room in your practice
as well." From this one editorial, one sees the physicians' greatest fears about competition: hospitals gaining power, loss of income, loss of patients, further intervention by the government,
and interference in the doctor-patient relationship.

A number of structural changes are imposed specifically on
physicians practicing in HMOs, which vary with the form of
HMO (Luft, 1981a). Indeed, change in practice patterns is generally confirmed by interviews in the Twin Cities.

The most notable change in practice patterns for all HMO
physicians is the decrease in hospitalization. The explanation
that follows is characteristic of the physicians' perspective on
that change:

> There is definitely less hospitalization. It used to be
> when I was in training that the [internist] spent his
> mornings making rounds on his patients in the hos-
> pital and his afternoons in his office, but now most
> of his practice is in his office. [As a result of the
> awareness in the Twin Cities] patients are now put-
> ting pressure on you to keep them out of the hospi-
> tal. Sometimes when you have a patient you are
> worried about who really should be in the hospital,
> they argue with you . . . they say they'll take their
> temperature every four hours, or they have a friend
> who's a nurse and can give the injections . . . it's
> turned around; patients used to want to be in the
> hospital when they were sick.

Of those physicians who had partial HMO and partial fee-
for-service practice, most noted that they had learned new patterns of practicing but that they did not treat their HMO patients

differently. Rather, the changes in HMO practice "spilled over" into their fee-for-service practice. These physicians reported that changes did not lessen quality of care, and often they improved it. One physician explained it was once routine to watch the progress of pneumonia cases using x-rays. "The plan said that was too expensive," so now the physicians watch the patient clinically (by physical exam), with an x-ray at diagnosis and one at follow-up. He continued, "all those x-rays weren't necessary, and, in fact, it is better for the patient not to have all that irradiation."

An HMO physician from a group model HMO added, [practicing in an HMO]

> allows us to look at ourselves systematically and when, for instance, we can do a surgical procedure on an ambulatory basis, that in the past has been a hospital based procedure, that saves people money and gives equal or better outcomes, then we change that for everyone. It gives us the incentive to think of the cost issue as part of the quality of health care.

In the IPA model, physicians reported that at first they practiced much as they always had, but now the HMO administration imposes controls. When asked if there was a difference for an HMO patient, one physician replied,

> Yes, it's coming to be so because of the pressures being exerted on me by the HMO organization. . . . I feel now that I am being pressured to reduce the amount of medical care that I give to my HMO patients.

This physician went on to describe what is a paradoxical effect of HMOs. He explained that as a member of an IPA he would be penalized if he received more than a certain amount per patient per year.

> This means that if I see a prolonged, difficult problem coming up, I'm motivated to refer them to somebody else. And since [the ceiling is on] office practice, I am actually motivated to do some things in the hospital that I might do in my office.

In spite of the pressures, practitioners are reluctant to drop out because of the competitive conditions. One physician, whose average fees were higher than others in his specialty, was asked to resign. He refused.

> So they said that if I did not want to resign that I
> could sign an agreement that I would undertake to
> repay them any amount above the average for their
> physicians group. I went along with them and did it.

This is an important point because the attitudes that physicians in Minneapolis-St. Paul recalled having in 1975 and 1976 are similar to those that Chicago physicians reported in 1983.

Chicago

It was already noted that the impact of physicians and HMOs in a community is reciprocal. It is consistently the case that where there has been little impact by physicians on HMOs, as in Chicago, there is also little impact by HMOs on physicians.

In Chicago, physicians were increasingly conscious, but often only abstractly, of competitive forces in medicine. Physicians there were thoughtful about HMOs but not threatened by them. In 1983, physicians were just beginning to think it might be becoming necessary to compete with HMOs.

In the 1970s, there had been scattered, hostile reactions to HMOs in the Chicago metropolitan area. However, as HMOs gained strength nationally, respondents reported that hostile physicians felt required to "back off." At one time, a county medical society attempted to hold hearings to oppose a developing HMO, but it was discouraged when a U.S. District Court passed a decree prohibiting a medical society in Florida from opposing an HMO there (Group Health Association of America, 1980). By 1981, *Chicago Medicine* ran a series about HMOs and IPAs, and a former president of the Chicago Medical Society, Clifton Reeder, M.D., said,

> Competition is the American way of life. HMOs do
> offer some competition to the fee-for-service. Within
> the fee-for-service system competition does not exist
> for all practical purposes. The current method of
> creating and marketing HMOs is cumbersome and
> not very effective. Innovation is needed. . . . Either
> the government or the threat of government will be
> on our backs until there . . . are sufficient . . . alter-
> natives . . . to create meaningful competition. Com-
> petition is much preferable to a government fi-
> nanced system with all the controls that it would
> entail. Let's keep medicine in the private sector.
> Meaningful competition will do it.

However, Chicago physicians do not yet see HMOs as significant competition. Chicago fee-for-service physicians did not report patients asking that their records be transferred to HMOs. Instead, reimbursement for public aid recipients was still considered the most pressing problem by Chicago physicians.

There are some issues of competition in Chicago that parallel concerns and patterns among Twin Cities physicians. For example, physicians in Chicago continue to view hospitals as major usurpers of power. One politically active physician spoke characteristically, "Hospitals, in my opinion, want to practice medicine. I think that's wrong!" But, he worried, "Doctors are lousy businessmen." Physicians' concern about hospital power is played out in classic battles between hospital administrators and their medical staffs, so admitting privileges are tightly guarded by Chicago physicians. In addition, teaching hospitals at a number of medical centers are demonstrating some response to competition. Some predict that in a competitive environment, teaching hospitals will "broaden their patient base" by adding primary care physicians (Ellwood and Ellwein, 1981). Indeed, primary care staff and clinics have been expanded at a number of teaching hospitals in Chicago to train students and house staff, and draw patients to the hospitals.

In addition, new programs and practices are being added by university physicians at teaching hospitals in direct response to private utilization review organizations developed to contain costs. For example, in January 1983, the Zenith Corporation in Chicago began the "Zenith Medical Services Advisory Program" for all its employees with Blue Cross-Blue Shield coverage. It requires that the employee "contact the Medical Services Advisor prior to any nonemergency hospital admission." As a result, a major university medical center affected by this innovation issued a memo about a new program "that will permit obtaining necessary laboratory tests, x-rays, and other studies before elective admission of a patient to the hospital." Furthermore, the staff was advised about the difference in cost between "routine" and "stat" laboratory tests and how to avoid additional charges. The memo concluded:

> Because of the concerns of external groups, as indicated in the previously distributed Zenith Medical Services Advisory Program, I wish to emphasize two points. 1. Any laboratory tests felt necessary for patients being admitted electively should be obtained on a routine basis preceding the time of elec-

tive admission for the patient. 2. Consideration should be given as to the medical needs/usefulness for any laboratory tests being obtained for a patient admitted electively.

Such occurrences suggest an increasingly competitive environment in the Chicago area. Most Chicago physicians, even some at hospitals sponsoring prepaid plans, are not yet acutely aware of competition, but many are accepting change. One respondent explained:

> HMOs have acquired respectability. I don't want to join an HMO, but I don't care if you do. What I say is that if an HMO can do a better job, then, damn it, we deserve to have them with us. If we can do a better job, well, then they'll go away.

At the end of 1983, they have not gone away, and some physicians are beginning to modify their practice styles to be more cost-competitive. Still others are joining HMOs as they accelerate their development in the Chicago area.

SUMMARY

The centrality of the doctor-patient relationship and the crucial importance of professional independence and autonomy have always pervaded any physician's relationships with other professionals and paraprofessionals. Referral patterns, specialization, and peer review are also important. These historic issues are seen to converge in HMOs.

An analysis of the topics that relate physicians and HMO development in these two communities reveals physicians who are similarly committed practicing in notably different communities. Most revealing in this study is the complex interaction between the medical community and the community as a whole. Dominant historic themes in American medicine continued to be expressed by the physicians interviewed in both communities. However, these physicians are citizens in communities with dramatically different characteristics. Although they share common understandings and similar professional attitudes and values, they also respond to the norms and values, as well as the important problems, of their own metropolitan areas.

In the Twin Cities, homogeneity reinforced trust and communication networks in an environment already predisposed to collectivism. Furthermore, HMOs were seen as relevant to the predominant health care problem of escalating costs, and group practice patterns were well established. Perhaps most important, in an environment rich with sources, communication patterns, and earlier successes, physicians took proactive leadership and management roles. In turn, because there is Twin Cities physician leadership, there is less fear among physicians of bureaucracies run by nonphysicians, which would threaten their professional autonomy. As a result, there is less cause for reactionary behavior in the medical community. In the Twin Cities, proactive physicians, such as those at St. Louis Park Medical Center, motivated other physicians by competition and leadership in the medical community.

In Chicago too, the community has strong, ideologically committed physicians who could provide leadership for HMO development. However, in this large, economically burdened, diverse, and fragmented environment where there was little experience with group practice, their efforts were isolated from citywide influence and confined to local success. In the absence of commonly recognized proactive medical leadership, alternative nonmedical bureaucracies developed. These in turn drew distrust and resistance from the Chicago medical community. In neither community did their professional attitudes and values enable the physicians to be initiators in changing the health care system. However, in the Twin Cities, which has an abundance of resources and history of cooperative decision making and problem solving, physicians responded not only as physicians but also as citizens of this unique community, and as a whole, they supported and were an important factor in the successful development of HMOs.

6

HMOs and Insurers

In both metropolitan areas there was early insurer involvement. HMOs were regarded not as competitors but rather as innovations to be observed and possibly incorporated. In the Twin Cities, HMOs have probably gained more at the expense of Blue Cross than at that of commercial insurers because HMOs made initial inroads into the large employer and public employer market. Only recently have HMOs made inroads in the small employer market in the Twin Cities. Blue Cross developed its own HMO; other insurers sold ancillary management services to HMOs or managed multiple choice plans for employers. In Chicago, Blue Cross market share is declining, but HMO market share is still too small to have much effect. Also, there is not much activity in "ancillary HMO services" by insurers, though Blue Cross, CNA, Prudential, and Aetna have developed alternative service groups. In both areas, there is heavy pressure for cost containment. In response, the distinctions between HMOs and fee-for-service insurers are beginning to blur as HMOs begin to install copayments, deductibles, and other cost-sharing devices and as fee-for-service insurers implement more utilization review programs, PPOs, etc., to gain increased leverage over providers.

Health maintenance organizations can be viewed as innovative market challengers to a mature health insurance industry. In response, many insurers have sought to protect their market shares or gain expertise by participating in HMO development

This chapter was written by Bruce W. Butler, Assistant Project Director.

activities. As HMOs grow, however, they not only reduce insurers' market shares but also present insurers with new problems such as risk pool fragmentation and adverse selection patterns in multiple choice health benefit plans.

Information in this chapter comes, in part, from the analysis of thirty-one interviews with respondents in the insurance sector, representing carriers and consultants.

BACKGROUND

The precedent for modern health insurance coverage emerged by the early part of this century as trade associations, employers, and insurance companies began to offer, on a group risk-sharing basis, cash benefits to cover wages lost due to accident or illness. As medical expenses became more significant components of the financial burden of sickness, cash payments for medical care were offered as add-on benefits to the early sickness benefit plans (Somers and Somers, 1961; Sheps and Drosness, 1961). Involvement of insurance companies in medical expense coverage was limited in this early period by caution regarding the underwriting feasibility of such coverage (Woodward, 1978).

The health insurance industry as it currently exists stems from the development of the Blue Cross system in the 1930s and 1940s. The underlying demand for the Blue Cross system emerged as hospital costs increased beyond levels that typical households could budget for in advance (Anderson, 1975). In addition, the depression economy exacerbated household financial problems and caused the failure of many labor-management benefit plans (Somers and Somers, 1961).

During and immediately following the Second World War, the inclusion of health insurance in employee benefits packages expanded greatly because of union pressures for broader benefits, court rulings expanding the scope of collective bargaining to include health and social insurance, favorable tax treatment of fringe benefits, and wartime attempts to limit inflation through the restriction of wage increases (Munts, 1967). By this time, Blue Cross plans for hospital services and Blue Shield plans for physician services were becoming fairly well established. However, commercial insurance companies responded to the increasing demand for health insurance and to the Blue plans' demonstration of the insurability of medical care by entering the market rapidly. Between 1942 and 1951, the number of insurance companies offering health insurance expanded from 37 to 212 (Woodward, 1978).

Historically, independent plans, such as HMOs, union trust funds, and employer self-insurance plans, have not held major shares of the health insurance market. Between 1972 and 1979, however, independent plans increased their share of total private sector premium income from 6.2 percent to 16.8 percent (Carroll and Arnett, 1981). The bulk of this gain was at the expense of the commercial insurers' aggregate share of premium income, which declined from 49.4 percent to 41.2 percent. The Blue plans' aggregate share of premium income also declined from 44.4 percent to 42.0 percent during this period. To some extent, however, these losses were compensated by insurers taking on the administration of employers' self-insurance plans.

Measured in terms of the proportion of the population covered, the health insurance market has reached or is at least approaching the point of saturation. Nationally, the proportion of the civilian noninstitutional population under sixty-five with some level of private health insurance coverage stood at approximately 84 percent in 1981 (Health Insurance Association of America, 1983). Approximately 99 percent of employees in companies with 100 or more workers are currently eligible for some form of health insurance benefits (U.S. Department of Commerce, 1981). Therefore, the most significant growth opportunities available to health insurers lie in expanded coverage, as well as replacement marketing to customers who are already being served by competitors.

Respondents in this study reported that the ability of fee-for-service health insurance to produce even marginal profits is severely limited now because of rapid cost inflation in health care. Representatives of some insurance companies reported that this was tolerable since health insurance is only one part of a larger package of more profitable types of fringe benefits. Others, though, described corporate policies that insisted that all lines of business should be self-sufficient and that low profit margins in health insurance were compensated by high cash flow volumes. All agreed, however, that an insurance company that did not offer health coverage would have a difficult time now competing for other segments of the fringe benefits market.

Traditional market channels in group health insurance have

consisted of either direct sales to employer and union decision makers or the payment of commissions to insurance brokers who perform comparative shopping and purchasing services for employer and union clients. Traditionally, the resulting contract between the insurer and the covered group has been exclusive. Consumer-oriented marketing has been unnecessary, therefore, since individuals within groups have not had the opportunity to choose among competing insurers.

Individual and family health insurance policies have traditionally been sold on a one-on-one agent-to-customer basis. This marketing method is more costly than group insurance methods. Individual and family premiums as a percent of total hospital-medical premium income for insurance companies declined from 33 percent in 1960 to 13 percent in 1980 (Health Insurance Association of America, 1982). Several major insurers have recently decided to phase out their individual and family health insurance lines.

TRENDS IN GROUP HEALTH INSURANCE

Respondents in this study generally agreed that there were three major stages in the development of demand for group health insurance: the expansion of benefits, the increased sophistication of benefits management, and the eventual demand for cost containment provisions and benefit reductions. A brief discussion of these trends follows. More extensive analysis of the demand for health insurance through employee benefit plans can be found in chapter 7.

Until the 1970s, strong demand for benefits expansion led to incremental increases in the scope of services covered and in the levels of reimbursement for covered services. For example, insurers competed with one another by introducing innovations such as major medical plans in the 1950s and dental insurance in the 1960s. Reimbursement levels for services, such as hospital room and board, tended toward 100 percent coverage.

By the middle 1970s, demand for benefit expansion began to wane. Informants in this study attributed this to the fact that employee satisfaction with health benefits had reached a level that made the expansion of other fringe benefits more attractive. In addition, nascent concerns regarding health care cost escalation began to inhibit employers' benefit expansion plans. In response to decreased interest, insurers began to compete by offering sophisticated cash-flow devices that allowed employers to retain the same benefit levels but for lower overall costs. For example, plans were developed in which an employer paid a discounted premium in advance. The balance was due only if the group's experience actually warranted additional payment. In the extreme, employers took on the entire risk for their employees' medical care and retained insurers only to perform claims processing or other administrative services. Concurrent with the trends outlined above, insurers reported an overall increase in the management sophistication of employee benefits departments. Benefits managers began to take a highly active role in benefit design and began to demand a wide range of individually tailored features for their companies. Thus, the speed, sophistication, and flexibility of financial management and data processing functions became increasingly important areas of competition in the health insurance industry.

During the late 1970s and early 1980s, concern regarding health care cost containment intensified demand for the cash-flow devices outlined above. In addition, many employers demanded a wide variety of cost containment features, such as coverage for outpatient surgery, preadmission testing, and second surgical opinions. Although these particular features are actually benefit expansions, many employers also began to demand benefit plans with restrictions that disallowed or penalized weekend hospital admissions, mandated outpatient surgery for certain procedures, and denied surgical claims unsupported by second opinions. Some employers have begun to request benefit plans with higher deductibles and coinsurance for employees. Finally, to evaluate the effects of all these provisions on health care costs, employers are demanding extensive, group-specific reports from insurers about utilization and cost.

In addition to developing services to meet the demands outlined above, insurers have attempted to alleviate cost escalation through public policy. The commercial health insurance industry has traditionally maintained that it does not possess sufficient market power over providers to stimulate cost-effective utilization patterns. The industry has in many cases, therefore, favored regulatory strategies ranging from the restriction of hospital bed supply to prospective reimbursement systems (Enthoven, 1980). In Chicago, an employer and insurer coalition was active in unsuccessful efforts to establish a prospective payment program in Illinois.

Increasingly, however, insurers are developing and implementing strategies for cost containment through increased influence over providers. Examples include the provision of data on provider-specific charges to employers, participation in private utilization review programs, and the development of alternative delivery and finance systems such as health maintenance organizations and preferred provider organizations.

DEVELOPMENT OF COMPETITION

HMOs represent a significant innovation in the health insurance industry in that they closely integrate financing and delivery functions. Therefore, they are at least in theory more capable than other organizations of directing provider behavior toward cost-effectiveness.

Despite their innovative nature, HMOs are nevertheless influenced by the same basic trends in demand that influence the health insurance market as a whole. As the focus of employer demand for health insurance plans has changed, the rationale for employer interest in HMOs has also changed. For example, in the early 1970s, many Twin Cities employers were interested in HMOs as a means of expanding benefits. Later, employers concerned about cost containment focused on the apparent capability of HMOs to reduce hospital use among their enrollees. With this increased interest in HMOs for cost containment purposes came skepticism regarding the possible role of self-selection processes in determining the different rates of utilization between HMOs and fee-for-service plans. In some cases, HMOs have also taken advantage of regulatory mandates giving them access to employees regardless of the level of interest exhibited by employers.

In general, identification of HMOs with general patterns of health insurance demand has been exhibited more strongly in the Twin Cities than in Chicago. Reliance on the mandate process has correspondingly been much more extensive in Chicago, though it has been a valuable tool in the Twin Cities as well.

The entrance of HMOs into the health insurance market significantly alters traditional marketing channels. To preserve employees' rights to choose their own medical providers, employers usually do not develop exclusive contracts with HMOs. Instead, employees are typically offered the choice of a fee-for-service plan and one or more HMOs. Therefore, consumer marketing strategies are becoming increasingly relevant in the group health insurance industry. New HMOs are at a disadvantage in the consumer's decision-making process because they are not well understood and because veteran employees must make an active choice to join an HMO but can retain fee-for-service coverage by default. To compensate, many HMOs have undertaken aggressive consumer marketing efforts. Methods have included group meetings with employees, mailings, and mass media advertising. Especially in the Twin Cities, employers have cooperated with these efforts because they feel that special efforts need to be made to familiarize employees with a novel and complex form of health delivery and financing.

In response to the development of competition from HMOs, established insurers may pursue one or all of the following strategies:

1. aggressive competition,
2. internal development of HMOs or similar organizations, or
3. development of exchange relationships with existing HMOs.

Interviews conducted for this study suggested that established insurers have not yet become aggressive in consumer marketing designed to retain enrollees in multiple choice plans. The reasons for this, suggested by various industry representatives, include the high cost of consumer marketing, the difficulty of changing established procedures, and the reluctance of employers to cooperate with the marketing of a product that their employees already understand. While examples of consumer marketing through employers and the mass media exist, direct competitive responses to HMOs by insurers have been generally limited to pricing and product design. It was reported that from the early to the middle 1970s some insurers expanded ambulatory coverage to compete with HMOs, but this strategy disappeared as price became the overriding issue later in the decade. While current efforts by insurers to contain premium costs may significantly affect HMOs, these efforts are not necessarily attributable to the presence of HMOs in the market. Given the great demand for cost containment by employers, it is likely that insurers would attempt to contain costs to compete among themselves, even if HMOs were not present. Visible confrontation aimed directly at HMOs is not common yet.

According to a representative of an industry-sponsored public relations agency, the insurance industry does not wish to present a confrontational image to the public, preferring instead to meet potential threats through negotiation, compromise, and adjustment of its own position. To a large extent, this nonconfrontational approach characterizes the response of the health insurance industry to HMOs. While interviews for this study suggested that there was some resentment toward HMOs in the early 1970s, this reaction did not come from corporate policy-making levels but rather from marketing representatives who were threatened with the loss of sales and commissions. At the policy-making level, insurers appeared to take a much broader perspective regarding the potential threat of HMO development. Rather than competing aggressively with HMOs, insurers sought generally to retain their positions in the marketplace by working with and through HMOs. As evidence of this strategy, in 1969 the Board of Directors of the Health Insurance Association of America accepted this recommendation of the association's Subcommittee on Health Care Delivery of the Committee on Medical Economics:

> That insurance companies [should] continue to remain abreast of developments in the prepaid group practice field and be prepared to conduct experiments, the purpose of which would be to determine the proper relationship of insurance companies to this concept. . . . It is important that insurance companies do not place themselves in the position of impeding any such sound developments (Health Insurance Association of America, 1969).

Individual insurers developed corporate policies that closely mirror this recommendation (Koncel, 1980). Insurers displayed a range of involvements with HMOs to implement these policies (Provence, 1981). For example, many insurers were leaders in offering multiple choice health plans to their employees. Insurers also actively provided administrative and financial services to HMOs, ranging from stop-loss insurance to administrative contracts for claims processing, actuarial, and marketing services. Insurers even became involved in providing venture capital for HMO development. Finally, a number of insurers developed or acquired HMOs as joint ventures or subsidiary corporations. The following section discusses specific examples of involvement by insurers in the development of HMOs in the Twin Cities and Chicago.

HMOs AND INSURERS: MINNEAPOLIS-ST. PAUL

Involvement of insurers in HMO development

The involvement of insurers in Twin Cities HMO development was extensive and represented the various types of experimentation, affiliation, servicing, and subsidiary development discussed above.

An early example of insurer involvement occurred in 1968 when a locally headquartered firm, Northwestern National Life, entered into negotiations regarding the development of a prepaid practice plan as a joint venture with the University of Minnesota Medical School Faculty. This project was not implemented, owing in part to projected high costs of hospitalization at university facilities and to difficulties in defining the exact nature of faculty participation. However, this project did provide Northwestern National Life with valuable experience in the HMO field as well as generating greater community interest in HMOs.

In 1969, the Equitable Life Assurance Company sent its medical director to the Twin Cities to explore a wide range of options for involving Equitable in HMO development. These options included an HMO network of Northern Pacific railroad hospitals in the Midwest and Northwest; a large Twin Cities HMO modeled after Kaiser-Permanente; and a central marketing and administrative services organization for a number of smaller Twin Cities HMOs. While none of these specific projects was implemented, this effort served as a catalyst for the formation, in the early 1970s, of the TCHCDP, a coalition of insurers and employers that was instrumental in raising the level of awareness regarding HMOs in the business community and in improving the legislative climate for HMOs.

Northwestern National Life was a key participant in the TCHCDP and was simultaneously active in the planning and early development of MedCenter Health Plan. Initially, the insurance company provided a range of administrative services on a contractual basis. As the HMO expanded, it increasingly assumed these functions internally. However, Northwestern National Life has been able to draw on its experience with MedCenter to develop consulting and administrative contracts with other HMOs in the Twin Cities and elsewhere.

Also in the early 1970s, Nicollet Clinic, another multispecialty group practice, began planning an HMO and received assistance from Blue Cross-Blue Shield of Minnesota. Blue Cross-Blue Shield did not seek operational involvement, so the HMO developed a contractual administrative relationship with another insurer. Blue Cross-Blue Shield then undertook the development of a subsidiary HMO, which entered the market several years later. Recently, Blue Cross-Blue Shield of Minnesota developed a preferred provider organization.

The St. Paul Companies, another locally headquartered insurer, provided venture capital and contractual administrative services to Physicians Health Plan. In addition, a retired executive from the St. Paul Companies was active in the early administration of Physicians Health Plan. As the HMO retired its debt to the insurer and developed its own management staff and administrative capabilities, formal relationships between the two organizations were not continued.

In addition to the relationships outlined above, many insurers served as leaders in the business community by offering HMOs to their employees. Northwestern National Life was one of those early leaders, and it developed a line of business providing other employers with management assistance for multiple choice health plans. These services included management of multiple payroll deductions, centralized payment of HMO premiums, and preparation of benefit comparisons for employees.

In general, insurer involvement in Twin Cities HMO development was greatest in the planning and early development stages. With the exception of the Blue Cross-Blue Shield, no insurers were heavily involved in HMO operations on a sustained basis. One possible reason for this pattern is that Minnesota legislation permits only non-profit HMOs, thus removing some of the incentive for HMO subsidiary development by for-profit insurers. Employers reportedly reacted negatively to the prospect of local HMO development that would be controlled by the insurance industry, particularly by outside insurers. Also, insurers were possibly reluctant to enter into direct competition with provider-sponsored HMOs. The operational involvement of insurers in HMOs that were developed by provider groups has generally been reduced over time by the preferences of the HMOs for performing all administrative functions themselves. Typically, contractual marketing services were the first things terminated as HMOs sought to establish independent identities. As HMOs grew in size, they also found it advantageous to internalize claims processing, billing, and actuarial functions. Insurers still provide stop-loss insurance to Twin Cities HMOs, but demand for this product by HMOs may also diminish as the HMOs grow larger and more capable of assuming unrestricted risk. The only long-term opportunity for insurer involvement in HMO ancillary services appears to be management of multiple choice plans for employers.

While the number of relationships between insurance carriers and HMOs appears to be diminishing in the Twin Cities, the number of relationships between insurance brokers and HMOs appears to be growing. In the early stages of HMO development, brokers and HMOs generally exhibited mutual disinterest. HMOs concentrated their initial marketing efforts on large employers, which are not heavily served by brokers. As HMOs saturated the large-employer market, however, they focused their efforts on smaller employers. This presents HMOs with potentially higher marketing costs per new enrollee and also places HMOs more directly in competition with brokers. Therefore, it is becoming increasingly advantageous for HMOs and brokers to develop commission relationships. To develop these relationships, several HMOs are currently conducting extensive marketing and education campaigns aimed at acquainting brokers with the process of offering HMOs to employers. HMOs reported that the response of brokers to these efforts has been "warming" in recent years.

HMO impact on insurers

The most obvious impact of HMOs is on insurers' market shares. In the Twin Cities, where approximately 25 percent of the total population is enrolled in HMOs and penetration rates run as high as 85 percent for some major employer accounts, health insurers naturally reported that their market shares were eroded significantly by HMOs. This also applied to the business of providing administrative services only, because HMOs drew many enrollees out of major self-insured plans. When asked to speculate regarding the upper limit of HMO growth in the Twin Cities, insurers and consultants named figures in the range of 40 to 50 percent of the population. Although actual and projected HMO market shares were reported to be extremely troublesome to sales personnel, a sense of strategic concern regarding HMO growth was conspicuously absent in most interviews with representatives of the insurance industry. For large firms with regional offices in the Twin Cities, this perspective may have reflected a strategic outlook based on the level of competition from HMOs on a nationwide basis, which is less significant than in the Twin Cities. In addition, some firms are active in HMO subsidiary development in other parts of the country. As discussed above, insurers that are more focused on the Twin Cities were the most active providers of local HMO ancillary service and subsidiary development.

Concern by Twin Cities insurers regarding the HMO market share per se was lower than might be expected. However, insurers and benefits consultants did report great concern regarding other factors related to HMO market share, such as risk pool fragmentation, adverse selection patterns, and HMO hospital discounts.

The introduction to multiple choice plans presented the health insurance industry with a new set of underwriting problems. At the simplest level, multiple choice plans can fragment employee groups, resulting in a smaller risk pool. For insurers that set experience-based rates, this can lead to higher premiums since the variability of experience is higher in a smaller group. This problem is most significant for groups that are small initially. In some cases, fragmentation of small employee groups resulted in discontinuation of coverage by carriers that considered their remaining portion of the group too small to be insurable.

While the absolute size of fragmented risk pools presented insurers with some underwriting problems, additional problems were caused by the employee selection patterns within multiple choice plans. According to insurers, benefits consultants, and some employers in the Twin Cities, younger and healthier employees tended to select HMOs disproportionately. A common explanation for this phenomenon was that HMOs offered a quick and easy way to become integrated into the health care system for those who were not already. Among those who were not integrated into the health care system previously, there was a high representation of persons who were young or who had never been seriously ill. Conversely, older persons or persons with prior illnesses were more likely to be integrated into the fee-for-service system and to remain there. In addition, the generous

ambulatory coverage available through HMOs appealed strongly
to families with young children, but this group did not make
heavy use of expensive inpatient services. For employees who
are responsible for paying a share of health plan premium costs,
premium differentials among competing plans also affected selection patterns. When HMO premiums were significantly higher
than fee-for-service premiums, selection tendencies are less
strong. HMOs in the Twin Cities, however, were generally successful at reducing or reversing such premium differentials. To
some extent, selection patterns may contribute to reductions in
premium differentials, leading to additional selection of low-risk
enrollees by HMOs.

Informants in the Twin Cities reported that the selection processes outlined above affected fee-for-service insurers' rate-making procedures in two ways. First, the disproportionate retention
of poor risks in fee-for-service plans results in correspondingly
higher experience-based premiums. Second, underwriters had
not yet devised accurate methods for predicting the nature and
extent of self-selection processes. Therefore, they were likely to
set overly conservative rates in a multiple choice situation. As a
general rule of thumb, several interviewees reported that underwriting procedures become disrupted when HMO penetration
rates exceed 15 to 20 percent of a given group.

In the opinion of several benefits consultants, these self-selection and underwriting problems were likely to worsen in the
near future as fee-for-service premiums increase to levels where
only persons who are strongly motivated because of ongoing
treatment regimens will remain in the fee-for-service system.
Eventually, however, this process was expected to stabilize as
HMO members grow older and as the expansion of IPA and network models allow more people to join HMOs without sacrificing
ongoing physician relationships. In addition, increased employee
cost-sharing provisions in fee-for-service plans may limit the selection processes discussed above.

Another major concern on the part of Twin Cities insurers
regarding HMO development focused on the ability of HMOs to
negotiate discounts from hospitals. Until recently, Minnesota
state insurance regulations prohibited insurers from negotiating
any special arrangements with hospitals other than roughly 4 to 5
percent discounts justifiable on a cash flow basis. Since HMOs
were under the regulatory jurisdiction of the Department of

Health, they were exempt from this restriction and were able to obtain larger discounts from hospitals. As a result, the fee-for-service insurance industry was concerned that HMOs exacerbated the hospital cost-shifting problems that they already faced because of public sector limitations on hospital reimbursement.

HMOs AND INSURERS: CHICAGO

Involvement of insurers in HMO development

As in the Twin Cities, insurer involvement in the development of several Chicago HMOs was extensive. In contrast to the Twin Cities, however, insurers were more extensively involved in the ownership and management of HMOs but less involved in the provision of ancillary services to HMOs.

In the early 1970s, CNA Insurance, a locally headquartered firm, funded a feasibility study for the development of Inter-Group HMO. Subsequently, CNA provided venture capital, management services, and management personnel in exchange for a percentage of the HMO's earned premiums. Later, CNA acquired the HMO as a subsidiary, but in 1982 new management decided to sell the HMO to Maxicare, Inc., an HMO owned by Fremont General, a California insurance company.

In the middle 1970s, Blue Cross of Rockford provided extensive capitalization and administrative services to NorthCare, a consumer-sponsored HMO located in the suburb of Evanston. Eventually, this assistance was insufficient to secure the plan's financial viability, and the HMO was sold to Prudential Insurance in 1981. Since that time, Prudential has financed extensive expansion of the plan, which is now called PruCare.

Blue Cross-Blue Shield of Illinois, headquartered in Chicago, was also an early participant in the HMO market. Illinois Blue Cross-Blue Shield developed an early HMO, CoCare, as an internal line of business. CoCare was a network-model HMO that contracted with several other developing HMOs as well as other provider groups. Blue Cross-Blue Shield later restructured the HMO as a subsidiary corporation, HMO Illinois, in compliance with federal qualification requirements that HMOs be separate corporate entities. Also, relationships established by CoCare with other HMOs were gradually eliminated.

More recently, John Hancock Insurance Co. was active in the

Chicago market through its HMO services subsidiary, Hancock-Dikewood. Hancock-Dikewood provided venture capital and an administrative contract to Cooperative Health Plan, a developing IPA model, in exchange for part-ownership of the HMO.

Another recent development has been the involvement of Aetna in the formation of Choice, a PPO. Choice offers incentives for primary care practitioners to refer patients to designated inpatient facilities where a discount has been negotiated. Although Choice does not conform to the typical HMO organizational forms, it has been licensed by Illinois to operate as an HMO.

Unlike the extensive administrative service relationships developed between insurers and HMOs in the Twin Cities, the involvement of insurers in HMO ownership in Chicago is likely to be sustained for as long as the insurers perceive their involvement as advantageous.

Other examples of insurer involvement with HMOs in Chicago were limited for the most part to insurers' offering HMOs to their employees and providing HMOs with fairly routine services such as stop-loss coverage. Insurer involvement in the HMO ancillary services market in the Chicago area was small, perhaps because most HMOs in Chicago were backed by large hospitals or the insurers themselves and did not need to purchase administrative services.

As in the Twin Cities, insurance brokers were not involved with HMOs during their early development. Because HMOs were a less powerful force in the Chicago health insurance market, broker involvement was not expanding as rapidly as in the Twin Cities.

HMO impact on insurers

Representatives of the health insurance industry interviewed for this study reported that HMO development had little or no impact on the industry in Chicago. Overall market shares remained low, and HMOs attained high penetration rates in relatively few accounts. Furthermore, the systematic selection patterns in favor of HMOs, which were widely reported in the Twin Cities, were apparently not present in Chicago. When asked to comment on selection patterns, insurers, benefits consultants, and employers offered mixed responses. In some cases, informants reported that poorer risks selected HMOs in Chicago. The most common explanation for this phenomenon was that the large premium differentials outweighed the usual tendency for younger persons to join HMOs. Another potential area of HMO impact, that of cost-shifting because of hospital discounts, has likewise not manifested itself in the Chicago area as yet.

Currently, HMOs in Chicago are displaying reduced premium differentials and increased growth rates. If this trend continues, market conditions may change rapidly in the Chicago area as HMOs attain market shares large enough to result in impacts on the health insurance industry similar to those observed in the Twin Cities.

SUMMARY

A pattern that is emerging clearly in the Twin Cities is that HMOs are maturing beyond the point where they can reasonably be regarded as experimental organizational forms by insurers. In the Twin Cities, HMOs have captured large market shares and are becoming integrated into traditional health insurance market channels, such as brokers. If HMO development patterns in the Twin Cities continue, and are duplicated on a nationwide basis, it is likely that fee-for-service insurers will exhibit much stronger competitive responses than they have in the past. While it is still too early to determine how closely HMO development patterns in Chicago will mirror those in the Twin Cities, there are some indications that market shares may ultimately be comparable.

In response to changing demand patterns, HMOs may need to make significant adjustments in their products. Strategies that have been implemented or considered by Twin Cities and Chicago HMOs include introduction of copayments, elimination of add-on benefits, and diminished benefits during the first year of enrollment for persons with preexisting conditions. The introduction of copayments by HMOs is particularly noteworthy since first-dollar coverage has been a major attribute differentiating HMOs from less-comprehensive fee-for-service plans.

As a result of many of the ongoing changes discussed above, the health insurance industry appears to be developing from the previous extremes of fee-for-service insurers and HMOs into a continuum of choices of alternative delivery and financing systems. This may be achieved both by the introduction of independent competing plans and by diversification toward middle ground by fee-for-service insurers and HMOs.

7

HMOs and Employers

The Twin Cities employer community tends to act decisively and in concert to implement community objectives. Twin Cities employers were active in HMO development activities in the early 1970s, more to "get involved in improving the health care system" than to "get involved in reducing benefit expenditures." Large corporate employers' support of multiple HMOs have been important factors in HMO development in the Twin Cities. Twin Cities employers, in the late 1970s and early 1980s, became much more concerned with reducing benefit expenditures and their health care activism is being reoriented in this light. Twin Cities employers now want to see documentation of alleged cost savings in HMOs, and they are becoming involved in a wide variety of other cost containment initiatives. Employers in Chicago are much less cohesive, and there has been very little HMO "boosterism." Employers tend to evaluate HMOs strictly as employee-benefit purchases, not as means to improve the health care system at large. In the late 1970s and early 1980s, high levels of interest and activity in cost containment developed. There is increased interest now in HMOs as a component of this broader concern.

Employers serve as purchasing agents for employee health benefits, so they constitute the major market entry point for competitors in the health insurance industry. To gain access to potential enrollees, HMOs must become suppliers of health benefits either through negotiation or through application of federal- or

This chapter was written by Bruce W. Butler, Assistant Project Director.

state-mandated offering provisions. Alternatively, employers themselves may become active in the process of HMO development.

Interviews with forty-four representatives of employers in the Twin Cities and Chicago metropolitan areas were the primary data source for this chapter. The majority of the interviews were with personnel and benefits administrators, ranging from middle management to vice president levels, of large private sector employers. Interviews were also conducted with representatives of public sector employers, small employers, business coalitions, and employee benefits consultants. Additional data sources included published research findings, survey results, and newspaper reports.

HISTORY OF EMPLOYEE HEALTH INSURANCE BENEFITS

Initial involvement of business organizations in health care delivery emerged during the late 1800s in the form of on-site medical services for projects in remote areas. During the early 1900s, employers began to develop benefit packages that included disability payments and industrial medical care. Motivations for expanded involvement included the improvement of employee and community relations as well as the desire to preempt union organization (Munts, 1967).

During the 1940s, federal government policies were important in stimulating the expansion of health benefits. Exemption of fringe benefits from wartime wage and price control guidelines provided strong incentives to introduce or expand health benefits. Shortly after World War II, an interpretation of the Wagner Act of 1935 encouraged the proliferation of union health insurance plans. This set the precedent for requiring employers to negotiate regarding social and health benefits. Previously, only wages and working conditions had been clearly established as mandatory collective bargaining issues (Munts, 1967).

Subsequent expansion of health benefits has been encouraged by continued pressure from organized labor, by efforts to forestall union organization, and by the desire to attract and retain superior employees. Furthermore, because of the economies of group coverage and the tax-exempt status of this form of compensation, health insurance benefits have been more valuable to employees than the equivalent amounts in cash (Ginsburg, 1981; Wilensky and Taylor, 1982; Morrisey, 1983). All of these conditions have contributed to the inclusion of health insurance as a customary component of compensation for the vast majority of employed persons. For the same reasons, the expansion of the proportion of workers eligible for health benefits has been accompanied by expansion in the scope and generosity of benefits. This has been accomplished through increases in the comprehensiveness of health insurance plans and reductions in mandatory employee contributions toward these benefits.

The nationwide market for employee health insurance benefits reached approximately $48.9 billion in 1980, representing 19.8 percent of total national expenditures for health (U.S. Department of Commerce, 1981a, 1981b). The rapid expansion of this market over time is illustrated by its doubling from 8.0 percent to 16.2 percent of total national health expenditures between 1960 and 1970, the same time period that large-scale public sector health programs were being put into place.

For employers reporting specific information on health insurance a recent Chamber of Commerce survey indicated that the average expenditure on health insurance across all industries accounted for 4.7 percent of total payroll. Respective high and low extremes were assigned to the primary metal industry with 7.8 percent of payroll, and the wholesale and retail trade with 4.0 percent of payroll (U.S. Chamber Survey Research Center, 1981). The same survey also indicated that 99 percent of respondent employers across all industries offered life and/or health insurance benefits to their employees. Consequently, the health benefits industry is characterized by a high degree of replacement marketing, with customers switching back and forth among competitors rather than entering the market anew.

Since 1970, employee health benefits have undergone significant change. The trend of benefits expansion, which had been continuing since the 1940s, slowed dramatically in the late 1970s. Also during the past decade, increasingly sophisticated data processing and financial management techniques, such as the retention of cash flows through company self-insured plans, have been applied to employee health benefits. Increasingly, benefit design techniques are being applied to reduce cost escalation. As a result of these developments, the role of employee benefits managers has also changed significantly. Benefits managers have traditionally been charged with developing packages that maximize the employer's abilities to recruit and retain well-qualified employees. Such packages are subject to budgetary constraints determined by executives and to strategic constraints that withhold some benefit increases for the future to demonstrate a continual stream of improvements. According to observers in the insurance industry and benefits consulting firms, however, recent increases in the sophistication of health benefits management and the importance of health benefit cost escalation have resulted in the development of a professional cadre of benefits managers with decision-making responsibilities that affect their companies' financial status and labor market competitiveness.

Concurrent with the trends outlined above, the expanded presence of HMOs has caused additional changes in the traditional health benefits management process. Previously, health insurers typically competed with one another for exclusive contracts with employers on a year-to-year basis. Benefit levels were determined by management or by collective bargaining. If employees made any decisions whatsoever, their choice was limited to a high-option or low-option plan with corresponding differences in payroll deductions. Since HMOs by nature entail some limitation regarding health service providers, they have proven to be infeasible as exclusive sources of health coverage in employee benefit packages. Consequently, the inclusion of HMOs in benefit packages requires that the practice of developing exclusive contracts be abandoned in favor of the simultaneous inclusion of two or more competing plans. From the point of view of the employee, a multiple choice option introduces an unprecedented decision in which individuals must evaluate the insurance value, the payroll deduction, and the health care delivery characteristics of competing plans. In addition, a multiple choice option introduces an unprecedented element of competition for insurers in that they must practice not only industrial marketing but also consumer marketing in their group insurance business.

Based on the characteristics of multiple choice options, a theoretical framework was developed suggesting that the introduction of HMOs into the health insurance market should curtail cost escalation in this industry (Enthoven, 1978; Ellwood, et al., 1981). The ideal health benefits structure on which this theoretical framework was based consisted of an employer who makes a fixed contribution toward an employee's choice among several health plans. The employee pays the difference if the full premi-

um cost of the chosen plan is higher than the employer's contribution. Alternatively, the employee might receive a rebate or
credit toward other benefits if the full premium cost of the chosen plan is less than the employer's contribution. Given this
structure, it was hypothesized that HMOs would be able to provide a more attractive combination of coverage and cost because
of the action of internal financial incentives on participating
physicians. Therefore, cost-limiting rate competition was expected to intensify, and insurers were expected to seek ways to
encourage less costly behavior patterns among fee-for-service
physicians as well.

   This framework predicted that departures from the ideal
benefits structure would detract from the cost containment potential of HMOs. For example, a fixed, limited contribution by an
employer toward an array of differently priced health plans is
thought to introduce cost-limiting consumer price sensitivity.
However, 100 percent payment of the full cost of any offered plan
would eliminate price as an element of competition for enrollees,
within whatever cost boundaries the employer would tolerate.
Thus, the cost containment potential of HMOs is determined not
only by the performance of the HMOs themselves but also by the
ways in which employers integrate them into their overall health
benefits structure.

CHARACTERISTICS OF EMPLOYERS

   The industrial composition of employers in each of the two
metropolitan areas studied is different. While the Twin Cities
workforce comprises a higher percentage of white-collar employees, Chicago has a larger proportion of employers in the
manufacturing industries. The Twin Cities also exhibit slightly
higher percentages of public sector and wholesale/retail workers
than Chicago. Other important contrasts between the two metropolitan areas involve the size and concentration of employers.
While there are roughly three times as many private sector employers in the Chicago area, large employers are slightly more
predominant in the Twin Cities when totals are adjusted for
population. In 1980, the Twin Cities SMSA had 39.7 employers
per million population with 1,000 or more workers (84 establishments), compared to 32.5 employers per million population in
Chicago (231 establishments). Likewise, the Twin Cities SMSA is

home to a disproportionate share of large corporations. Five "Fortune 100" companies are located in the Twin Cities area compared to seven such companies in the Chicago area, which is more than three times larger in population.

As would be expected from nationwide surveys, both metropolitan areas exhibit high proportions of employees who are eligible for health insurance benefits. According to the Bureau of Labor Statistics' periodic Area Wage Surveys covering establishments employing 100 or more workers, 99 percent of both plant and office workers in the Chicago metropolitan area are eligible for some form of health insurance benefits, while 96 percent of plant workers and 99 percent of office workers in the Twin Cities are eligible for such benefits. Despite the slightly lower coverage in the Twin Cities, benefits levels there are somewhat more generous relative to Chicago, as indicated by higher percentages of workers who are eligible for various types of noncontributing health insurance plans (see tables 1.21 and 1.22 on pages 57 and 58). One explanation for this experience is that unemployment rates have historically been lower in the Twin Cities, possibly representing a more competitive labor market.

Minneapolis-St. Paul

In the Twin Cities, respondents pointed out that community business leadership is tightly knit, both professionally and socially. Leadership is derived from approximately twenty chief executives of large locally headquartered firms, with representation from some of the founders (or their descendants) of leading Twin Cities corporations. According to key informants, this leadership group is small enough to facilitate effective working relationships, yet it represents sufficient resources to exercise considerable influence over community affairs. Indeed, the Twin Cities business community has exhibited a pattern of successful cooperative involvement in activities such as the improvement of downtown shopping areas and inner-city housing, and the provision of subsidized loans for small businesses. Corporate involvement is also prevalent in traditional charitable causes, arts and culture, social services, and education. Whereas the national average for corporate giving is approximately 1 percent of pretax profits, at least one major Twin Cities corporation established a pattern of donating 5 percent of pretax profits to charity ever since this amount was first allowed as a tax deduction in 1939. In

1976, a recognition program entitled the "5% Club" for corporate giving was formed in the Twin Cities and has since spread elsewhere. A "2% Club" followed in 1978, and the two clubs have each gained approximately forty-five Twin Cities members.

On a more formal level, two business organizations have been formed to advance corporate activism in community affairs. The Minnesota Project on Corporate Responsibility focuses on internal education regarding social responsibility within participating companies, and the Minnesota Business Partnership attempts to represent corporate interests and to foster cooperation between community organizations and government. Both organizations grew from an annual retreat of Twin Cities business leaders in 1976 that focused on society's decreasing esteem for private enterprise. Both organizations have successfully retained the interest and participation of many high-level executives.

The community of people responsible for making decisions regarding employee benefits parallels the tightly knit character of the business community as a whole. According to employee benefits consultants, there is a "benefits network" consisting of approximately 100 key decision makers representing major employers, insurance carriers, and insurance brokers. Within this network, senior personnel and benefits administrators represent the same group of companies whose chief executives constitute the leadership of the overall business community. Reportedly, communication is extensive within this network and new concepts and developments diffuse rapidly.

Chicago

The Chicago business community is fragmented and scattered because of its size and diversity. Key informants in the Chicago area reported that no single group of business leaders speaks for the interests of the business community as a whole or is involved in a broad range of civic affairs. Instead, a wide variety of ad hoc groups has formed, some more successful than others. Chicago United, a coalition of executives and minority-group leaders, has focused on issues such as race relations and the management of the public school system. The Chicago Association of Commerce and Industry has marshalled the participation of several thousand executives in its community affairs committees. However, an attempt to form a "5% Club" for contributions was largely ignored. In general, coordination and communication within the Chicago business community are inhibited by its own scale, while the relatively intractable nature of many of the area's urban problems has prevented business from assuming a highly visible role in community development activities.

As in the Twin Cities, the people responsible for employee benefits decision making reflect the characteristics of the business community as a whole. While some informants reported extensive communication with their counterparts in other firms, no communitywide network has emerged in the Chicago area. Specific to health benefits, however, several Chicago area employer coalitions are working to counteract this fragmentation. These efforts will be discussed extensively in the following section.

THE DEVELOPMENT OF COST CONTAINMENT EFFORTS

Current concern

Almost unanimously, respondents from the employer sector responded that cost escalation was the most pressing issue in health care facing their organizations. Furthermore, almost all reported that their firms had undertaken specific cost containment measures and were actively considering further measures for the near future. In many instances, these cost containment measures represented significant changes in the organization's health benefits structure and management policies.

These findings contrast sharply with a study conducted in the late 1970s that concluded that "corporations were neither greatly concerned nor strongly motivated to do much about their health care costs" (Sapolsky, et al., 1981). Several possible explanations can be advanced for the discrepancy between studies. First, respondents for this current study reported that actual magnitudes of cost escalation have increased much more rapidly since 1979 than in prior years. It is reasonable, therefore, that higher levels of concern were observed now than in earlier studies. Also, the interviews for this study were conducted in the midst of a deep recession, during which employers were likely to be cutting costs in all operational areas, including employee benefits (Juffer, 1982). The level of authority of people interviewed may also be an important factor contrasting the two studies. In the Sapolsky study, a wide range of executives were interviewed, but there was clearly strong representation from chief executive officers. In this study, respondents were personnel and benefits administrators, ranging up to the vice presidential level. These administrators indicated that their level of concern about health costs was higher than that of the chief executives, who were naturally concerned with a wider range of operational and strategic issues. However, the administrators reported that top executives "raise their eyebrows" or "bluster" at certain milestones of cost escalation, such as increases of annual health insurance premiums exceeding 20 percent without benefits improvement, or the decline of pension costs to second place behind health care as the most expensive fringe benefit. Rather than becoming directly involved in the design or implementation of specific solutions to these problems, top management has typically expressed its concern by issuing open-ended directives to manage health costs more effectively and by allocating increased staff and data processing resources for health benefits management.

Historical basis

The new concern for health benefits cost containment appears to stem from two major types of nascent concern from the 1970s. The first type can be labeled "strategic." This type of concern entailed viewing health care cost escalation as a long-term problem for both the community and the corporation. This concern generated activism in community affairs and the development of innovative benefit policies that did not conflict with an overall pattern of gradual benefits expansion. The second type of concern can be labeled "operational." Included in this category is the development of innovative management practices such as self-insurance and other devices for improving cash flow. Typically, these changes in management practice did not have direct effects on employees' interests.

Informants in the Twin cities reported that strategic concerns regarding health care costs began within the business community as early as the late 1960s. At this time, concern focused not on the absolute level of health expenditures but on the belief that the health care system as a whole was allocating its resources inefficiently by duplicating capital investments and overemphasizing tertiary care. As a result of the general activism of Twin Cities employers in community affairs, these concerns began to be expressed publicly during the early 1970s. One example was the formation of the TCHCDP, a group of employers and insurers that advocated the development of health maintenance organizations on the grounds that HMOs would deliver health care more efficiently than the fee-for-service system. Also during the early 1970s, the Citizens League expressed interest in limiting cost escalation through management of the hospital bed supply. After much controversy regarding the implementation of this strategy, the Citizens League developed an alternative position, also adopted widely within the business community, that competitive system reform provided a more appropriate and effective means for stimulating the reorganization of the health care system around HMOs and other providers. Many Twin Cities employers conformed to the general nationwide trend toward self-insurance to use the health benefits cash flow and avoid premium taxes.

In the Chicago area, employers generally did not exhibit early interest in strategic health care issues. One exception, the Loop Bank Task Force, was formed by personnel executives as a proactive response to the passage of the Employee Retirement Income and Security Act. This group actively monitored and commented on policy developments pertaining to national health insurance in the mid-1970s, but the group disbanded when serious consideration of national health insurance ended. Regarding early operational concerns, however, Chicago employers were at least as involved as Twin Cities employers, and possibly more so. According to several Chicago informants, employers there were among the national leaders in the trend toward self-insurance during the 1970s.

Both strategic and operational aspects of early health care cost containment served to increase employers' familiarity with and expertise regarding health care issues. This early familiarity and expertise provided a foundation for more extensive involvement later on. Some of the major types of cost containment strategies that developed during the 1970s and early 1980s are discussed below.

Health promotion

Although the traditional role of business in health care has been to fund the delivery system, the idea of health promotion has captured the interest of many employers during the past ten years. Defined as "a process of educating individuals in adopting more healthful lifestyles," specific applications include programs in stress management, smoking cessation, hypertension screening, physical fitness, and treatment of alcohol and drug abuse (Sehnert and Tillotson, 1978). The relevance of health promotion programs to cost control is subject to debate. Proponents maintain that these programs offer lower overall health care costs by reducing serious illnesses as well as increased worker productivity through lower absenteeism and improved worker morale. The actual impact of health promotion programs on costs and productivity is difficult to measure conclusively, at least so far.

Several leading Twin Cities employers are strong advocates of health promotion, and there is a fairly high level of interest in the concept among Twin Cities employers in general. This interest, however, developed at a time when benefit expansion in general was still common. Therefore, it is difficult to determine whether these programs were adopted primarily as cost containment programs, as paternalistic devices to improve employee well-being, or as methods of attracting and retaining employees who share the growing popular interest in disease prevention. It is possible that health promotion programs may have been adopted by some firms regardless of cost containment concerns, but that the logical potential of such programs to reduce costs provided employers with additional incentive.

In the Chicago area, several employers had extensive health promotion programs, and many respondents showed at least some enthusiasm for the cost containment potential of disease prevention programs. The overall level of adoption of health promotion programs, however, seems considerably lower than in the Twin Cities. A possible explanation for this difference is that widespread interest in health promotion may have developed later in Chicago, at a time when benefit expansion was less feasible. Among heavily unionized firms, however, several people reported that they were implementing or planning health promotion programs since these were the only cost containment options open to them, given that benefit design was locked in by collective bargaining.

Benefits design

Employers are reluctant to disrupt employee relations by requiring employees to absorb greater shares of their health care costs (Sapolsky, et al., 1981). One person from this study reported that a special effort was made to prepare employees for the news that there would be no health benefits improvements in 1983. A large number of respondents reported that their reluctance was being overcome by the necessity to take action against what they perceive as an acute operational crisis in health benefits costs since 1979.

Employers reported that increasing the employee share of premium costs provided "the quickest fix" for rising health care costs but could conceivably backfire since employees might then be motivated to "get their money's worth" out of health benefits. In contrast, increased deductibles and coinsurance payments were perceived by employers as highly effective since they not only reduced premium costs but also encouraged employees to be more price-sensitive consumers of health care. Restrictions, such as disallowed weekend hospital admissions, were also favored. The implementation of benefit restrictions and increased employee premium shares, deductibles, and coinsurance was widespread, even among firms that operate in competitive labor markets of highly skilled people with generous benefits packages. Some employers reported substituting one type of cost-sharing for another to lessen the impact of benefit redesign on employee relations. For example, one employer replaced a 100 percent-coverage hospitalization plan requiring employee premium contributions with an 80 percent-coverage plan that required no employee contributions.

Employers also reported widespread implementation of improved coverage for alternative services perceived as cost-effective. These services have been included on their own merits and to provide employees with a "trade-off" for increased cost-sharing. Examples include coverage for preadmission testing, second opinions regarding the necessity of surgery, and outpatient surgery. In general, however, employers reported that measures such as these were ineffectual unless strong incentives were established for employees to use them. Examples of such incentives include higher cost-sharing rates for inpatient versus outpatient services, full or partial denial of surgical claims unless supported by a second opinion, and "medical services advisory plans" that require employees to receive advice regarding less costly alternatives prior to hospitalization. Other benefit design innovations include "health incentives plans" that reward employees who receive low-cost health care.

Examples of many of these benefit design strategies exist in both the Twin Cities and Chicago, although strategies that involve actual reductions in benefit levels appear to be somewhat more prevalent in Chicago. Possible explanations for this difference include a higher degree of paternalism among Twin Cities employers and an industrial composition less vulnerable to recession than Chicago's.

Coalition activities

While the strategies outlined above can be undertaken fairly easily by individual employers, strategies that involve attempts to disseminate information to other employers or to influence the behavior of providers, insurers, and government, or that necessitate comparative data bases, are most readily achieved through employer coalitions. Following is a brief overview of some of the various coalition activities that have developed in the Minneapolis-St. Paul and Chicago areas.

The earliest example of a formal health care coalition in either of the two areas was the TCHCDP, which focused on HMOs. The activities of this coalition will be discussed further in this chapter. The Midwest Business Group on Health (MBGH), formed in 1980, was based on prior experience with the Chicago Loop Bank Task Force and was modeled loosely after the Washington Business Group on Health. MBGH has chapters in cities throughout the midwest, including Chicago and Minneapolis-St. Paul. It can be characterized as action-oriented, with major projects in developing private utilization review contracts, improving members' health care cost and utilization information systems, sharing cost and utilization information, educating hospital trustees who are affiliated with member firms, and education programs. To implement the improvement and sharing of cost and utilization data, MBGH members have organized around several "insurer user groups" in which the customers of specific carriers negotiate for the release of aggregate and company-specific data on which to base future cost containment decisions. A subgroup of MBGH, the Chicago Health Economics Council, is working with providers and insurers to establish a private utilization review program.

Reflecting the size and diversity of the Chicago business community, a fairly large amount of coalition activity is being conducted simultaneously, with varying degrees of overlap. The Lake County Business Coalition, which formed independently of MBGH at the same time, shares roughly the same interests and has a high degree of overlapping membership with MBGH. The Illinois Coalition on Health Care Costs consists primarily of insurers and employers, and it actively supported legislative efforts for prospective hospital reimbursement in Illinois. This effort was not successful. The group now focuses on the education of the public regarding cost shifting from public sector health care payors to private sector payors. The Municipal Advisory Council, a group of public sector employers, acts as an information dissemination agent and a Blue Cross-Blue Shield consumers' group. Currently, a health planning group is being formed with the participation of the Chicago Association of Commerce and Industry and the Chicago Hospital Council.

In the Twin Cities, the formation of the Minnesota Coalition on Health Care Costs was initiated by the state medical society and has been characterized as more of an information-sharing group among employers and providers than as an action group. However, the Minnesota Coalition and its employer members, who also belong to the MBGH, were instrumental in the development of a private utilization review program in the Twin Cities. The Twin Cities chapter of MBGH has also been successful in extending the consumers group concept to HMOs.

While there appears to be greater formal coalition development in the Chicago area, the implementation of coalition activities seems to meet with more rapid success in the Twin Cities. As an example, private utilization review was implemented in the Twin Cities in 1981, but it is still in the preoperational stage in Chicago. According to a Chicago coalition representative, this difference in implementation rates is a reflection of the large number of employers in Chicago, each with a small proportionate share of influence. A much higher "critical mass" of coalition involvement must therefore be reached before results can be achieved. In contrast, the tightly knit nature of the Twin Cities business community facilitates the implementation of coalition activity and may to some degree actually preclude the necessity for formal coalition activity since a great deal can be accomplished through long-standing informal networks.

EMPLOYER INVOLVEMENT IN HMO DEVELOPMENT

The business community at large did not show an early interest in Group Health Plan, the first HMO in the Twin Cities. Not until the 1970s did Group Health Plan attract widespread favorable attention from private sector employers. Instead, union groups and public sector employees provided the plan's early enrollment base. The efforts of some unions to have Group Health Plan offered through major employers were strongly opposed by management, which was in some cases influenced by corporate medical directors as well as fee-for-service insurers who threatened to terminate coverage if Group Health Plan was offered.

Employer interest in HMOs was catalyzed in 1971 and 1972 by the formation of the TCHCDP. This project grew out of efforts by Dr. Leon Warshaw, Medical Director of Equitable Life Assurance, to organize employers and insurers in the Twin Cities around a single organization, which would operate as an HMO or at least provide management services to affiliated HMOs. While the centralized concept was rejected by business leaders, this effort was nevertheless instrumental in convincing an influential group of business leaders that prepaid health care offered significant advantages over the fee-for-service system and that employers should participate in a formal organization to promote HMOs. As discussed earlier, employer interest in the health care system at this time was oriented more toward improving efficiency than toward cost containment. Employers were not greatly disturbed by the amounts of money that they were spending on health care, but they were uncomfortable with what they perceived as waste within the system. In the eyes of some of the early organizers of TCHCDP, HMOs provided a means to reduce this waste. TCHCDP seems to be an exception to the general finding of this study that high-level executives are not likely to become closely involved in health benefits issues. However, the nature of TCHCDP is consistent with the tendency of high-level Twin Cities executives to become involved in community affairs in general. TCHCDP may be characterized more accurately as a corporate responsibility and community affairs initiative than a health benefits management initiative.

Two of the key sponsors of TCHCDP, General Mills and Northwestern National Life, participated in the planning and development of MedCenter Health Plan, and they became the first major firms to offer an HMO to their employees. In general, though, the involvement of TCHCDP with specific HMO development efforts was quite limited. Instead, the major accomplishments of the project included the familiarization of the Twin Cities business community with the HMO concept and the provision of a forum for employers and health care providers to discuss HMO development. TCHCDP was not successful in securing passage of state HMO-enabling legislation that would have allowed the development of proprietary HMOs and the offering of individually tailored HMO benefit packages. The compromise legislation that resulted was important nevertheless in granting unambiguous legal status to HMOs.

In the Chicago area, one major bank conducted a feasibility study from 1973 to 1974 regarding the development of its own HMO, but this effort was abandoned prior to the implementation stage. Management considerations for employee benefits contributed to the decisions of two major teaching hospitals to form HMOs, but as a rule Chicago employers did not become involved in the early planning and development of HMOs. While some employers did serve as highly responsive initial customers for developing HMOs, these employers were quite atypical. The few firms that did exhibit early enthusiasm for HMOs either did not attempt or were unable to convince others.

FACTORS INFLUENCING EMPLOYER RESPONSES TO HMOs

Once HMOs were beyond their early developmental stages, they continued to elicit contrasting patterns of response in the respective market areas of Minneapolis-St. Paul and Chicago.

The magnitude of positive employer responses in the Twin Cities stands in sharp contrast to the experience of most other metropolitan areas. According to the Bureau of Labor Statistics Area Wage Survey, 46 percent of plant workers and 64 percent of office workers in the Twin Cities were eligible for HMO coverage in January 1981. In a 1981 survey of 64 large employers in the Twin Cities, 87 percent of the employers surveyed offered at least one HMO, with three or more HMOs offered by 64 percent of the employers (see table 1.21 on page 57).

In contrast to the Twin Cities, the responses of employers in the Chicago area have been generally less favorable to HMO options. The Bureau of Labor Statistics Area Wage Survey indicated that only 22 percent of plant workers and 38 percent of office workers were eligible for HMO coverage in May 1980 (see table 1.22 on page 58).

A nationwide survey of employers located in areas served by HMOs indicated that the main advantages that employers thought they would gain from HMOs were, in order of importance, cost containment, improved health of employees, and reduced claims processing burdens (Lou Harris & Associates, 1980). Regarding cost containment, the largest number of employers who believed that HMOs were effective in containing costs attributed this ability to "undefined reasons," with "stimulation of competition" and "provision of preventive medicine" as the second and third most often mentioned reasons. When asked how current HMO offerings had affected their organization's health benefit costs so far, 70 percent of the respondents reported "no effect" or "too soon to tell," with the remainder almost equally split between "increased costs" and "decreased costs." Major obstacles to employer acceptance of HMOs were, in order of importance, concern about financial stability in HMOs, disapproval of government involvement in HMOs, high cost to employees, and lack of prior experience with HMOs.

Given this national background, survey and interview data focusing on the Twin Cities and Chicago provide additional insights into their individual patterns of response to HMO development. Following are brief descriptions of major sets of factors that influenced employer responses to HMOs in the two areas.

Prior familiarity with the HMO concept

The TCHCDP played an important role in familiarizing employers with the HMO concept by formally disseminating information and by showing examples of enthusiastic involvement with HMOs by several high-profile sponsoring organizations.

Another influence on employers regarding HMOs in the Twin Cities came from InterStudy. Although InterStudy's agenda was national in scope, Paul Ellwood and Walter McClure addressed many local business meetings and luncheons, providing the conceptual framework of HMOs as a way to increase the efficiency of the health care system without sacrificing quality.

As a result of these influences, HMOs in the Twin Cities benefited from a pool of employers who did not require extensive additional familiarization with the concepts of prepaid health care or multiple choice benefit plans. TCHCDP participation in the political process leading to state HMO legislation may have also defused some of the suspicion of government involvement in HMOs that employers have exhibited on a nationwide basis. In addition, the fact that many of the TCHCDP participants were fairly high-level executives undoubtedly facilitated HMO development because policy changes could be implemented more quickly from above.

In the Chicago area, the DuPage County Comprehensive Health Planning Agency, a Health Systems Agency precursor, made an attempt to catalyze employer interest in HMOs prior to 1973. Although the agency sponsored several forums for employers, little interest was generated. An informant, who was involved in this effort, reported that much of the difficulty in generating employer interest stemmed from a fairly high level of satisfaction with existing fee-for-service benefit plans. Opposition from physicians was expressed through social networks and was also a factor. As was mentioned previously, the early positive responses by some Chicago employers did not spread to other firms. Thus, HMOs developing in Chicago were faced with the challenge of marketing to a large, diverse employer community that possessed very little familiarity with the HMO concept.

Since 1980, the Executive Service Corps, an organization of retired executives, has developed a project with several full-time staff members that is designed to eliminate some of the barriers to HMO development. Efforts of the Executive Service Corps in this regard have included developing various generic advertising efforts, conducting meetings and forums on HMOs for high-level executives, and advocating the HMO concept through the extensive professional networks still available to the organization's retired volunteers.

Prior involvement with carriers, brokers and self-insured plans

As mentioned above, satisfaction with fee-for-service insurance coverage contributed to the lack of interest with HMOs in Chicago. Likewise, this factor was mentioned to explain why many Twin Cities employers, some of whom had been involved extensively in TCHCDP, delayed offering HMOs.

Commitment to the status quo appeared to have been stronger in both areas among employers who had invested resources in self-insured plans. Such employers considered themselves "out of the market" for health insurance, and they were perhaps biased toward their own product.

Companies that depended on insurance brokers to design their benefit plans were also relatively slow to develop relationships with HMOs. HMOs have been relatively slow to develop relationships with brokers. Small firms rely heavily on brokerage services and have tended therefore to remain isolated from HMO marketing efforts. Small employers are also more vulnerable to risk pool fragmentation and, in some cases, are in danger of losing their status as insurable groups (in the eyes of fee-for-service insurers) if they develop multiple choice plans. While these factors have tended to limit the involvement of small employers with HMOs, several other factors indicate nevertheless that small employers may provide a potential market to HMOs. As HMOs become more established and exhaust their growth opportunities with large employers, it will become increasingly beneficial for HMOs and brokers to develop relationships with one another. In addition, small employers are often subjected to unstable premiums because of experience-rating by insurers. HMOs are in some cases providing a more attractive alternative for small employers since they are in effect pooling the risk of small employers in community-based rating structures.

Additional factors that affect the willingness of employers of any size to supplement satisfactory and established fee-for-service health insurance plans with HMO options involve perceptions regarding the cost containment potential, benefit quality, administrative complexity, and union approval of HMOs. Ultimately, some employers offer HMOs only in compliance with the mandate provisions of the federal HMO act. These and other factors are discussed further below.

Premium costs and cost containment potential

In both metropolitan areas, HMO premiums at the time of their introduction were considerably higher than most fee-for-service premiums. Reasons for these initial differences may have included the obvious factor of more comprehensive benefits as well as economies of scale for large established plans and the cash flow and premium tax advantages of self-insured plans. Competition with self-insured plans may be particularly difficult for HMOs in high-cost medical care markets, such as Minneapolis-St. Paul and Chicago, since some employers average the utilization and cost experiences of their nationwide operations to develop a base cost per employee.

During the course of HMO development, HMO premiums have tended to increase more slowly than fee-for-service premiums. Consequently, premium differentials are shrinking or reversing. This process appears to have occurred more rapidly in the Twin Cities, where very few employers reported significant premium differences by 1982. In Chicago, responses were more mixed. Employers reported generally that HMO premiums have decreased relative to fee-for-service premiums in recent years. Many reported, however, that significant differences remain.

Twin Cities HMOs may have some advantage over HMOs in other areas regarding premium competitiveness because of a relatively comprehensive and expensive benefit package mandated for fee-for-service carriers in Minnesota. The mandated benefit package eliminates some of the traditional differences in coverage between HMOs and fee-for-service insurers, thus increasing the ability of HMOs to compete favorably on price. Fee-for-service insurers in the Twin Cities have had particular difficulties controlling the costs of mandated mental health and chemical dependency coverage, but HMOs have managed these costs by developing innovative capitation agreements with outpatient counseling centers.

Premium cost differentials are most salient for employers who pay a high percentage of health benefit costs because of collective bargaining agreements or employee relations policies. Even for employers who contribute a fixed-dollar amount toward premiums, however, the total premium costs of HMOs are perceived as a signal regarding the plausibility of HMOs as cost containment devices.

In the Twin Cities, appearances suggest that employers disregarded initial premium differentials in favor of the cost containment logic of the HMO concept introduced to them through the familiarity-building channels outlined above. In other words, employers seemed willing to invest higher initial premium costs on the promise of future reductions. Indeed, Twin Cities employers generally exhibited a strong belief in the concept that HMOs have greater cost containment potential than fee-for-service medicine because of incentives for preventive medicine and utilization control. A smaller group of employers articulated the concept of cost containment through alternative delivery system competition. When pressed to discuss the critical motivations behind the actual management decision to offer HMOs, however, many of the Twin Cities respondents reported that cost containment considerations were secondary at most. Instead, HMOs were offered by many Twin Cities employers in the early and middle 1970s based on the perception that HMOs were a "better value." Employers were interested in expanding their benefits packages and HMOs provided a relatively economical way of doing this. For some employers, HMOs were attractive simply because they offered the promise of better health care for their employees with little or no consideration of costs. In summary, early premium differentials were apparently a relatively small issue for Twin Cities employers because of their perceptions of HMOs' efficiency, value, quality, and future cost containment potential.

In the Chicago area, those employers who believed that HMOs had greater cost containment potential than fee-for-service coverage credited the same factors as their Twin Cities counterparts—preventive medicine and internal utilization control. However, Chicago employers showed greater emphasis on and expectation of the preventive medicine factor. Very few Chicago area employers articulated the idea that HMOs are instrumental in stimulating competitive reform systemwide.

While selected Chicago employers expressed the cost containment perceptions outlined above, Chicago employers in general exhibited relatively low acceptance of these concepts. Only a few employers expressed strong belief in the cost containment potential of HMOs, and an additional group expressed favorable but tentative perceptions. A large number of informants in Chicago did not attribute any particular cost containment properties to HMOs other than the need to be price-competitive with other forms of health insurance. Likewise, Chicago employers in general were less enthusiastic about the benefits and health care attributes of HMOs. As a result, objective premium differentials have probably been a more important issue for Chicago employers than for Twin Cities employers.

As the acuity of cost containment concerns has increased and the range of premium differentials has diminished, Twin Cities employers have become more interested in the prospects of objective cost savings from HMOs. For the same reasons, increased numbers of Chicago employers have become interested in developing relationships with HMOs. Employers are uncertain, however, of the ability of HMOs to retain their current competitiveness in the face of fee-for-service premium cutting efforts, such as increased deductibles and copayments.

Quality of benefits and health care delivery

To evaluate the attractiveness of HMOs, employers tended to focus on the following factors: reputation of affiliated providers, convenience of delivery site locations, value of HMO benefit structures of their employees, and the medical care delivery structure of HMOs. Ultimately, employers are concerned that HMOs serve as positive employee relations tools, or conversely, that HMOs not create employee dissatisfaction that would reflect poorly on the company.

The attitudes of fee-for-service physicians have had a negative impact historically on the reputations of HMO-affiliated providers. In the Twin Cities, however, possible reservations that employers might have had regarding HMO providers were eliminated early by the association of St. Louis Park Medical Center with MedCenter Health Plan. MedCenter's location was also thought to influence employers, since many key decision makers resided in the vicinity of St. Louis Park. Location factors were rarely regarded as drawbacks by Twin Cities employers since small travel times and the willingness of Twin Cities residents to go outside their neighborhoods for medical care allowed HMOs to develop satisfactory networks of delivery sites rapidly. If an employer found that a single HMO could not adequately serve the geographic distribution of employees, one or two additional HMOs were usually sufficient.

In the Chicago area, the credibility of technical quality in HMOs was increased by the early involvement of respected teaching hospitals in HMO development. However, the inner-city location of these hospitals limited their acceptability as primary-care providers. Although the hospital-based HMOs undertook satellite clinic development efforts and two network-model HMOs developed affiliations with geographically dispersed medical groups, the size of the metropolitan area and the existence of numerous medical submarkets inhibited the HMOs' efforts to develop a delivery infrastructure that satisfied employers' desires for uniform availability to all employees. Another factor that has limited the willingness of Chicago employers to offer HMOs is a perceived relationship of "clinics" and "health centers" with low-quality welfare medicine.

Employers in both areas who were satisfied that HMO providers were of acceptable quality tended to develop corporate policies in favor of multiple choice plans based on the principle that employees should have free choice among health care delivery systems. Ironically, the logic behind the policies was sometimes expressed in a fashion that closely paralleled arguments against HMOs on the grounds that they restricted free choice of physicians.

Employers in both areas recognized that comprehensive first-dollar coverage in HMOs would be particularly attractive to certain types of employees. Categories most often mentioned were young persons with small children and persons with chronic health problems. As mentioned earlier, employers were in some cases attracted to HMOs as a structural improvement over fee-for-service medicine. The potential advantages perceived included preventive medicine (also a cost containment factor) and coordination of care.

Positive perceptions regarding benefits and medical care quality were stronger and more prevalent in the Twin Cities. In Chicago, improved medical care delivery structure was rarely attributed to HMOs. Instead, Chicago employers tended either to have no opinion on the medical care delivery structure of HMOs or to use negative labels, such as "bureaucratic" or "impersonal." Regarding benefits structures, Chicago employers were well aware of the comprehensive first-dollar coverage of HMOs. Chicago employers, however, were generally satisfied with opportunities for benefit improvements in the existing fee-for-service structure.

Administrative efforts and costs

Employers in both areas agreed that the initial development of multiple choice health benefits plans required a significant administrative investment and that the subsequent management of multiple choice plans required great effort during open enrollment periods. Employers also agreed that HMOs reduced claims processing and day-to-day paperwork. Most employers reported that there are no systematic differences in the number of employee complaints between HMOs and fee-for-service insurers.

In the Twin Cities, these advantages and disadvantages were recognized by major employers but were not considered to be important factors in the initial decision to offer HMOs. In Chicago, administrative efforts and costs appeared to have slightly greater importance, but they were not mentioned as decisive factors for major employers. Several employers mentioned the concern that administrative efforts to develop multiple choice plans would be wasted if very few employees subsequently enrolled in HMOs.

For small employers, benefits consultants reported that the administrative considerations outlined above take on greater importance since small employers often devote less than one full-time employee to benefits administration. The administrative tasks associated with multiple choice could be prohibitive, yet the decreased claims administration burdens associated with HMOs could be attractive.

An additional factor affecting the administrative complexity of multiple choice health plans for some employers is the nature of union response to HMOs. This topic is considered separately in chapter 8, but it is relevant that HMOs introduced additional complexities into the collective bargaining process. Employers with unionized workforces may be discouraged from offering HMOs because of the additional negotiating efforts required.

Federal qualification

Three major factors regarding federal HMO qualification were mentioned by employers: government evaluation of HMO financial stability, government evaluation of HMO quality, and the ability of federally qualified HMOs to activate legislation requiring employers with twenty-five or more workers to offer HMOs in their benefit plans. Employers tended to fall into several distinct categories regarding the level of importance that they placed on federal qualification, ranging from supporting the HMO concept regardless of federal qualification to reluctantly offering HMOs only in compliance with legislation.

For the group of Twin Cities employers who included HMOs in their benefit plans during the early 1970s federal qualification was obviously not an important issue. At this time, no Twin Cities HMOs were federally qualified.

A smaller group of Chicago employers also fell into this category, offering HMOs before they became federally qualified. Several Chicago employers, who later offered federally qualified HMOs in response to mandates, stated that they would have offered HMOs eventually in any case.

Another major category of employers showed neutral or positive attitudes regarding HMOs but offered only federally qualified plans. Typically, firms that adopted this policy were large and decentralized, with large workforces scattered across the country. Such employers were apparently not willing or able to expend the great effort required to evaluate the quality and financial status of many independent HMOs in multiple locations. Federal qualification was used as an indicator of acceptability. As benefits managers increased internal familiarity and expertise with HMOs and with health care in general, employers seemed to be more confident of their ability to evaluate HMOs independently. Several informants reported that while they had offered only federally qualified HMOs in the past, they were now considering exceptions to this policy. Since the risk of HMO bankruptcy and subsequent employer liability for claims was mentioned as a primary reason for offering only federally approved HMOs, employers may be willing to accept the backing of large financially stable HMO parent organizations in lieu of federal qualification status.

In the Twin Cities, a significant number of major employers refrained from offering HMOs in the early 1970s. These firms were not necessarily unfamiliar with or skeptical of HMOs, since several had been active participants in the TCHCDP. In 1976, SHARE Health Plan obtained federal qualification and activated mandating procedures for many of the reluctant employers. As a result, by the late 1970s, almost all major Twin Cities employers offered HMOs. Many of the mandated employers then evaluated the local HMO market as a whole, and they concluded that it was necessary to offer one or several HMOs in addition to SHARE so that employee residence patterns would be uniformly served and so that employees could choose from a variety of plans. Thus, competition among HMOs was also increased by the mandating process.

The response of Twin Cities employers to the mandating process stands in contrast to other metropolitan areas in which considerable antagonism resulted. A possible explanation for this atypical reaction is that Twin Cities employers in general had a favorable attitude toward HMOs whether they offered them at the time or not. At the very least, the federal mandate process was apparently applied mainly to employers that fit this description. Several employers, who did not offer HMOs until they were mandated, reported that they followed this course out of conservatism, preferring to observe the experiences of other employers rather than having a trial experience themselves. Since the reports of firms that had early HMO experiences were generally favorable, it was not a significant disruption for the reluctant firms to be forced by regulation to abandon their conservatism.

Faced with a more adverse set of market conditions, Chicago HMOs undertook correspondingly more aggressive mandating policies in the middle to late 1970s. The various responses of employers to this strategy reflect employers' wide range of prior exposure and attitudes regarding HMOs. Employers that exhibited the most favorable responses to mandating were large national firms, which had experienced favorable relationships with HMOs in other parts of the country or had monitored the federal HMO legislation and had decided to comply with the law. Attitudes expressed among such firms included relatively enthusiastic HMO advocacy statements, e.g., "Given that we were required by law to offer HMOs, we decided to do the best job we could of offering them." The responses of these firms to mandates resembled patterns in the Twin Cities in that multiple HMO offerings often resulted from a single mandate.

Another characteristic group of Chicago employers regarded HMO mandates as just another government intervention in the already heavily regulated activity of providing employee fringe benefits. Employers in this category expressed indifference toward HMOs, which was often reinforced by extremely low rates of HMO enrollment among their employees.

Finally, a small group of employers expressed great antagonism toward the mandating process. Several employers reported that their initial reactions to receiving mandates in the mail consisted of shock, confusion, annoyance, and quick telephone calls to colleagues or consultants in an effort to learn what an HMO was. While some employers, who were taken by surprise by the mandate process, subsequently developed positive or at least tolerant attitudes, others retaliated by threatening to preempt mandates by offering competing HMOs instead of the mandate initiator, collaborating with unions to take advantage of the unions' option to exclude their members from mandated HMO offerings, restructuring fee-for-service benefit plans to provide employees with strong disincentives against enrolling in HMOs, and generally adopting an attitude of noncooperation with HMOs.

FACTORS INFLUENCING EMPLOYEE PARTICIPATION AND SATISFACTION

After employers choose to offer HMOs or are required to do so by mandates, the response of employees to HMO options assumes primary importance in determining HMO development patterns. Factors determining the response of employees include prior exposure, HMO marketing efforts and the extent of employer cooperation with these efforts, premium costs and the insurance value of covered services, convenience of delivery sites, perceptions regarding HMO technical quality and ambiance, and the degree of employee commitment to the fee-for-service system.

Prior familiarity with the HMO concept

Although the existence of Group Health Plan in the Twin Cities prior to 1970 was not generally regarded as an important factor in the formation of employer attitudes toward HMOs, several benefits consultants reported that prior familiarity with Group Health Plan in the public at large had a strong influence on early employee responses toward HMOs. Informants reported that generally high levels of commitment and satisfaction among early Group Health Plan members resulted in favorable word-of-mouth endorsements regarding the HMO concept among the public at large. Several employers also reported that employees were influenced by media coverage surrounding the Twin Cities Health Care Development Project and made inquiries of their benefits departments regarding the possibility of joining HMOs at that time.

In Chicago, the familiarity of the general public with HMOs remained at a fairly low level. Benefits managers often reported that relatively few employees have working knowledge of the definition of an HMO. Early media coverage of HMOs in Chicago was limited.

HMO marketing and employer cooperation

Traditional group health insurance marketing was not consumer-oriented since employers and/or unions determined the coverage and communicated the outcome to employees. With the advent of HMOs and multiple choice plans, however, consumer marketing has entered the group health insurance field, using media advertising, group presentations, brochures, and mailings. With the exception of media advertising, employer cooperation is essential for HMOs to gain access to employee audiences. Since employees have traditionally received all of their health insurance information from benefits managers or union representatives, the actual participation of these individuals in the HMO marketing process was reported to be an important implicit endorsement, which allayed employee reluctance to experiment with HMO enrollment.

As an expression of their overall positive attitudes toward HMOs, Twin Cities employers cooperated with efforts by HMOs to market to their employees. Examples include group meetings on company time with participation from benefits officers, the provision of employee mailing lists to HMOs, and in-house documents and films describing and comparing HMOs. While this cooperation often reflected active strategies to encourage HMO enrollment, it was also recognized by neutral employers that multiple choice health benefit plans were a radical departure from the standard procedure of offering a single package that required no evaluation by employees. Extensive employee education programs were instituted to avoid misconceptions and oversights, particularly regarding emergency room usage and self-referral limitations in HMOs.

Employers in the Chicago area exhibited a wide range of cooperativeness regarding HMO marketing efforts. Several employers reported that they actively advocated HMO enrollment among their employees. One firm, which had originally offered HMOs to comply with the HMO act, actively promoted HMOs among its employees when it discovered that, contrary to the experience of most other Chicago employers, HMO premiums were lower than the costs of its self-insured plan. In general, however, active promotion of the HMO concept was rare among Chicago employers and the tolerance of extensive contact between HMO marketers and employees was low in comparison to the Twin Cities. Many employers made conscientious internal efforts to communicate the nature of HMO options to their employees, but others applied very little effort at all. A few employers stated that it was inappropriate for them to cooperate with marketing efforts or conduct their own communication efforts since these activities would imply favoritism. While Chicago employers were less uniformly enthusiastic than their counterparts in the Twin Cities regarding the communication of HMO options to employees, even those Chicago firms that undertook extensive efforts experienced HMO penetration rates far below typical Twin Cities levels. This was confirmed by the experience of several firms with operations in both metropolitan areas. These firms reported drastically different results in the two areas despite standardized policies and procedures toward HMOs. When asked to speculate regarding factors that account for low HMO penetration rates in Chicago, respondents pointed to premium cost, facility location, and quality perceptions.

Cost and coverage differentials

When evaluating the cost of joining an HMO, employees are responsive to the magnitude of their share of the premium as well as the expected effect that the level of coverage in an HMO will have on their out-of-pocket medical expenses (Berki and Ashcraft, 1980). The magnitude of employee premium share is determined by the total premium cost and the policies of individual employers regarding cost-sharing. The relative importance of cost and coverage for individual employees is influenced by factors such as number of dependents, discretionary income, and expected future medical care utilization. When employers pay a very high percentage of premium costs, the relative comprehensiveness of an HMO constitutes an unqualified cost advantage to employees, provided that provisions like restricting emergency room use and out-of-plan self-referrals are accepted.

In the Twin Cities, employers reported that early premium differentials between HMOs and fee-for-service plans did not have a significant negative impact on HMO enrollment patterns since the differences were not great enough to outweigh coverage advantages and other attractive features. HMO penetration rates have expanded further, and HMO premiums have decreased relative to fee-for-service plans. Still, informants generally did not perceive a causal relationship between these two trends. If anything, decreased premium differentials were thought to be caused by increased HMO size.

In contrast, Chicago employers speculated that high premium differentials between HMOs and fee-for-service plans were at least partially responsible for low initial HMO penetration rates, and that recent reductions in the premium differentials were at least partially responsible for later increases in HMO enrollment. Even employers that paid 100 percent of all premium costs, however, did not experience dramatically higher levels of HMO enrollment. This suggests that factors other than cost were at least as important in determining employee response patterns.

Convenience and quality

Perceptions garnered from hearsay and other sources affect employees' willingness to enroll in HMOs, and actual experiences after enrollment affect employees' willingness to remain enrolled as well as influencing the type of information they pass on to others. As reported by benefits managers, on behalf of their employees, perceptions regarding quality incorporated not only technical capabilities of providers but the attractiveness of facilities and personalization of services as well. Perceptions regarding convenience included the location of facilities, amount of paperwork involved, length of lead time for appointments, amount of time spent in waiting rooms, and the ability to obtain multiple services at a single location.

Twin Cities employers reported that many of the early "risk-taking" HMO enrollees had been fee-for-service patients at the medical groups initially affiliated with HMOs. Thus, many of the early enrollees were already satisfied with many of the factors listed above. Later, employers reported continued high levels of employee satisfaction, particularly with locations and the lack of claims and bills to process. Negative experiences were rare, and they tended to focus on problems obtaining appointments.

Experiences in Chicago were much more diverse. As in the Twin Cities, prior relationships with participating providers encouraged employees to join HMOs. For other employees, benefits managers reported some reluctance because of inconvenient locations and perceived possibility of being treated by foreign medical graduates. Once employees were enrolled, their satisfaction was limited in some cases by long waiting lines, impersonal service, and site closures. Employers were also disturbed by the turmoil that resulted from site closures between open enrollment periods. Negative perceptions and experiences were far from universal, however, and many employers reported that favorable attitudes regarding HMOs are building among employees because of the same positive attributes mentioned above in regard to Twin Cities HMOs. It should be noted that benefits administrators generally regarded location as the most important of any of the convenience or quality factors mentioned above. Increased HMO enrollments in recent years were strongly associated by employers with the development of additional delivery sites.

Commitment to the fee-for-service system

In both metropolitan areas, employers reported that reluctance to abandon existing relationships with fee-for-service physicians inhibited some employees from joining HMOs. Some employees were also reluctant to give up the option of receiving care at "medical meccas," such as the Mayo Clinic, or at well-known universities in the event that they developed severe, life-threatening conditions. Similarly, benefits managers occasionally reported that employees interpreted the emphasis of HMOs on cost containment to mean that their access to high-technology medical care would be limited. As might be expected, employers reported that the expansion of IPA and network models allowed more employees to join HMOs without changing physicians.

In the Chicago area, an interesting case illustrating these issues was reported by a municipal employer. This agency employed a workforce with an extremely high average age, and its experience-rated fee-for-service premiums were correspondingly high. To alleviate this problem, the agency offered several HMOs, but very few employees enrolled. To encourage employees to join, the agency began to require employee contributions to fee-for-service premiums, but HMO premiums were paid in full by the employer. Still, very few employees enrolled. Finally, the agency added $1,500 deductibles to their fee-for-service plan. At this point, there was widespread HMO enrollment. Thus, reluctance to exit from the fee-for-service plan may be impervious to relatively small financial incentives, but it is ultimately responsive to cost.

The tendency of employees to retain fee-for-service use patterns even after enrolling in an HMO provided employers with difficulties in both metropolitan areas. Anecdotes regarding the burden of mediating reimbursement conflicts between HMOs and employees who "did not understand that they could no longer go running off to emergency rooms all the time" were fairly common.

Employers with well-established self-insured plans reported some degree of employee reluctance to abandon fee-for-service coverage out of loyalty to the company. Employees who had been with a company for a long time developed a strong allegiance to the "company plan" and thought it inappropriate to switch, particularly if they knew that the company was offering HMOs in compliance with federal regulation.

Selection patterns

Many of the consumer decision factors outlined above affect not only the overall rate of HMO enrollment growth but also the greater selection of certain groups into HMOs. While some Twin Cities employers reported no significant differences in selection patterns between HMOs and fee-for-service, most informants reported some or all of the following patterns. Groups considered most likely to join HMOs included young persons and new hires from out-of-town, employees with young families, and persons who had already been fee-for-service patients of HMO-affiliated medical groups and physicians. Groups thought less likely to join HMOs included older persons who had established long-term doctor-patient relationships or other habits favoring fee-for-service medical care and insurance.

In addition to the above factors, Chicago employers mentioned that HMOs were particularly attractive to people who were risk-averse because they had little discretionary income and to people who expected great need for medical care for themselves or their family members because of chronic illness. Several employers reported that the tendency for young families to join HMOs was affected in Chicago by the slow development of HMO delivery sites in parts of the metropolitan area where young families tend to reside. One benefits manager in a firm that actively promoted HMO enrollment reported that the company's relocation assistance department typically placed newly hired professionals with families in a far-west suburban area that had no HMO delivery sites.

HMO IMPACT ON EMPLOYERS

In general, the impact of HMO development on employers is related to the proportion of employees within the company or in the community at large who actually enroll in HMOs. Major categories of impact include employee relations, administrative effort and cost containment.

Employee relations

In the Twin Cities, HMOs were originally thought to have positive employee relations effects because of their comprehensive coverage and perceived quality. As a larger proportion of the population enrolled in HMOs, they nearly became a necessity for employers who wished to be competitive in the local labor market. One benefits consultant illustrated this point by reminding employers that they could expect that one out of four people hired from the local market in 1982 would be an HMO enrollee and would probably wish to remain with a particular HMO. Employers are encouraged, therefore, to offer several or all of the available HMOs.

Chicago employers reported that HMOs are well liked by a small proportion of the workforce. However, HMO development has not yet affected the labor market to the point that employers are pressured by employees to offer HMOs.

Administrative efforts

Some fixed administrative investments, such as the development of multiple payroll deductions and employee education efforts, are required for the employer to be able to offer HMOs, but the payoff in terms of reduced claims processing workloads is related to enrollment levels. However, employers in both areas reported that while administrative factors were noticeable, they were not extremely important.

Cost containment

Since most employers reported that health care cost escalation was the most pressing issue in health benefits management, the effects of HMOs on health care costs assumed a central role in most interviews.

Employers in the Twin Cities exhibited continued enthusiasm for the role of health maintenance organizations in cost containment, and they cited the ability of HMOs to lower their premiums to levels equal to or less than fee-for-service premiums. However, many employers qualified their enthusiasm by pointing out that the effects of HMOs on health care costs may be more complex than comparisons of premium costs indicate.

First, some employers expressed concern that HMOs were not providing premiuim cost savings to the fullest extent possible. Instead, it was reported that when HMO and fee-for-service premiums became roughly equivalent, HMOs began to compete for enrollees by expanding their range of covered services rather than seeking to undercut fee-for-service premiums. HMOs felt this strategy would be advantageous since few employers offered their employees any incentive for enrolling in plans that cost less than the company's base premium contribution. In response to this strategy, employers reported only limited negotiating power over HMOs that had already enrolled large numbers of their employees. While changing fee-for-service health insurance would have little or no effect on employees, changes in HMO offerings could be highly disruptive for employees. Therefore, employers threatened to terminate an HMO's access to their employees only in extreme cases. Despite this concern, very few employers reported that they were considering any structural changes in their benefit plans that would eliminate the incentive for HMOs to compete in this manner. One method, the development of flexible benefit plans in which employees would receive credit toward other benefits in exchange for choosing a less expensive health plan, was being implemented by a small number of Twin Cities employers. In general, however, employers were skeptical of the large investment in management information systems and employee communications that would be required to run such a program.

Twin Cities employers also expressed concern regarding the impact on total costs of employee self-selection between fee-for-service plans and HMOs. Since HMOs often appealed more strongly to young persons, employers were uncertain whether HMO premiums represented cost-effectiveness or merely healthier risk pools. If in fact low-risk employees were joining HMOs while high-risk employees remained in fee-for-service plans, employers would find their higher risks in a self-insured or experienced rated plan, with lower risks in plans that might be fully or partially community-related. Thus, employers would be paying fee-for-service premiums for a known high-risk group, but they would have no way of knowing if their HMO premiums truly reflected their group experience, or instead might include a cross-subsidization factor from another employer with high-risk HMO enrollees.

Most Twin Cities benefits consultants expressed the opinion that self-selection problems will eventually work themselves out as HMO members age and greater proportions of physicians affiliate with HMOs. In the short run, however, employers were sufficiently concerned about self-selection and competition through coverage expansion, and they were making strong demands for company-specific utilization data from HMOs. The local chapter of the MBGH was serving as a central negotiating agent in this effort, and it raised the possibility of collective termination of HMO offerings for plans that did not comply. Reportedly, HMOs were complying reluctantly since the divulgence of how risk is spread across groups may disrupt their rate-making procedures.

Chicago employers, with a few exceptions, reported that HMOs were having little or no impact on their health care costs because HMO premiums were still higher than fee-for-service premiums and because HMO penetration rates were not high enough to create problematic selection patterns. When selection patterns were discussed in Chicago, the migration of unfavorable risks into HMOs was mentioned at least as often as the migration of favorable risks. Explanations of adverse selection into HMOs centered on premium costs and included the argument that if an HMO were extremely expensive to an employee, only persons in dire need of more comprehensive coverage would enroll. Furthermore, employers generally agreed that any adverse selection into HMOs occurring already would probably be intensified by the trend toward increased coinsurance and deductibles in fee-for-service plans because these measures penalize high utilizers and increase premium differentials. Because of these market conditions, several benefits consultants and insurers speculated that employers would increasingly seek cost savings by "dumping" high-risk employees into community-rated HMOs. This topic was touched on by only one benefits manager, who reported that he would counsel employees with chronic illnesses to avoid deductible and coinsurance provisions by joining HMOs. Thus, HMOs in Chicago may be having a greater impact on employee health benefit costs than is apparent from premium cost comparisons, but only because of a process that is disadvantageous to the HMOs themselves. In response to these market conditions, several HMOs were considering the development of low-option plans with deductibles to minimize premium differentials believed to be responsible for their adverse selection problems.

SUMMARY

The growth of health maintenance organizations is highly dependent on the response of consumers in the health insurance benefits market. This market is two-tiered, with employers making decisions regarding HMOs' access to group accounts, and employees making the actual enrollment decisions.

Health benefits consumers in Minneapolis-St. Paul and Chicago exhibited markedly different patterns of response to the introduction of HMOs. To some extent, these differential patterns may be due to differential attributes of the HMOs themselves. However, this study delineates a number of characteristics of health benefits consumers themselves that may contribute to differential response patterns. These characteristics include the employer communities' levels of cohesiveness and geographic dispersion, the existence and effectiveness of HMO advocates within the employer community, and the nature of demand for health benefits in general.

The cohesiveness and moderate size of the Twin Cities business community suggest that new concepts, if perceived as advantageous by opinion leaders, are likely to gain relatively quick widespread acceptance. Not only were HMOs perceived as advantageous by some Twin Cities employer community opinion leaders, but several major employers pursued activist policies promoting HMOs. As a result, Twin Cities employers tended to offer HMOs to their employees relatively early, and exhibited a relatively high degree of cooperation with HMOs. Employment and residence patterns in the Twin Cities made it relatively easy for Twin Cities HMOs to develop delivery site networks convenient to most employees. Minnesota employers were required by state law to offer a comprehensive set of health benefits, making it easy for HMOs to compete with fee-for-service plans on a premium basis. The Twin Cities labor market is relatively competitive, which may also have stimulated the provision of comprehensive benefits. Federal mandate provisions were used selectively in the Twin Cities and did not have significant negative repercussions, perhaps because of the high level of prior familiarity with HMOs even among employers who were ultimately mandated. In general, Twin Cities employers adopted an active role as HMO consumers, participating in development efforts, responding enthusiastically to their presence in the health benefits market, and often taking the initiatives to develop relationships with HMOs.

In contrast, the Chicago employer community exhibited a number of characteristics that probably inhibited HMO development. The large, fragmented, and diffuse nature of the Chicago business community suggested that it would be relatively difficult for any new product or service to gain a large share of industrial markets. While Chicago employers occasionally pursued activist policies on community issues, such as education, mass transportation, and race relations, their involvement in health care was relatively conservative until recently. Few if any employers promoted HMO development in the community, and those employers who adopted the HMO concept early did not have strong influence over other employers. Employer coalitions, which later came to play important roles in the health care system, adopted neutral roles in HMO development in accordance with the priorities of their constituents. Commuting patterns in the Chicago area and the existence of numerous medical submarkets made it relatively difficult for HMOs to develop delivery site networks convenient to the majority of employees. The overall comprehensiveness of health benefits appeared to be lower in the Chicago area than in the Twin Cities, at least for the nonunion workforce. This may be due to a less competitive labor market or less vigorous regulatory requirements regarding mandated benefits. The use of federal mandates by HMOs in Chicago had mixed results, with the most favorable reactions coming from large national firms with prior HMO experience and the least favorable reactions coming from smaller local firms for whom mandates provided an initial introduction to the HMO concept. In general, Chicago employers adopted a passive role as HMO consumers. They responded to HMO mandates and marketing efforts but rarely made an effort to "shop" for HMOs.

8

HMOs and Organized Labor

In general, unions have been more responsive to HMOs in the Twin Cities than in Chicago, probably because HMOs are more widely known and accepted by the public at large in the Twin Cities. In specific cases, unions have encouraged or participated in several HMO development efforts in both the Twin Cities and Chicago, including Group Health Plan, Anchor, Michael Reese Health Plan, and Union Health Service. Many unions are supportive of the HMO concept in principle, but the added complexity of offering multiple choice plans through the collective bargaining process can deter HMOs from being offered to unionized workforces at a local level.

Labor unions exert significant influences on employers' decisions regarding health benefits, either directly through collective bargaining or indirectly as employers seek to satisfy nonunion employees and forestall further organization. In addition, labor unions have played major roles in the development of several HMOs in the two market areas covered in this study. Once HMOs are operational, labor unions continue to have a strong effect on the HMOs' abilities to sell themselves effectively to employee groups that are covered by collective bargaining agreements.

Interviews with fifteen representatives of labor organizations in the Twin Cities and Chicago metropolitan areas are the primary data sources for this chapter. Additional data sources include published research findings, conference proceedings, pub-

This chapter was written by Bruce W. Butler, Assistant Project Director.

lished speeches, survey results, and news media coverage in the two cities.

HISTORY

Historically, organized labor has played an important role in the provision of health insurance benefits to workers (Munts, 1967). Many of the trade unions that were formed in the 1800s were designed to serve primarily as risk-sharing societies that provided workers with various social and health insurance benefits. As many of these trade unions developed, however, objectives shifted rapidly in favor of widespread organization to build bargaining power. Given these objectives, member-financed social and health benefits came to be regarded by some leaders as at worst a detriment to membership growth because of the high dues necessary to support such programs, and at best costly instruments for retaining member loyalty during recessionary times. Thus, the financial involvement of employers was welcomed, but employer-initiated programs were recognized as possible sources of erosion of employee loyalty to the union. Organized labor therefore developed the stance that while funding for social and health benefits should come from sources other than union dues, such benefits should continue to be identified directly with union efforts. This position was implemented on a large scale shortly after World War II when a court decision interpreted the Wagner Act of 1935 to require employer participation in collective bargaining for social and health benefits. The result has been a proliferation of collectively bargained health insurance plans and a dramatic increase in the proportion of the population covered by health insurance.

The strong interest of organized labor in health benefits has not subsided. In recent years, there have been several major disputes between management and organized labor focusing on this issue (*Business Week*, 1977, 1983). One explanation of the importance of health benefits in labor negotiations is that while tax laws and other market conditions cause both employers and employees to receive advantages when nonwage compensation is offered, the optimal percentage of nonwage benefits is lower for employers than for employees because of the high administrative costs of obtaining such benefits on an individual basis (Mabry, 1979). The difference between the two optimal percentages pro-

vides the basis for labor-management conflicts. Another explanation is that negotiations for fringe benefits can increase the status
of union leaders within their own organizations since a newly
won benefit might have more emotional appeal than an equivalent wage increase amounting to only a few cents per hour (Sapolsky, et al., 1981). While bargaining for health benefits may
have a highly pragmatic value for unions, the modern labor
movement has continued to exercise its social philosophy regarding health care by supporting the concept of universal national
health insurance whenever the subject enters the political arena.
Since this union support has not been successful in the past and
is not likely to be in the near future, the primary arena for union
involvement in health care issues continues to be the collective
bargaining process.

The threat of unionization is a significant factor in management decision making even though current union organization is
limited to a relatively small number of industries and involves
only approximately 20 percent of the nation's workers (Sapolsky,
et al., 1981). For employee groups that are not yet organized, the
provision of attractive health benefits has historically been seen
as a method of maintaining the status quo even if large expenditures are involved. At least until recently, many firms have followed careful strategies designed to provide nonunionized workers with benefit packages that are equal or superior to those
secured by unions. The preferences of organized labor can be
implemented, therefore, not only directly through collective bargaining, but also indirectly through the implicit threat of unionization.

THE COLLECTIVE BARGAINING
ENVIRONMENT

Two major forms of collective bargaining for health insurance have emerged. In the most prevalent type, a level of benefits
is negotiated, and the employer then provides these benefits from
a health insurance carrier or a self-insured plan. The extent to
which these benefits are known to be replacements for wage income depends largely on the sophistication of particular unions
and their insistence on full information. In the second major type
of plan, a dollar amount is negotiated, and a trust fund for health

benefits is established. The dollar value of union health insurance is naturally more explicit in a trust fund.

Historically, the goal of organized labor regarding health benefits has been simply to remove the financial barrier between workers and health care. To accomplish this goal, unions have attempted to minimize explicit employee cost-sharing in the form of payroll deductions for premium costs or of deductibles and copayments levied at the time of health care delivery. In addition, unions have sought gradual expansion in the scope of services covered by negotiated health plans. According to union representatives interviewed in this study, the highest priority in collective bargaining for health benefits is the avoidance of cost-sharing. Explanations for this emphasis include the high visibility of cost-sharing provisions such as payroll deductions from the workers' point of view, as well as concern that copayments and deductibles might discourage workers from obtaining appropriate health care.

Many of the union representatives reported that health benefits have historically been easier to win than concessions on wages or working conditions. While employers have been fairly willing to accept union demands for better health benefits, unions have often not sought an active role in the management of these benefits. For example, one respondent reported that in the past, collective bargaining for health benefits had often been characterized by an attitude of "negotiate a first-dollar coverage package and walk away," leaving the details to the employer and the insurance carrier. Exceptions to this pattern, of course, are provided by unions that perform an active role in the management of trust funds.

Given current conditions in the employee health benefits market, many of the patterns discussed above are changing rapidly. In general, the bargaining position of unions was weakened by economic recession. Job security became a high-priority issue for workers. At the same time, respondents in this study reported a growing recognition on the part of union negotiators of the problems surrounding the disproportionate escalation of health benefit costs. These problems developed as employers became less willing to expand health benefits because of the open-ended nature of costs, and as increasing resources were devoted to the maintenance of constant levels of benefits. Union negotiators increasingly concluded that health benefit cost escalation was eroding their ability to bargain for wage increases.

In response to this changing environment, union leaders reported widespread reorientation of historical union goals regarding health benefits. In contrast to prior efforts for the expansion of health benefits, union leaders indicated that now they can realistically attain, at best, the preservation of current benefit levels. Recent efforts for expansion, if any, have been directed at lengthening the period for which laid-off employees are eligible for group health insurance coverage.

To preserve current benefit levels, executives in heavy industry who were interviewed in this study reported that many major unions approach bargaining sessions with the position that cuts in health benefits are nonnegotiable. It is noteworthy that this stance is taken when several major unions have accepted significant wage concessions. While there have been exceptions to this posture, the pattern is one of union inflexibility regarding cutbacks in health benefits (*Business Week*, 1983).

Union leaders are also paying more attention to strategies for increasing the cost-effectiveness of current benefit levels. The cost containment methods favored by unions, however, are generally different from some of the methods currently favored by employers and government, such as cost-sharing, flexible benefits, and taxation of premium expenses.

Union leaders are adamantly opposed to cost containment strategies that are based on increases in cost sharing in the form of deductibles and copayments. Typically, cost sharing is considered an unacceptable erosion of benefits rather than a viable cost containment strategy. Union leaders view these strategies as merely a form of cost shifting rather than cost savings. They are skeptical that consumer behavior incentives can have a significant impact on health care utilization rates unless the incentives are so severe that workers are discouraged from receiving appropriate care. In effect, the union position is that there is some health care that is appropriate and some that is overutilization; copayments and deductibles are thought to have little effect on reducing overutilization, and they run the risk of discouraging appropriate utilization. It is also reported that increases in cost-sharing would be extremely difficult for elected union officials to justify to their constituencies since they involve tangible increases in out-of-pocket expenses and represent the loss of a previously secure bargaining prize.

While increases in copayments and deductibles are typically not acceptable to unions, one representative stated that in some cases the extent of covered services is an area in which unions are more willing to make concessions. The reason for this flexibility is that the extent of covered services is less tangible for the rank and file. In cases where particularly rich benefit packages have been negotiated in the past, some union leaders are willing to concede benefits that they do not consider vital to the welfare of workers. One respondent referred to "fringe fringes," such as optical and dental benefits, that could be conceded to preserve basic benefit levels.

In many cases, employers have tried to introduce increased copayments and deductibles and/or narrower coverage by offering these plans as options to employees in exchange for lower payroll deductions. Although such strategies allow employees to remain with their original coverage, they are generally not preferred by unions because of uncertainty regarding the outcome of consumer decision-making processes. Union leaders expressed concern that if persons made accurate predictions of their future health status and selected a high-option or low-option plan accordingly, risk pools would become fragmented, and the value of insurance as a means of spreading financial misfortune over a large group would be defeated. Union leaders were also concerned with the opposite problem—persons who made poor predictions of their future health status might suffer grave misfortune in the long run.

In addition to the prevalent private sector cost containment initiatives mentioned above, union leaders were also opposed to those public sector initiatives that involve the attenuation of tax-exempt status for health benefits. Their concern was that these strategies would intensify pressures for benefit reduction from employers, and would place the tax-exempt status of Taft-Hartley trust funds in question.

The discussion above delineates the types of cost containment initiatives that unions are not likely to support. However, unions are becoming active in other forms of health care cost containment. In general, labor leaders exhibited great interest in initiatives designed to increase levels of accountability on the part of providers and insurers. In support of this emphasis, respondents offered many examples of physician overprescriptions, hospital overcharges, and lax claims administration by insurers. The most common theme of these complaints was that insurers exercise insufficient control over fraudulent, inappropriate, or incorrect claims. For example, one reported instance involved an outlandishly high hospital charge, caused by a keypunch error in the hospital's billing system. This claim was paid without investigation by an insurer, but was noticed by the patient who brought the matter to the attention of a union benefits representative.

With great regret, some leaders also expressed doubt regarding the continued viability of fee-for-service coverage that allows free access to high-cost providers and/or self-referrals of questionable appropriateness. One person reported that his union had recently closed a loophole in its benefits structure that allowed some workers to enjoy "free vacations" in another part of the state at the expense of the union's alcoholic rehabilitation program. Others foresaw that in the future, unions might be forced to install restrictions on access that would be much more difficult and sensitive, such as disallowing self-referral to subspecialists. While such measures were seen by some union leaders as ultimately necessary, they were also viewed as undesirable since they would restrict access to the "best" health care available.

To achieve tighter control of health insurance plans and greater cost-effective benefit structures, union leaders reported a tendency toward addressing complex benefits management issues during collective bargaining sessions, with increasing emphasis on obtaining assurances that the benefits provided by the employer represent the best value available and are efficiently managed. In some cases, insurers have been brought into bargaining sessions to respond to union demands for changes in administrative practices or coverage. It was reported that employers have historically opposed union requests for three-way negotiations of this sort, but the growing desire of employers to exercise greater leverage over insurers has softened this opposition.

While union leaders in general supported at least some cost control efforts, it was also reported that the potentially negative impact of cost control efforts on organized health service workers was a drawback to active union involvement in such efforts. Thus, unions that represent large numbers of health service workers are likely to be particularly conservative regarding cost containment efforts.

Union representatives interviewed for this study generally approved of HMOs as means to increase the accountability of providers and third-party payers regarding health care costs. This capability was attributed generally to the structure of HMOs, which was believed to tie utilization patterns to financial viability more closely than in the fee-for-service system. Consumer choice between HMOs and the fee-for-service system was considered necessary to avoid restrictions in access unacceptable to workers, but choice was not considered valuable in stimulating cost control through competition among alternative delivery systems. Union representatives in general seemed favorably inclined toward variations of the HMO concept, such as IPAs and PPOs, as means of accomplishing cost containment with minimal restrictions in access.

A subset of union representatives can be classified as active HMO advocates. They favor an increase in consumer control over health care delivery, which they think can be achieved with HMOs, particularly staff model HMOs that are organized as consumer cocperatives. These HMO advocates, unlike union representatives in general, tended to be strongly opposed to concepts such as IPAs and PPOs on the grounds that they retain the fee-for-service system's unacceptable level of domination by providers' interests.

UNION INVOLVEMENT IN HMO DEVELOPMENT

Several of the most important national labor organizations strongly favor the concept of prepaid group practice over the traditional fee-for-service, individual practice method of health care delivery. In 1955, the founding convention of the AFL-CIO passed a resolution calling for "a program of federal aid, such as grants and low-interest loans, to further the development of non-profit, direct service, prepayment medical care plans, based on group practice" (Kirkland, 1975). While the passage of the Health Maintenance Organization Act of 1973 undoubtedly reflected the interests of other groups as well, this legislation closely resembled the long-held AFL-CIO position described above. Exceptions to the AFL-CIO position included the extensions of the legislation to involve for-profit HMOs and IPA models.

Examples of direct union involvement in HMO development are numerous. For example, the United Auto Workers acted both independently and in cooperation with Ford Motor Corporation to aid the development of HMOs in the Detroit area (Shelton, 1979). Other labor organizations or affiliates that have been actively involved in the development of prepaid group practices, at least on the local level, include the Teamsters, the United Steel Workers, the United Mine Workers, the Amalgamated Meat Cutters, the Hotel and Restaurant Employees and Bartenders International, the Retail Clerks International, the International Brotherhood of Electrical Workers, and the American Federation of State, County, and Municipal Employees (AFSCME) (U.S. Council on Wage and Price Stability, 1976).

The impetus for this support came largely from concerns regarding consumer control over quality and accessibility of care. In general, union HMO advocates argue that fee-for-service medicine does not serve consumer interests adequately. The traditional health care delivery system has been described as "a piecework system of paying doctors . . . encouraging the production of more pieces," rather than encouraging the production of well patients because "the sicker you are the more the doctor makes" (Seidman, 1980). In prepaid group practices, it is claimed these incentives are reversed. According to this point of view, prepaid group practices consisting of physicians who are employees of a consumer-controlled organization are highly desirable. Early HMO plans, organized as consumer cooperatives, received strong union support.

Minneapolis-St. Paul

The formation of Group Health Plan in the early 1950s is an example of the early involvement of trade unions in HMO development. This involvement included ideological and financial support in the plan's early stages. Actual enrollment of union groups occurred later. Several leading Twin Cities union officers "were enthusiastic and supportive even though their unions did not join the plan in its early stages" (Uphoff and Uphoff, 1980). To raise initial capital, the plan issued $100,000 of investment certificates, the majority of which were purchased by local labor unions. By the early 1960s, union support for Group Health Plan grew in the form of enrollment from both union-managed plans and negotiated company-managed plans. Accounts from the United Auto Workers, AFSCME, and local teachers' unions provided the plan with a significant enrollment base. In addition, union representatives served on the plan's consumer-elected Board of Directors.

In the early 1970s, AFSCME representatives from Ramsey County participated with the Ramsey County Commissioners, St.

Paul-Ramsey Hospital, and consultants from Group Health Plan to form Ramsey Health Plan (now Coordinated Health Care). Union members have subsequently served on the board of this HMO and several other Twin Cities HMOs as well.

Union representatives in the Twin Cities also noted that organized labor has been active politically in support of HMOs, most notably by supporting the passage of state HMO legislation in 1973. This act included a mandate provision that required all employers with more than one hundred workers in Minnesota to offer an HMO if they were approached by an HMO. While this mandate provision was rarely, if ever, activated by HMOs, union representatives interviewed for this study suggested that voluntary compliance with this regulation by employers contributed strongly to HMO growth. Organized labor also supported provisions of the act that required Minnesota HMOs to incorporate as non-profit organizations.

Another major aspect of health insurance legislation that was supported by organized labor, the Minnesota Comprehensive Health Insurance Act of 1976, may have indirectly aided HMO development because it required an extensive set of mandated benefits by fee-for-service insurers, which diminished the ability of insurers to offer lower premiums than HMOs.

Chicago

Labor unions in Chicago were also involved in the early development of prepaid group practices. The first plan in Chicago, Union Health Service, was established in 1952 by the Service Employees International Union (SEIU). Union Health Service provided prepaid ambulatory care for SEIU members and contracted with fee-for-service insurers for hospitalization coverage. In the early 1970s, Union Health Service began providing services to other union groups and also began functioning as a provider group for other HMOs. In 1957, the Amalgamated Clothing and Textile Workers Union (ACTWU) established the Sidney Hillman Health Center, a prepaid group practice limited to the provision of ambulatory care for ACTWU members.

While union involvement in these prepaid group practices was much more direct than the simultaneous union involvement in Group Health Plan in the Twin Cities, union-sponsored prepaid group practices in Chicago did not evolve into major competitors in the health insurance marketplace as did Group Health

Plan. Instead, the union-sponsored prepaid group practices in Chicago tended to limit themselves consciously to a fairly narrow enrollment base. Currently, however, Union Health Service is undergoing efforts to expand its role in the marketplace.

Two other Chicago HMOs, formed by tertiary medical centers, were founded in the early 1970s as means of satisfying the demands of the medical centers' unionized employees for ambulatory health care coverage. Subsequently, both of these plans developed into full-fledged HMOs and marketed their services successfully to employers at large.

UNION RESPONSES TO HMO DEVELOPMENT

Despite organized labor's strong ideological support for the prepaid-group-practice concept and their increasing concern about higher health benefit costs, HMOs have, in some cases, unsuccessfully penetrated the market for health benefits in bargaining sessions. While there may be a positive relationship between unionization and early HMO development in a large sample of SMSAs (Luft, 1981), case studies of HMO development in the Chicago and Philadelphia SMSAs concluded that there were significant obstacles involved in marketing HMOs to unionized groups (ICF, 1980a, 1980b). Mirroring the two-stage process of marketing HMOs to any employee group, obstacles to union enrollment may arise not only in formalizing the HMO offering to the group but also in encouraging enrollment of individual employees.

Amendments to the federal HMO act in 1975 required that the decision of an employer to offer an HMO be subjected to collective bargaining. Therefore, an employer must gain union approval before offering an HMO to employees covered by an existing labor contract. Union approval must also be gained for mandated HMO offerings to be valid for the unionized portion of an employer's workforce.

Union leaders interviewed in this study pointed to a wide variety of factors that may inhibit the implementation of HMO offerings in negotiated benefit plans. At the general level, one respondent commented that the nature of the collective bargaining process itself tends to permit only incremental changes in existing benefit structures. HMOs represent a significant departure from the status quo, and the conditions of their inclusion are therefore unlikely to be readily agreed upon by both sides. This problem was thought to be particularly acute in situations where the HMO concept is poorly understood by one or both parties in the bargaining process, resulting in an even greater atmosphere of caution. In extreme cases, there is reflexive opposition by one party to any initiative proposed by the other party.

A significant proportion of union contracts are negotiated at the local level rather than the national level, and those representatives we interviewed suggested that much of the positive opinion regarding HMOs on the part of national leadership has not trickled down to local negotiators and business agents. A major area of uncertainty for local union negotiators is the effect HMO offerings might have on consumer satisfaction. Negotiators are unlikely to accept HMOs, let alone to push for them, until they are firmly convinced that such a change will not create dissension among the rank and file. Of particular concern is the limitation of choice of medical care providers in HMOs. While it is recognized that dual choice provisions would protect workers who might be dissatisfied with HMO providers, negotiators are nevertheless wary of including options that might be held in less than the highest regard by workers. Several representatives generalized that the more negotiations are conducted closer to the local level, the more negotiations focus on "safe" increments rather than politically risky innovations.

Another major obstacle to offering HMOs in union health benefit plans involves premium differentials between HMOs and fee-for-service plans. When HMOs are more expensive than existing fee-for-service insurance plans, unions are reluctant to institute the increased payroll deductions that would be necessary, in many cases, to gain employer acceptance for an HMO. In such a situation, unions that have negotiated fee-for-service plans with no payroll deductions are particularly reluctant to develop HMO offerings, to avoid setting a precedent in favor of cost-sharing.

When labor unions and employers are able to agree in principle regarding an HMO, administrative difficulties may still inhibit the implementation of such an agreement. Often, proposals to offer specific HMOs on a local basis are referred to the union's headquarters for an exhaustive review of the HMO's organizational viability, benefit structure, and quality (Kovner, 1977). According to a respondent in this study, the turnaround time for reviews such as these may be as long as six months.

From the point of view of employers, the prospect of complex negotiations regarding HMOs may significantly limit their enthusiasm for offering them. According to employers interviewed for this study, when a single organization must negotiate contracts with multiple trade unions, the task of offering an HMO to all or most of the workforce becomes so difficult that only employers who are firmly committed to the HMO concept will expend the effort necessary to implement such a plan. Likewise, an employee group that is segmented among multiple trade unions presents a relatively difficult marketing task to HMOs. Each HMO's services must be sold to a larger number of decision makers than would be the case in a nonunion or single-union workplace.

In Taft-Hartley trust funds, the administrative difficulties surrounding HMO plans may be particularly acute when a single trust fund handles health benefits for many union locals, each of which operates under a separate collective bargaining agreement and may represent only a small percentage of the trust's total beneficiaries. Such trust funds typically self-insure or retain a single carrier to provide coverage to all locals. Given the potential administrative difficulties involved with offering unique multiple-choice options to various locals, trust funds are not likely to be leaders in the process of encouraging union involvement with HMOs. As an example, a representative of one large trust fund stated that the fund approved of the HMO concept in principle and would attempt to accommodate any local that desired a multiple-choice plan, but the trust fund would in no way advocate that locals become involved with HMOs.

The familiarity and attitudes of the union rank and file regarding HMOs are important determinants of the marketing success of HMOs in unions. As mentioned previously, local union officials are likely to be cautious about advocating ideas that risk disapproval or apathy among the rank and file. If local officials are not familiar with or supportive of the HMO concept, they are not likely to undertake efforts to persuade their members that HMOs would be beneficial. Moreover, national and regional officials who are in favor of including HMOs in union benefit plans are reluctant to "go around" the authority of local leaders to influence the rank and file. Therefore, the process of building familiarity among union workers could be blocked because union members are likely to depend upon local officials for benefit information, but local officials tend to reject positions that the rank and file do not already support. According to several people in this study, one way that HMOs have overcome this problem has been to secure an offer to salaried employees and then to wait until union members demand equal treatment. The success of this strategy, of course, depends highly on the HMO's ability to attract and satisfy enrollees from the salaried workforce. Reportedly, this strategy has been effective in the Twin Cities. In Chicago, however, several benefits managers reported that HMOs have been slow to gain acceptance among salaried workers but might appeal more strongly to union members if only they were more familiar with HMOs. Another way that HMOs can overcome these obstacles is through mass media advertising directed at union members and the public at large. In the Twin Cities, mass media advertising by HMOs has been extensive. In Chicago, such efforts are building, and several benefits managers felt that further efforts would be crucial to HMO growth.

Minneapolis-St. Paul

While all of the problems discussed above have been apparent in both of the metropolitan areas covered by this study, each area has displayed some unique characteristics with regard to the union environment and the relationship between unions and HMOs. In the Twin Cities, labor leaders reported that the general union membership is relatively skewed toward highly trained or white-collar workers, that benefits are perhaps more generous than elsewhere in the country, and that labor-management relationships are relatively cordial. An example of cooperative relations by labor and management is provided by jointly sponsored job training programs for Southeast Asian refugees. Labor unions in the Twin Cities appear to be atypically active in health issues in general: occupational health programs, mandated benefits, and HMO-enabling legislation. While Chicago labor leaders who were involved in health issues tended to express some disappointment regarding the lack of interest among their peers, labor leaders in the Twin Cities expressed disappointment in their national organizations, which were not as involved as they had perceived themselves to be. While many of the problems mentioned above occur in the Twin Cities, informants also pointed to several examples of extremely favorable union responses to HMOs, ranging from the involvement of unions in the early development of Group Health Plan to the active participation of some local union leaders in HMO marketing efforts. For example, when one large employer was mandated by an HMO, the local president of the employer's major union sent out letters to all members urging them to join. In subsequent collective bargaining sessions, this union requested that other HMOs be offered as well. In other cases, union leaders have assisted HMO group marketing meetings in union halls.

With the exception of union involvement in Group Health Plan, informants reported that unions have not taken a leadership role in HMO development, nor have they actively opposed HMO development. Rather, union members and leaders have tended to mirror the generally receptive attitude of the Twin Cities community to HMOs. This attitude has reduced the inherent difficulties of marketing HMO services to unions in the Twin Cities.

Chicago

In the Chicago area, informants familiar with the labor market reported that the composition of the union workforce is fairly typical of most metropolitan areas, including strong representation from heavy industry and blue-collar occupations. Labor representatives reported a wide range of benefit packages in place, ranging from the all-inclusive and company-financed plans obtained by historically strong unions such as the Steel Workers, to largely employee-financed plans with limited benefits that are available to workers in many small shops and plants.

Positive responses by unions to HMO development have been limited in the Chicago area. In the absence of any strong movement in favor of HMOs from within unions or of any groundswell of approval from the general public, the inherent problems of marketing HMOs to unions seem to be somewhat more restrictive in the Chicago area than in the Twin Cities. To counteract this situation, efforts have been undertaken recently by the suburban HSA and the Executive Service Corps' HMO Project to build familiarity with HMOs among union leaders. Also, the newly formed metropolitan Chicago Labor Health Council advocates that its member organizations strongly consider the negotiation of alternative delivery systems, including HMOs and PPOs. If such efforts, along with continued marketing efforts by the HMOs themselves and increasing acceptance of HMOs among the general public, are able to overcome the inertia that currently limits the response of unions to HMOs, the penetration rates for HMOs may increase significantly in the future.

SUMMARY

Health insurance benefits became an important aspect of collective bargaining negotiations after World War II. The historical goal of labor organizations has been to remove financial barriers between workers and health care. In recent years, action has focused on retaining current benefit levels and opposing increases in cost sharing, e.g., copayments and deductibles. Union representatives generally approve of HMOs to increase the cost accountability of providers and third-party payers. In specific cases, in both metropolitan areas, unions were directly involved in the development of HMOs. In other cases, though, administrative difficulties and lack of familiarity worked against union involvement. Local unions in the Twin Cities have generally reacted more positively toward HMOs than have those in Chicago.

9

HMOs: A View from Inside

Analysis of the formation, administration, medical delivery, and marketing of the HMOs in the two study areas demonstrates that the HMOs and the markets in Minneapolis-St. Paul and Chicago are in different stages of development. Although the HMOs began at similar times and their organization and operation are similar, HMOs in the Twin Cities had two vital supports that appeared to be absent in Chicago. Some were sponsored, and all were facilitated by the presence of multispecialty group practices, which were respected and well suited to HMO development. Futhermore, HMOs in the Twin Cities marketed to employers who were for the most part informed, receptive, and supportive. In contrast, HMOs in Chicago had to develop where multispecialty groups were largely unknown and unwanted. The HMOs also had to market products to employers who were resistant. Now, in 1984, the Minneapolis-St. Paul market is leveling off, and the Chicago market is developing rapidly.

Health maintenance organizations (HMOs) have moved from the periphery of the health care system to a central position. HMOs are now being embraced by both purchasers and providers of health care. In addition, HMOs have come to occupy prominent positions in health care policy proposals. In fact, the term HMO was coined in the context of a national health policy proposal. In recent years, HMOs have been the centerpiece of several proposals for health care reform. Most recently, HMOs have interested

This chapter was written by Terry E. Herold, Project Director.

policy analysts for their potential to introduce competition into the health care system.

An HMO integrates the financial and health care delivery functions into one entity (Zelten, 1979). As such, HMOs are seen by some observers as a next step in the evolution of health care organizations (Starr, 1982). Where most health care organizations perform one or the other of these functions—health care delivery or financing—HMOs combine them.

This basic organizational characteristic of the HMO, which unites the flow of dollars with services, can result in a cost-effective system. Many purchasers of health care, in both the private and public sectors, have adopted the HMO as one means to contain escalating health care costs. On the micro-level, extensive research documents these savings (Luft, 1981a). Less research has investigated the organizational processes and structures that produce these savings. On the macro-level, many people question the ability of HMOs to introduce changes that will result in beneficial competition between health care providers and insurers (Luft, 1981b).

Over the past few years, the HMO industry has undergone notable growth in terms of both the total number of HMOs and the number of members enrolled in HMOs. From its infancy in the 1970s, the industry is now maturing. This presents a new set of circumstances as challenging as those faced by the developing industry.

This chapter examines internal aspects of HMO development and issues regarding the development of the HMO industry. Like preceding chapters, this chapter's perspective is processual and dynamic, attempting to understand how HMOs develop and change over time. This longitudinal analysis of HMOs and their environments contributes to an understanding of the organizational life cycle of the HMO and of HMO-environment interaction and adaptation.

This chapter is based on case studies of all of the HMOs in the two areas. The data were gathered until spring 1983 from the HMOs' own records and publications and from sixty-six interviews with directors, administrators, and other staff members of the HMOs. To suggest the most important aspects of the HMO case studies four distinct but interwoven topical areas will be examined: 1) HMO formation, 2) administrative and organizational development, 3) medical delivery system development, and 4) marketing development.

BACKGROUND

The initiation sequence of HMOs in Minneapolis-St. Paul and Chicago was very similar. Most of the HMOs were introduced between 1971 and 1975, with one HMO in each of the markets existing prior to this time. In each of the markets, there was a variety of sponsors for the HMOs. In addition, the HMOs in each area represented all of the ideal types of medical delivery structure (see the table on page 6).

The growth in the membership in HMOs has been quite different in the two areas. The HMOs in Minneapolis-St. Paul were significantly larger than those in Chicago. The overall market penetration was also significantly greater in Minneapolis-St. Paul than in Chicago. Tables 9.1 and 9.2 display membership growth, growth rates, and overall market penetration for the HMOs in each market through 1981.

HMO FORMATION

The first HMO in any market paves the way for subsequent HMOs in several ways. First, legal and regulatory issues are generally identified, addressed, and resolved. Second, the first HMO plays a significant role in the education of health care providers, consumers, and purchasers concerning the HMO concept. Although in some new markets HMOs are seen as radical innovations (Lewis, 1977), subsequent HMOs are no longer viewed as "foreign" entities. Finally, the first HMO often serves as an example for subsequent HMOs, less in an organizational sense than in the sense of successfully making and implementing a plan.

Interviews with HMO administrators demonstrate that sponsors play critical roles in the formation of HMOs. Several attributes of sponsors seem to be important in the formation of HMOs. The commitment of the sponsor is critical. Second, the medical and administrative resources possessed by the sponsor are important in relation to the chief functions of the HMO—delivering and financing medical care. In addition, general organizational, operational, and mangerial skills are imperative. These resources are particularly important in less receptive markets, such as Chicago. A final attribute is the sponsor's reputation and perceived legitimacy vis à vis physicians, employers, and consumers.

TABLE 9.1 Minneapolis-St. Paul HMO Market

Enrollment	1970	1971	1972	1973	1974	1975	1976	1977	1978	1979	1980	1981
Group Health Plan	35,996	42,879	52,230	59,172	66,638	76,883	91,375	107,517	121,184	130,810	153,869	181,328
Coordinated Health Plan			1,715	1,945	2,184	2,941	3,578	3,985	4,025	4,459	4,922	5,243
Medcenter			1,000	4,233	7,049	10,090	17,591	31,797	46,706	61,278	70,616	90,282b
Nicollet-Eitel Health Plan				441	1,853	2,370	3,179	5,491	8,485	14,957	20,984	27,373b
SHARE				2,846	3,299	9,189	12,130	17,121	21,862	27,449	33,898b	37,486b
HMO Minnesota					1,725	2,914	3,368	6,400	12,170	26,195	48,309	49,511b
Physicians Health Plan						53	9,708	14,227	26,422	45,240	85,173	95,141b
Total	35,996	42,879	54,945	68,637	82,748	104,440	140,929	186,538	240,854	310,388	417,771b	486,364b
% Growth		19	28	25	21	26	35	32	29	29	35	16
Metro Population	1,874,400	1,883,100	1,891,600	1,899,200	1,914,900	1,912,500	1,924,100	1,931,500	1,945,600	1,959,800	1,985,700	1,989,600
% Metro Population	1.9	2.3	2.9	3.6	4.3	5.5	7.3	9.7	12.4	15.8	21.0	24.4

a--Seven county metropolitan area.
b--Includes Medicare Demonstration Project Enrollment.

TABLE 9.2 Chicago HMO Market

Enrollment	1972	1973	1974	1975	1976	1977	1978	1979	1980	1981
Union Health Service	13,188	13,547	12,266a	10,838a	23,933a	31,679a	21,780a	21,990a	25,619a	22,536a
ANCHOR	4,580	4,843	4,925b	6,411b	6,707b	9,224c	25,609	33,984	43,395	51,079
Intergroup/Maxicare	181	5,413	7,193	6,451	20,069	10,740	13,959d	22,456d	38,788d	51,354d
HMO Illinois	1,800e	2,002e	12,374e	20,319e	22,913e	28,726f	30,609f	36,544	46,157	58,429
Michael Reese/ Health Plan	4,282	5,029	6,665	8,984	10,795	11,789	13,194	15,620	24,404	34,983
NorthCare/PruCare				5,519	7,565	10,485	15,292	22,769	28,162	30,649g
Roosevelt/Chicago HMO					1,105	2,466	2,182h	2,301h	2,463h	3,093h
Total	24,031	30,834	43,423	58,522	93,087	105,109	122,625	155,664	208,988	252,123
% Growth		28	41	35	59	13	17	27	34	21
SMSA Population	7,084,600	6,999,900	6,971,400	6,982,900	7,006,400	7,016,600	7,035,200	7,069,200	7,103,600	7,111,900
% SMSA Population	0.3	0.4	0.6	0.8	1.3	1.5	1.7	2.2	2.9	3.5

a--Excluding Intergroup and Co-Care/HMOI members.
b--Excluding Co-Care members.
c--Excluding Co-Care/HMOI members.
d--Excluding members outside SMSA.
e--Co-Care members.
f--Co-Care and HMOI members.
g--NorthCare and PruCare beginning 6/81.
h--Excluding HMOI members.

What commitments precipitate the formation of HMOs? Some HMOs are formed for ideological reasons. These include expanding benefits, increasing consumer access, increasing the coordination of care, focusing on preventive care, increasing efficiency, and containing costs. Other rationale for forming HMOs, especially for recent ones, are market oriented. Market stimuli may result in proactive or reactive behavior. Proactive behaviors emanate from a sponsor's perceived opportunities. The sponsor may be addressing internal problems and concerns or may be taking advantage of market opportunities. HMOs are seen then as a way of taking advantage of these opportunities. Reactive behaviors relate to competition or costs. These two types of behavior essentially mirror the HMO as a marketing tool.

Changes in health care markets have been occurring rapidly. Competition is surfacing in nearly every health care market. Certain supply and demand characteristics tend to hasten market competitiveness (Morrisey and Ashby, 1981). For example, a health care market with excess resources and decreasing demand may heighten competition and lead health care providers to seek out HMOs as an avenue toward increasing their market shares. A proactive response on the part of one HMO sponsor, though, may lead in time to a reactive response from other sponsors.

Some market factors help facilitate HMO formation. Knowledge of and support for the HMO concept among consumers, employers, and health care providers tend to facilitate HMO formation in health care markets, and market factors can precipitate their support. Oversupply and overcapacity in the health care system may lead providers to examine and support HMO formation. These market conditions coupled with declining utilization tend to increase the competitiveness of the health care market as well.

A host of groups have sponsored HMOs. Health care consumers played a significant role in sponsoring early group health plans. Some consumer-sponsored plans, including Group Health Plans in Washington, D.C., St. Paul, and Seattle, are among the largest and oldest in the country. These plans were formed during a period when HMOs were seen as a means of increasing consumer access, benefit coverage, coordination of health care, and consumer control over health care. Sponsorship by consumers has decreased in recent years. The strength and early contribution of consumer-sponsored HMOs was a consequence of their ideological underpinnings and perserverance. However, consumer-sponsored plans are heavily dependent on others for capital and for financial, managerial, and technical expertise. Consumers' inability to operate effectively in complex health bureaucracies is discussed in chapter 3.

Health plans sponsored by employers or unions share many of the goals of consumer-sponsored plans. The roots of the Kaiser health plans and the Sidney Hillman health centers reflect these goals. These sponsors possess large financial and membership resources, but they have not played a significant role in the proliferation of HMOs. In recent years, these groups have sponsored HMOs more for reasons of cost and control than for benefit enhancement. While employers and unions are increasing their activities in the health care sector, there lingers a reluctance on their part to involve themselves in the delivery of medical care.

A major group of sponsors for HMOs are health care providers—hospitals and physicians. An obvious strength of these sponsors is their control over medical delivery resources. However, they often lack expertise in the managerial, operational, and insurance aspects of HMO development. Over time, these sponsors are increasing their knowledge in these areas in response to the changes in their immediate operating environment.

Until recently, few hospitals have been interested in HMO sponsorship. A large part of this reluctance has been a result of the implicit functional territories of the hospital vis à vis physicians. Hospitals have not wanted to compete with physicians. The relationship between physicians and hospitals has undergone significant changes in recent years, which has changed the perspective of hospitals regarding HMOs.

Physician sponsorship has historically come from multispecialty groups and from IPAs sponsored by county medical societies. Both these groups are still quite active in HMO sponsorship. A major concern of multispecialty groups has been the effect that HMO sponsorship might have on their traditional referral patterns. IPAs sponsored by medical societies have historically formed in response to competition from existing HMOs.

An interesting trend is emerging in that hospitals and physicians are combining their efforts and resources to sponsor HMOs. The hospital, serving as the focus for organizing physicians with staff privileges, is an adaptation to increasing competition; it provides both with opportunities for HMO sponsorship or affiliation. Non-profit and for-profit national hospital chains are also becoming involved in HMOs and other alternative delivery systems.

HMO sponsorship by insurance carriers has been growing in recent years. HMO sponsorship has been considered as a logical endeavor for health insurers for some time. Health insurers possess the necessary organizational skills and technical expertise to form and develop HMOs. In recent years, prominent indemnity insurers, such as Prudential and CIGNA, have made major commitments to HMO development in anticipation of and response to cost containment pressures from major health insurance purchasers. HMOs are also perceived as a means of protecting and building their market shares. Blue Cross and Blue Shield plans have also been very active in HMO development for many of the same reasons.

A more recent phenomenon has been the sponsorship and development of HMOs by existing HMOs. Several national development companies have formed for the sole purpose of developing HMO networks nationwide. These firms usually sponsor the HMOs themselves or jointly develop an HMO, usually with health care providers. While some sponsors lack the technical expertise necessary to develop an HMO, these national companies have developed such expertise. They are still largely dependent upon health care providers for delivery resources, but with increasing physician supply and decreasing inpatient utilization, this does not represent a formidable problem. These general characteristics and problems of HMO formation were echoed in the interviews of both areas, although distribution and emphasis vary.

Minneapolis-St. Paul

In the Twin Cities, a number of critical factors precipitated the formation of HMOs: 1) an early HMO served to lay the legal foundation and provide essential education to the community, 2) the participation of prestigious, well-known, and respected physicians in prepaid health care, and 3) organizations and individuals activated the interest and support of the employer community, demonstrating a market for HMO services. These three aspects provided a fertile environment in which HMOs grew and prospered. The reception, which the earlier HMOs received, indicated to others that they should participate, or they would be left out. So it was that Blue Cross-Blue Shield and the Hennepin County Medical Society decided to sponsor HMOs.

HMOs grew rapidly in the homogeneous community. Except for Group Health Plan, all of the HMOs were begun between 1972 and 1975. Since 1975, no new HMOs have entered the market, partially because of the success of the existing HMOs and because of a perception that the market for prepaid alternatives is reaching maturity. The following are examples of sponsorship and introduction of HMOs in Minneapolis-St. Paul.

The earliest HMO in Minneapolis-St. Paul, Group Health Plan, paved the way for other HMOs. Its origin can be traced to 1937, when consumers, in this case credit union leaders, tried to establish a plan for group health care to mitigate the financial burdens of health care for their members (Uphoff and Uphoff, 1980). At the time, however, they were blocked by the attorney general's opinion that formation of such a plan would violate laws forbidding the corporate practice of medicine. Following years of lobbying and education, the attorney general's opinion was changed. In 1957, Group Health Plan was incorporated. In spite of hostility and opposition, it served to familiarize and educate health care providers and purchasers about prepaid care.

In 1972, physicians at two prestigious clinics expressed interest in sponsoring HMOs. Physicians at St. Louis Park Medical Center sponsored MedCenter Health Plan. They saw opportunities to expand their practice, to fulfill their mission, and to prepare for what they believed was the imminent arrival of national health insurance. A premier multispecialty medical group, St. Louis Park played the important role of legitimizing prepaid medicine to the mainstream medical community. Almost simultaneously, physicians at Nicollet Clinic developed a prepaid plan, again underscoring the legitimacy of physician-sponsored HMOs.

Employers also had a crucial role in the early development of HMOs in the Twin Cities. They organized the TCHCDP, composed of influential health care and business leaders, to promote health care reform and achieve efficiency through prepaid alternatives. The TCHCDP educated employers about the HMO concept, and it demonstrated to the HMOs that a market existed for their products. When HMOs did become operational, the employer community was primed to offer them as options for their employees.

Several of the HMOs in the Twin Cities had ties with local

hospitals that hoped to broaden their patient base. SHARE Health Plan was established by the railroad workers union to revitalize a railroad hospital. Ramsey Health Plan was introduced to widen the patient pool in a public hospital following the "release" of its traditional patient base as a result of the Medicaid and Medicare programs. Ideological county commissioners also played an important role in initiating this plan. Eitel Hospital's joint sponsorship of the Nicollet-Eitel Health Plan included the desire of the hospital to receive additional patients and thus expand its services and facilities.

The most recent HMOs in the Twin Cities, such as Blue Cross-Blue Shield's HMO Minnesota, formed in response to competition from the earlier HMOs. HMO Minnesota provided Blue Cross-Blue Shield with a mechanism to participate in prepaid health care.

The Hennepin County Medical Society sponsored Physicians Health Plan to provide individual practitioners with a means to participate in prepaid medicine and to protect a share of the market that was being increasingly invaded by medical groups, the business community, and hospitals. Physicians' competitive responses are discussed more extensively in chapter 5.

Chicago

The issues of sponsorship and formation in Chicago were similar to those in the Twin Cities. The burden of responsibility was somewhat different, though, and the distribution of sponsors was very different. Unions motivated by ideology were among the first to develop prepaid plans. Although some physicians tried to initiate prepaid plans, there was very limited interest and considerable resistance within organized medicine or among the predominant private practitioners. Those who were interested turned to insurance carriers for help. In Chicago, hospitals were more often the focus of HMO development. The lack of HMO activity meant there was little sense of competition. The most notable difference between the two research sites was in the employer community (see chapter 7). There was little or no support for or understanding of HMOs among Chicago employers. Most were unfamiliar with the HMO concept. Among those who were knowledgeable, there was a lack of consensus about the utility of HMOs.

Many employers who were interviewed in Chicago said that there was little demand for HMOs because most employers were content with their health insurance plans. This inertia of employers was difficult to overcome.

However, since 1980, several factors have activated the interest of employers and other groups in HMOs. First, rising health insurance costs have precipitated employer interest. Second, attempting to control costs in the state Medicaid program, the Illinois Department of Public Aid has solicited proposals for Medicaid prepayment. Finally, in efforts comparable to those in the Twin Cities ten years earlier, several organizations have defined their mission as increasing the knowledge of employers and consumers regarding HMOs. For example, Chicago Executive Services Corps HMO Project, the Surburban Cook-DuPage County HSA, and the Illinois Association of HMOs have increased the public's knowledge about and support for HMOs.

As the research was being completed, one new HMO, Cooperative Health Plan, was established but had not yet enrolled members. Also, national HMO firms and local organizations were considering developing HMOs in the Chicago metropolitan area. Examples of sponsorship and formation of HMOs in Chicago follow.

The first prepaid plan in Chicago, Union Health Service, was sponsored by union leaders concerned about problems relating to the financing and delivery of health care. They saw a prepaid plan as one solution. They struggled with regulatory limitations because no statute explicitly sanctioned the formation of a prepaid plan. Union leaders lobbied vigorously and were instrumental in the passage of an early statute enabling prepaid plans in Illinois. Until the passage of an HMO act in Illinois some years later, HMOs were incorporated under this first statute.

At Rush-Presbyterian-St. Luke's Medical Center, leaders of the union for hospital employees requested more comprehensive health care coverage, including outpatient care. Administrators considered their concerns an opportunity to organize a prepaid plan as part of the medical center's long-term development. In addition, the medical center had prepayment experience as part of a federal neighborhood health center program. The HMO that resulted from their efforts was formed in 1971.

In the early 1970s, Michael Reese Hospital and Medical Center realized it had to move toward delivering more ambulatory care. Money from a benefactor was used to study the possibility of an ambulatory care program with a prepayment component. This study, the hospital's interest in avoiding an expensive employee health center, and significant pressure from the hospital employees' union precipitated the formation of Michael Reese Health Plan in 1972.

Roosevelt Health Plan (later changed to Chicago HMO) was formed later in 1976 by Roosevelt Hospital. Like some HMOs in the Twin Cities, Roosevelt Health Plan was formed to protect its market—a Medicaid population. Intergroup (now Maxicare/Intergroup) was the only HMO in Chicago initiated by physicians. The physicians explained that as members of a multispeciality group practice, they wanted to provide more comprehensive medical care to eliminate financial barriers to cost-effective medicine. These physicians sought a major health insurer as a cosponsor, and CNA Insurance expressed an interest. CNA saw prepayment as a natural area for the future involvement of a health insurance carrier. They could use existing corporate resources for the development of the HMO, and they saw the possibility of integrating the HMO and group insurance accounts. CNA underwrote a feasibility study, then capitalized and developed Intergroup.

Illinois Blue Cross-Blue Shield also became involved, partially in response to Intergroup. In the late 1960s, the health insurer began studying prepaid plans. In the early 1970s, it adopted a corporate policy to develop alternative delivery systems, and it pledged to provide developmental assistance to groups interested in developing plans. Based on prior HMO experience in southern Illinois, Blue Cross-Blue Shield decided to form a prepaid program—Co-Care—in Chicago. They offered it as an alternative to their regular health insurance plans.

NorthCare (now PruCare) was characteristic of those consumer-sponsored HMOs based on ideology. Four women from Evanston were dissatisfied with the lack of access to and coordination of health care in their community. After researching a variety of health care alternatives, they started forming a prepaid health plan with lay control. With support from federal grants, the Illinois Regional Medical Programs, Evanston Hospital, and several philanthropic foundations, the consumers group founded by these women hired administrators, staff, and a medical director. Their HMO began operations in 1975. Like other consumer-sponsored HMOs, though, they did not have plentiful capital or medical delivery resources.

ADMINISTRATIVE AND ORGANIZATIONAL DEVELOPMENT

HMOs are among the most complex of health care organizations. This derives largely from the fact that HMOs combine health care delivery and financing functions. As a result, these functions become interrelated, and a change in one part of the organization can affect other parts of the organization.

HMOs are still young organizations. The majority of HMOs have been established since 1970. Because of this, they offer a unique opportunity to study the life cycles of such organizations. (Kimberly, et al., 1980) We are able to examine the various stages that HMOs go through from their birth to maturity.

HMOs are constantly monitoring and adapting to their environment. Vast changes have occurred in the health care industry over the past ten years. HMOs have been an integral part of this change and have also had to adapt to these changes, like other organizations.

The medical delivery structure is the prime determinant of the administrative structure of the HMO. A key decision is whether the HMO owns or purchases medical services and facilities. If the HMO employs its physicians and owns its facilities (e.g., staff model), it resembles functionally a health care organization involved primarily in delivering medical care, such as a hospital or clinic. An HMO that purchases or contracts for medical services (e.g., IPA model) functions more like a conventional insurance organization.

The size of the medical delivery structure also affects the administrative structure of the HMO. As the number of physicians groups and hospitals that are affiliated with or employed by the HMO grows, the staff devoted to medical delivery grows proportionately. Likewise, the way that an HMO pays for medical services is administratively important. Employing physicians obviates claims payment. Similarly, capitation payments are administratively easier than reimbursement. HMOs that are based on fees for service, primarily IPAs, require a large claims processing staff and a sophisticated management information system (MIS), which integrates diverse financial, utilization, and membership information.

Increasingly, successful HMOs are differentiated by their management information systems. The medical delivery structure affects these systems greatly. Information is critical for control, so the decentralized HMO models require extensive data to monitor and control the medical delivery functions. Staff and group models have since implemented and refined information systems, but great differences still exist in their sophistication and scope.

As HMOs develop, structural differentiation occurs. Size appears to be the driving force behind structural differentiation. HMOs are similar to other organizations in this respect. HMOs start administratively as small, undifferentiated entities. In the beginning, it appears that HMOs are run by a small number of people who do everything. With growth and time, various functions in the HMO become differentiated.

Over time, HMOs also grow more bureaucratic in their structures and procedures. Formal policies are established to deal with a variety of common issues. In some HMOs, standard operating procedures are developed.

Managerial expertise was once considered a major barrier in the development of the HMO industry. Experienced HMO managers were in short supply, and federal HMO studies identified this as a major problem. As a result, management training programs were developed at the federal level. HMOs introduced new problems and responsibilities and it was difficult for individuals with traditional health administration or insurance backgrounds to perform at their highest potential. In retrospect, these individuals were too specialized for the HMO. Early HMOs either purchased services, when they existed, or developed expertise internally.

A particular area of services that were commonly purchased involved marketing. HMOs, particularly those that were sponsored by providers, contracted with insurance groups for marketing services. Unfortunately, in many cases, insurance organizations did not fully understand the complexities of HMOs, so they did not perform effectively. Insurance organizations performed much better in the more generalized areas of claims processing and payments, group billing, membership, and enrollment accounting.

In the early 1970s, very few organizations existed that provided general management services. In geographic areas where these services were available, they were used. The federal government played an important role in disseminating management, marketing, and financial information in the early days of the industry. Expertise also developed along with the industry. In most areas of HMO administration, new technologies and techniques had to be developed.

As HMOs developed experience, services that had once been purchased were internalized. It became more efficient for HMOs to perform these functions themselves, financially as well as for stability and control. HMOs that contracted for these services gained insights and knowledge about how best to perform them.

Recently there has been a greater availability of experienced HMO managers. As explained above, this results from 1) government programs aimed at developing such skills, 2) greater numbers of HMOs, 3) growing experience and functional specialization of the industry, and 4) interest in careers with HMOs. The increasing availability of managers has assisted the development of the HMO industry. However, supply has just barely kept up with demand.

Along with the increasing managerial skills and talent, there is a growing corporatization of HMOs. During the past five years, the industry has seen the emergence of at least ten companies that specialize in national HMO management and development. An interesting phenomenon is occurring. HMOs that previously focused on local markets are now becoming national corporations. Likewise, national corporations are acquiring, starting, or managing HMOs. These organizations succeed in concentrating management expertise, labor, and financial resources. National HMO development companies are also stockpiling experienced managers and are training functional specialists.

In addition, the industry is undergoing a transformation from a traditional non-profit industry to a for-profit industry. For-profit HMO companies are gaining equity capital in a variety of forms. Access to capital is presently one of the primary limitations to the development and expansion of HMOs. This is particularly true since the federal government has ended its role as the venture capitalist for the HMO industry. Whereas management expertise was once a barrier to HMO development, access to capital is now becoming one. The ability of national HMO companies to acquire and concentrate the scarce financial and technical resources required for developing HMOs greatly increases their success and position in the industry.

The HMO industry is now characterized by a high degree of business acumen and can attract top management talent from a variety of industries. With the degree of experience and resources that are now possessed by the HMO industry, HMOs can now be developed with a higher degree of success and much more rapidly than in the early days of the industry. Standardized systems, trained managers, and the ability to select markets that are conducive to HMO development have all accelerated the rate at which HMOs can be started.

Another interesting result of the corporatization of HMOs is that the corporate culture of the industry is undergoing changes. The early HMOs were relatively small organizations with strong leaders. A small group of people with close face-to-face interaction were the pioneers of the industry. Many of these individuals saw HMOs as a public good. With the industrialization of the industry, an increasing business orientation, and large, complex, bureaucratized organizations, the complexion of the industry has changed. Whereas informal controls bound together the HMO during its infancy, formal control mechanisms and bureaucracies are increasingly prevalent.

The relationship between the HMO and its sponsoring organization also changes over time. In its infancy, the HMO was quite dependent on the sponsor for its success, but as it developed, there was a growing independence of the HMO from its sponsor. In many cases, we are now seeing a growing dependence of the sponsor on the HMO.

Minneapolis-St. Paul

The rate of development of an HMO depends largely on the availability of necessary resources. One important factor for the growth of HMOs in the Twin Cities was committed sponsors. Ramsey Health Plan (now Coordinated Health Care) was developed in a relatively short time (six months) because St. Paul Ramsey Medical Center provided the necessary administrative and medical delivery resources. Less capital was needed because valuable administrative functions were donated.

When sponsors lacked necessary resources, development was much more difficult. The implementation of MedCenter Health Plan, which had the medical delivery resources, was lengthened by the need for consensus among the physicians of the sponsoring medical group about the structure of the health plan. Likewise, the sponsors did not have the expertise necessary to administer a prepaid health plan. Nicollet-Eitel Health Plan also encountered difficulties with administration. The sponsors made a decision quite early to have the plan administered by a third party experienced in health care financing and marketing, i.e., by an insurer. When it came time to implement the plan, Blue Cross of Minnesota, which had assisted in assessing the feasibility and planning, was asked to administer the plan. They declined because of internal debate regarding their role in HMO development. Nicollet-Eitel eventually found administrative services elsewhere.

Some plans suffered because they lacked sufficient commitment from their sponsors. HMO Minnesota, sponsored by Blue Cross-Blue Shield of Minnesota a year after Nicollet-Eitel began, was heavily dependent on the staff resources of the sponsor. The lack of complete commitment by corporate leaders slowed the plan's development. Likewise, SHARE lacked the complete backing of the board of the railroad workers' beneficial association. The board was concerned about the loss of control involved in opening up the health plan to the whole community.

Most HMOs in the Twin Cities received some outside assistance in their development or operation. Group Health Plan operated initially with the administrative and financial assistance of its sponsor, Group Health Mutual. After encountering financial difficulties during its first two years, Group Health Plan formalized its relationship with the mutual. The plan was run as a cooperative with a consumer board. Capital was provided through shares purchased by members. At this time, the plan hired an experienced manager for operations.

Coordinated Health Care received assistance during its initial development from Group Health Plan. Group Health Plan, through a grant from the federal government, provided Coordinated Health Care with technical assistance in administration, development, and marketing. Group Health Plan assisted in marketing the plan until Coordinated began to compete for Group Health Plan's accounts.

InterStudy was an important advocate of HMOs in general, and it supported certain HMOs in particular. It provided staff assistance to MedCenter Health Plan using a government grant. This assistance was important because the sponsoring physicians did not have the expertise or the time to work out the details of implementing a health plan. Later, MedCenter contracted with InterStudy for administrative services and with Northwestern National Life Insurance Company for marketing services. Over time, these contracted services were internalized, but one of the administrators later headed a firm managing Physician's Health Plan. SHARE Health Plan contracted for management services with InterStudy in hopes of securing the plan's survival during their dispute with the board of the railroad workers' beneficial association. Under the contract with InterStudy, SHARE incorporated independently of beneficial association. Eventually, the InterStudy management team joined the plan as employees. SHARE was the only Twin Cities HMO to receive extensive financial assistance from the federal Office of Health Maintenance Organizations and from the Family Health Center program. Money from the Family Health Center program was used to expand operations and to provide services to poorer people.

Other plans turned to insurers for assistance. HMO Minnesota has been mentioned as an example. Physicians Health Plan was developed by the Hennepin County Medical Society, but its marketing services were provided initially by Western Life, a subsidiary of The St. Paul Companies. The St. Paul Companies also added to the financial assistance provided to the plan by the medical society. Similarly, Nicollet-Eitel Health Plan contracted with Aetna for marketing functions. Both arrangements were terminated several years later because they attempted unsuccessfully to market the plan through agents.

As HMOs in the Twin Cities matured, their organization and management has adapted. Group Health Plan has evolved from a small organization with a strong and charismatic leader and a high degree of ideological commitment to a large, complex organization with new management that emphasizes decentralized decision making. HMO Minnesota has undergone several organizational changes. In 1976, new management at Blue Cross-Blue Shield of Minnesota made a strong commitment to the HMO. At the time, the HMO's functions were removed from the operating divisions and centralized. Since 1980, HMO Minnesota's management has been evaluating each function to determine whether it is performed best by being integrated or separated from the parent company's operating divisions.

The size of the administrative component of all the health plans has expanded with growth in membership. Coordinated Health Care is the smallest and most undifferentiated. Group Health Plan has the largest and most differentiated administrative structure. This is largely a function of the growth of its clinic sites. MedCenter Health Plan has remained administratively lean despite its assumption of functions that were previously performed by contract with outside vendors.

The relationships between the HMOs and their sponsors have generally grown more formal over time. Provider sponsors, such as St. Paul Ramsey Medical Center, St. Louis Park Medical Center, Nicollet Clinic, and Eitel Hospital, have benefited from their HMOs by learning cost containment technologies and marketing skills. In addition to these secondary benefits, the HMOs provided their sponsors with patients. HMO Minnesota has become increasingly important to Blue Cross-Blue Shield as a marketing mechanism. SHARE terminated its relationship with its initial sponsor to develop a viable plan. Physicians Health Plan has grown independent of its initial sponsor, the Hennepin County Medical Society, for legal reasons and on principle. Physicians Health Plan was competing against some of the society's members who were physicians associated with other HMOs.

The corporatization of HMOs nationwide discussed earlier is manifest in some HMOs in the Twin Cities. SHARE Health Plan created a for-profit management corporation, SHARE Development Corporation, which agreed to manage the plan. The employees of the health plan became employees of the management corporation. The management corporation is able to attract capital from private investors. This enables it to manage or own HMOs in other areas of the country. The corporation that manages Physicians Health Plan is also developing other HMOs nationally. Nicollet-Eitel Health Plan has taken its expertise to Wisconsin to develop and manage several HMOs there.

Chicago

HMOs in Chicago relied heavily on their sponsors for administrative and management expertise. Union Health Service was closely tied administratively to its labor sponsor. Anchor drew on the resources and personnel of its hospital sponsor and received financial assistance from foundations and the federal government. The development and operation of Anchor was guided by an experienced HMO administrator and medical director.

Michael Reese Health Plan was first developed as an outpatient clinic for employees. During the first several years of its operation, the plan lacked an experienced administrator, and it encountered severe financial and organizational problems. However, the sponsoring medical center reaffirmed its commitment to the health plan by hiring an experienced manager to provide the plan with financial stability.

Chicago HMO also turned to its sponsor, Roosevelt Hospital, for management and medical delivery resources. CNA initially funded a feasibility study for Intergroup. When it was decided to form an HMO, CNA provided capital through a loan. Intergroup also tapped the administrative and insurance expertise of its sponsor. HMO Illinois (formerly Co-Care) counted on the extensive financial and administrative resources of its sponsor, Illinois Blue Cross-Blue Shield. To develop a plan in Chicago, the insurer hired someone who had played a major role in developing Intergroup. Some years after Co-Care began operations, an independent corporation was formed for the HMO. This was required to receive federal qualification.

NorthCare did not have a corporate sponsor, so it relied heavily on federal and foundation grants and loans for its funding. It suffered from inexperienced management in its early years. The health plan developed a relationship with Rockford Blue Cross for administrative services and some funding. Management skills were developed by the medical and administrative directors as the plan grew.

Several of the HMOs in Chicago made organizational decisions different from those in the Twin Cities. HMOs in Chicago served limited populations before actively marketing to private employers. Anchor and Michael Reese Health Plan operated for several years as employee health clinics without marketing to private employers. Union Health Service served only union trust fund members for several years, and Chicago HMO served only Medicaid recipients for several years. In addition, Union Health Service and Anchor were provider groups for some network models that performed their own marketing functions. All of these mechanisms allowed these organizations to gain experience as HMO providers and to work on operational issues before they became responsible for their own marketing.

As in the Twin Cities, the relationships between HMOs and their sponsors in Chicago have changed over time. Some relationships have become closer, others more distant. Initially, Union Health Service operated largely under the direction of officials of the union trust fund. However, poor communication seriously inhibited decision making. Eventually, an administrator was hired who was given authority to make decisions for the health plan. In recent years, there has been a revitalization of the commitment of the union sponsor to the health plan.

Michael Reese Health Plan has experienced differing levels of commitment from the hospital under different administrations. In recent years, it has been an increasingly important part of the medical center, and it uses the hospital for a majority of its inpatient services. HMO Illinois operates under an administrative agreement with Illinois Blue Cross-Blue Shield. The functions of the health plan have always been integrated with the operating divisions of the parent. The HMO is becoming an important part of Illinois Blue Cross-Blue Shield for marketing purposes. As the HMO has grown in importance it has become easier to tap the financial and managerial resources of the corporation.

In contrast, Anchor has always been an important part of Rush-Presbyterian-St. Luke's Medical Center. With significant growth over the past few years, the health plan is becoming increasingly important to the medical center. The health plan purchases some administrative and medical services from the medical center. It uses the hospital for most of its tertiary inpatient care, and it uses the medical center's medical staff for referral services. The health plan is also an important part of the teaching program at Rush Medical College.

Chicago HMO initially had a very close relationship to its sponsoring hospital. When it became evident that Medicaid in Illinois was not going to be exclusively prepaid, the hospital became more distant. Their relationship has grown formal. Initially, the health plan purchased the majority of its administrative and medical service from the hospital, but now the health plan has internalized the majority of the administrative functions. It also contracts with medical providers not affiliated with the hospital.

The most dramatic administrative and organizational changes occuring in HMOs in Chicago have been the result of acquisitions. Both Intergroup and NorthCare were acquired by national HMO firms. Intergroup, initially a small non-profit entity in a large for-profit insurance company, didn't require extensive capitalization. In 1979, though, Intergroup launched a nationwide expansion project. It also decided to develop a new management information system. Both projects required extensive funding from CNA. As a result, CNA formed a for-profit holding company and converted Intergroup into a for-profit subsidiary. A short time later, the health plan was not becoming profitable, and it still required additional funding. At this time, competition was increasing among HMOs in Chicago and nationwide, and the group health business at CNA was experiencing financial problems. In addition, the top management of CNA was not totally committed to the HMO. As a result, a decision was made by the top management to divest the corporation of CNA Health Plans. Soon, Intergroup was sold to Maxicare Health Plans, a national HMO firm headquartered in California, which owns health plans in several large markets.

NorthCare has both changed the relationship with its sponsor and become part of a national corporation. After the maximum amount of money was borrowed under the federal HMO act, the health plan still wasn't profitable and required additional funding for expansion plans. The management was unsatisfactory, and the health plan was in debt both to the federal government and to Rockford Blue Cross. A consultant's study suggested several measures to solve some of the plan's organizational and operational problems. One suggestion was to add corporate representation to the consumer board. This polarized business-oriented management and the less pragmatic and more ideological consumer sponsors. When the consultant's recommendations were implemented the health plan continued to operate at a deficit and to need additional capitalization. It was decided that one way to obtain the needed capital was by associating with another organization. After negotiations with several potential buyers, including Kaiser, PruCare offered to purchase the plan. The decision to approve the sale of the health plan split the board but passed. PruCare is a subsidiary of Prudential Insurance Companies, which owns and operates HMOs in several metropolitan areas across the United States.

MEDICAL DELIVERY SYSTEM DEVELOPMENT

The medical delivery system of an HMO comprises two primary components—physicians and hospitals. These two components are responsible for the delivery of medical services to the plan's members. The medical delivery structure helps define the HMO's cost containment potential (Wolinsky, 1980) in terms of 1) control and selection of enrollees and 2) ability to effect changes in physician practice styles. Therefore, the medical delivery system has implications for the overall financial viability of the organization.

The terms of physician organization are the most varied and extensive. In most discussions of physician organization four types are referred to: staff, group, network, and IPA. There are two important dimensions to consider in physician organization: 1) the mode of practice and practice setting—either group practice or individual practice and 2) the financial relationship between the HMO and the physician. Either physicians are employees of the HMO or the HMO simply contracts for their services. In physician contracts, two dominant forms of financial relationships exist, capitation and modified fee-for-service reimbursements. In the capitation method, the HMO reimburses the physician a fixed amount per person, per specified period of time for a prescribed set of health care services. The other type usually reimburses physicians a set fee for each service rendered. Different financial incentives are implicit in the various reimbursement methods, encouraging either more or fewer services.

In a staff model, the physicians generally practice in a group setting, and they are salaried employees of the HMO. In a group practice model, a medical group affiliates with the HMO to deliver medical services. Reimbursement is generally in the form of a capitation payment. Group practice models are primarily multispecialty groups; however, this is changing, as will be explained later. A source of variation in group practice HMOs is whether the group exclusively renders prepaid services or also sees patients who are not HMO members on a fee-for-service basis. The network model is a variation of the group practice model. It is simply two or more groups that have affiliated with the HMO.

The IPA model has several variations. The traditional IPA was structured so that individual group practitioners joined an association, which in turn contracted with the HMO. One variation on this scheme is the HMO that contracts directly with individual physicians without an intermediary. IPA physicians usually practice out of their own offices and are reimbursed on a modified fee-for-service basis. For the majority of IPA physicians, only a small part of their practice is composed of HMO members.

In addition to the great variation that already exists in the ways physicians relate to HMOs, there is an increasing trend for HMOs to organize delivery systems that are eclectic. They take the best parts of the various types and put them together in new configurations. There has been much experimentation during the past decade in structuring delivery systems. This is continuing. No model appears ideal for all markets. Interestingly, in spite of the trend toward mixed models, established HMOs display great tenacity with respect to maintaining their chosen delivery models.

The primary advantage of the staff model is control and integration of medical delivery services. The concept of "one-stop shopping" for medical care applies to this form of organization. Another advantage of staff model HMOs, which is increasingly important, is their ability to integrate expensive referral physicians into their staffs as patient volume grows. This is critical to achieving a fully rationalized delivery system.

The primary disadvantage of this model is that such HMOs generally own and operate their own medical facilities. Since it is financially difficult for them to expand as rapidly as decentralized models, where the HMO contracts with providers who use their own facilities, these HMOs suffer from limited geographic accessibility. In addition, during periods of rapid growth, overcrowding becomes a problem. Financial constraints and overhead have been obstacles to accelerated development of the staff model for HMOs.

A problem that plagued staff models in the early days of the industry was staffing. In the period before 1975, HMOs were seen as radical innovations in health care delivery. The established medical community was hostile, and physicians in private practice questioned the quality of medical care delivered in HMOs. Private practitioners looked upon their colleagues in HMOs with disdain. As a consequence, physician recruitment was very difficult. This was also a period when physicians were generally busy and there was talk of a physician shortage.

A related problem is that staff models require a certain number of physicians regardless of the patient volume. Therefore physicians on staff are not always busy. On the other side, when the HMO experienced rapid growth, physicians complained about being overworked. A staff model HMO is susceptible to swings in physician workload.

Another problem for staff models is physician productivity. Since the physician is on salary, there are few incentives for productivity. A situation develops in which the physician can demand more from the health plan without increasing productivity. To adapt to this problem, administrators are developing incentive systems for staff physicians. Largely, these systems have fallen short of the expectations of plan administrators. In addition, administrators have to be careful to avoid accusations that they reward underservice.

With growth in the number of staff physicians, many administrators claim that new physicians working in HMOs are different from colleagues who practiced in HMOs early on. The early HMO physicians were seen as "outlaws" by their colleagues in private practice, and this bound the HMO physicians together. In addition, physicians who practiced in early HMOs were, administrators claim, ideological. They had a distinct mission. For the new physicians, HMO practice is less a result of ideology than of economic necessity. Thus, the informal control mechanisms and incentives that contributed to the productivity of early HMO staff physicians are not as important to the new generation of physicians.

Staff models are also introducing formal utilization control programs. The peer controls that helped establish a cost-effective practice style earlier are not as effective in organizations where there are literally hundreds of physicians. Formal controls are now needed to accomplish the same ends.

In staff models, antagonism often develops between physicians and management. This results because physicians generally prefer professional autonomy to staff employment. In many staff models, physicians have formed separate professional organizations to represent their collective interests. These organizations were often precipitated by issues of physician workload. Now issues of control over physician practice styles seem to precipitate their formation. In some situations, these physician organizations evolve into independent legal entities, which contract with the HMO.

Staff models are not dependent on existing medical resources in the community to the extent of the other models of HMOs. Instead, staff models are dependent on supply and demand characteristics of physician services. In the early days of the HMO industry, staff models had difficulty recruiting physicians. Now, however, with physician services in oversupply, recruitment is not a problem.

Several of the national HMO development firms are committed to establishing staff models because they maximize control and facilitate expansion. Sometimes it is easier and quicker to hire physicians than it is to affiliate with existing medical groups in the community. This is particularly true in areas that have not been touched by health care competition. With adequate capitalization, which many of the national HMO development firms have, a staff model is often the most expeditious route.

HMOs that are based on the group practice model face different circumstances. A primary advantage of the group practice HMO is that their practice style is generally conducive to the goal of cost-effective medical practice. Group practices are generally more outpatient oriented. Multispecialty medical groups provide coordinated care at primary, secondary, and tertiary levels. This combination of outpatient orientation and coordination accounts for a style of care that is cost-effective.

Another advantage of the group practice model is that the delivery system is built around established, functioning medical groups. Thus, developmental costs can be lower. In addition, building the HMO around an existing group practice offers the HMO a certain amount of legitimacy early in its development. Also, patients of affiliated medical groups often join the HMO with which the group affiliates.

However, the distribution of medical groups in the United States is uneven. In some areas, medical groups are not the prevalent form of practice. There are also issues of location when affiliation with existing groups is in question. Many times groups are not located in optimal locations from the HMO's perspective.

A seemingly insignificant but important fact is that physicians of the group practice model are not employees of the HMO. They are members of a professional corporation, which contracts with the HMO. This relationship preserves the autonomy of the physician and provides a buffer between individual physicians and the HMO.

The capitation form of reimbursement helps limit the HMO's need for utilization controls over primary care services. The group practice is financially responsible for providing all primary care services for the members. The responsibility for controlling services outside normal levels is that of the group. The group is the sole beneficiary of controlling such unnecessary service. The HMO can concentrate its efforts on controlling referral and inpatient utilization because its liability for primary care services is fixed contractually.

Several trends are developing with respect to group practice HMOs. Nationally, HMOs are now more frequently affiliating with existing groups than forming new, independent medical groups. Where there are few existing groups, though, HMOs sometimes form new groups. In most cases, it is not the intent of the HMO for these medical groups to provide only prepaid services. In some areas, HMOs exert control over the placement of satellites with groups that already affiliate with them. Since most of the multispecialty groups have already affiliated with HMOs, HMOs are turning to affiliation with primary care groups. There is an accompanying interest in HMOs on the part of single-specialty groups.

Finally, HMOs are increasingly attempting to share the risk for inpatient hospital services with affiliated medical groups. In the capitation contracts the medical groups are at risk for physician services. HMOs attempt to shift some of the risk for inpatient care through utilization controls.

Network models are established when HMOs affiliate with a number of medical groups. Because HMOs need to expand their geographic accessibility, HMOs that affiliate with only one group are now a minority. However, HMO affiliation with several unrelated groups is unwieldly. Each of the groups has its own interests, and they may not cooperate for the good of the HMO. A network model HMO may not achieve a fully integrated delivery system because the groups either will not refer to each other when possible or will not hire specialists to reduce outside referrals.

IPAs are becoming a prevalent model for HMOs. The IPA has the advantage of providing extensive accessibility. However, because individual physicians practice out of their own offices, standardization and supervision are difficult to achieve.

IPA models were initially organized by medical societies as a competitive response to increasing market shares of other HMOs. They provided a means for individual practitioners to become involved in prepayment alternatives, and they provided them with a marketing tool.

The majority of the IPA models are reimbursed on a modified fee-for-service basis, so there remains an incentive to provide extra services. Without adequate controls, this basic element of an IPA can present significant problems. Earlier, IPA models started with few controls over the practices of their affiliated physicians. After experiencing some financial difficulties, HMOs added controls over inpatient utilization. As the proportion of an affiliated physician's practice that is comprised of HMO members increases, the easier it becomes to introduce utilization controls in other areas, such as ambulatory care and diagnostic tests. Many of the early IPAs were open to specialists as well as to primary care physicians. In addition, many IPAs allowed members to refer themselves to any physician in the panel. Both of these factors opened the HMO to the possibility of adverse selection. In addition to selection problems, IPAs that allowed free choice of physician also had difficulties in controlling ambulatory utilization.

More recently, some HMOs have developed IPA models that incorporate a *gatekeeper* concept to circumvent the control problems produced by the free choice of physician. The gatekeeper concept requires a member to choose a specific physician, who is then responsible for coordinating the member's care, and for referring the member when necessary. The HMO maintains two networks of physicians—one primary care, the other specialist. Members of such IPAs can only elect to receive care from the primary care panel, and they are usually unaware of the specialist panel. The primary care physicians coordinate the member's care, and if necessary, they can refer the member to a physician from the specialist panel. Such variations are cost effective in two ways—reducing unessential referral care and retaining referrals within the organization.

In addition to the structural variations of IPA models, many of the primary care network models are changing the reimbursement schemes customarily found in IPAs. Traditional IPAs reimburse physicians on a fee-for-service basis. The primary care network models generally reimburse physicians on a capitation basis, thus putting the physician at risk for primary care medical services.

While many of the first IPAs were formed around county medical societies, there has been a trend recently for hospitals to be the focal points for IPAs. From the IPA's standpoint, the hospital's admitting staff provides an organizational focus that can greatly reduce the organizational effort needed to form a medical delivery system. Certain advantages also accrue to the hospital. These will be discussed later.

The majority of physicians now become affiliated with HMOs for economic reasons, rather than ideology. HMOs are one means for physicians to cope with increasing competition and with federal and state policies dictating the direction of medical care financing and delivery. HMOs offer a private sector solution that enables physicians to compete and to benefit from the marketing expertise that is becoming so important in health care.

While some physicians say that HMOs were initially seen as a defensive strategy by physicians, many see them now as an offensive strategy. Some respondents reported that physicians are viewing prepaid medicine as just another "line of business" that allows them to benefit from an expanding segment of the health care market.

The other major component of the HMO's medical delivery system is the hospital. HMOs have two options regarding inpatient services for their members. They may own a hospital or they may contract services from existing community hospitals. Most HMOs have chosen the latter option.

In selecting a hospital with which to affiliate, an HMO employs several criteria. One important criterion is service. Does the hospital provide the major types of hospital services that will be required by the HMO's members? Another important consideration is the marketability of the hospital. Marketability has a number of dimensions: image, both to consumers and to physicians; location; reputation for quality; and the hospital's relationships with the business community are the most important ones. Another important criterion is cost. The HMO is interested in selecting a cost-effective hospital whose financial position compares favorably with those of other institutions in the community. The HMO is also interested in affiliating with hospitals that are willing to establish a favorable financial relationship.

HMOs establish a variety of financial arrangements with hospitals. These arrangements include reimbursements for full charges, discounts of charges, per diem charges, per case charges, and risk-sharing arrangements. A variety of factors affect the type of financial arrangement that the HMO and the hospital settle on.

The model of physician organization in the HMO affects both the type of arrangement and the number of hospitals with which the HMO affiliates. Because volume is the primary determinant of the financial relationship, the ability to concentrate patients at particular institutions and the absolute number of HMO members are critical variables.

Staff models have the greatest ability to concentrate their members who need hospital services at particular hospitals. They are also most able to determine where their physicians have hospital privileges. Group practice and network models are generally able to focus patients depending where their physicians have admitting privileges. IPA models generally have the least ability to focus patients at any one institution. However, as the number of IPA members in a physician's practice increases, the IPA can increasingly affect the physician's hospital affiliations.

As their market share increases, HMOs have been able to negotiate more favorable financial relationships with hospitals. HMOs usually begin by negotiating relationships based on reimbursement of full charges. Later, these relationships can evolve into more favorable arrangements based on discounts, per diem or per case charges, or risk-sharing arrangements. The centralized HMO models can generally negotiate more favorable financial arrangements more quickly than the decentralized models because of their ability to concentrate patients.

Objective market conditions are extremely important to both physician models and hospital relationships. Geographic conditions of the HMO's service area may affect the number of relationships with hospitals and the most appropriate type of physician organization. Supply and capacity characteristics of the health care market have an immense effect on the willingness of physicians and hospitals to affiliate with HMOs. An oversupply of physicians and declining occupancy and utilization in hospitals have led to a perception of competition that has had a tremendous effect on the willingness of these sectors to participate in HMOs.

Minneapolis-St. Paul

The discussion of medical delivery issues above reveals a partial but important explanation for the vigorous development of HMOs in the Twin Cities. The Minneapolis-St. Paul medical delivery system in the early 1970s was already sophisticated about coordinated care through multispecialty group practices. The providers also had similar training and backgrounds. They respected each other and communicated readily. However, even in that environment, change in professional practice was accepted very slowly.

During the early years of operation, Group Health Plan was viewed with contempt by the medical community in the Twin Cities. As was discussed in chapter 5, the health plan was not formally censured by either the Hennepin or Ramsey County medical societies. Still, physicians associated with the plan were viewed by their colleagues as being outside the mainstream of medical practice. While the early physicians had a strong ideological commitment to prepaid practice, which helped them weather the storm, medical staff recruitment and management was an ongoing problem. Group Health Plan created an independent advisory board of prestigious academic physicians to validate their medical procedures and the qualifications of their staff. Nevertheless, the plan had trouble getting specialists outside the plan to accept referrals of Group Health members.

Until 1977, Group Health experienced recruiting, staffing, and workload problems. These problems, coupled with a perceived lack of physician input into decision making, led to a rift between the plan's administration and physicians. To provide greater communication, a coordinating committee of physicians and administrative staff was created. Later, physicians formed a physicians association to represent their interests.

Since 1980, Group Health has been concerned about physician productivity, motivation, and incentives. In addition, the health plan evaluated the merit of converting to a group practice model. More recently, to increase accessibility, the plan has begun affiliating with existing medical groups.

Like Group Health, SHARE began as a staff model HMO, and they experienced problems in physician recruitment. However, physician recruitment there was facilitated by the fact that the staff was led by two prominent, well-known physicians in the Twin Cities. In 1979, to expand more rapidly, the health plan began to affiliate with existing medical groups. Shortly thereafter, its medical staff formed an independent professional association, which completed a contract with the health plan.

Coordinated Health Care began by contracting with the Department of Medicine at the St. Paul Ramsey Medical Center to provide primary care services to plan members. Consulting services were provided by the other academic departments at the medical center. Over time, the staff of the medical center has formed a professional association and established several satellites. In addition, the health plan has affiliated with other existing medical groups.

MedCenter Health Plan and Nicollet-Eitel Health Plan each began with their sponsors acting as sole providers of medical care. Over time, the Nicollet Clinic has remained the sole provider for the Nicollet-Eitel Health Plan. It has established satellites throughout the metropolitan area. St. Louis Park Medical Center remains the largest provider for MedCenter Health Plan, but the health plan has affiliated with other existing medical groups in the area, including a federation of primary care groups in the east metro area. These affiliations are exclusive and subject to approval by the medical center. St. Louis Park Medical Center had grown by establishing satellites. Health plan members make up an increasing portion of the medical center's business. Originally, the medical center had expected a greater number of referrals from MedCenter's affiliated medical groups. Later, obtaining more accessible and convenient referral care became more important.

HMO Minnesota's medical delivery network is a combination of several models. The health plan began providing medical services through a network of multispecialty groups. Later, they added several IPAs. An increasing number of primary care groups have affiliated with HMO Minnesota. First, HMO Minnesota added several IPAs organized around hospital medical staffs. Also, the Ramsey County Medical Society formed an IPA that affiliated with HMO Minnesota. Currently, the plan affiliates with over 1,500 physicians in the Twin Cities. When the plan experienced utilization control problems, they instituted controls. They changed to a primary care gatekeeper concept. As a result of financial and utilization controls, several medical groups and IPAs terminated from the plan.

When Physicians Health Plan was organized by the Hennepin County Medical Society, the plan arranged contracts directly with physicians. Plan members can select care from any of the 2,000 physicians participating in the plan and can switch participating physicians as often as they like. In organizing the health plan, the administrative staff had difficulty convincing independent practitioners to join the health plan because physicians were generally busy and were experiencing only slight competition from other HMOs. In addition, the health plan was asking them to accept discounted payments for their services and to undergo utilization review. However, physicians reported that the endorsement of physician leaders in the Hennepin County Medical Society and the concerns about possible competition, particularly from hospitals, convinced many to join. Utilization and financial controls have been instituted gradually. After a contingency fund, voluntary controls, and peer review all failed to reduce utilization problems, mandatory hospital controls and mental health/chemical dependency controls were instituted. Currently, the health plan is reviewing physicians' office practices and establishing controls based on practice norms.

A variety of affiliations and financial arrangements exist between hospitals and HMOs in the Twin Cities. Several hospitals, such as Eitel Hospital and St. Paul Ramsey Medical Center, have risk-sharing arrangements with their affiliated HMOs. Most of the HMOs have been able to negotiate favorable financial arrangements with hospitals, such as discounts, per diem charges, or per stay charges, among others. The growing market share of the HMOs make such affiliations attractive for hospitals.

In this increasingly competitive market, some of the HMOs put their hospital services out to bid. In recent years, Group Health Plan has taken an aggressive stance in negotiations with hospitals. The plan can focus its inpatient needs at several hospitals. It wishes to affiliate with several strategically placed hospitals, who are willing to share the financial risks, and to align the incentives of the hospital with those of the health plan. The plan has been evaluating the feasibility of controlling or purchasing its own inpatient facility if it is unable to reach favorable agreements with existing hospitals.

On the other hand, Physicians Health Plan, which initially received no discounts from hospitals, is now in a position to negotiate per diems or per stay arrangements with its participating hospitals. If the hospital is unwilling to negotiate, it is removed from the list of participating hospitals, and its affiliated physicians are unable to admit. Hospitals are willing to negotiate because of the fear that if participating physicians are unable to use their hospital for HMO patients, they will also not use their facility for other patients.

Chicago

In Chicago, HMOs have had similar experiences with medical care delivery. Some problems, particularly concerning physician opposition and physician recruitment have been more persistant and widespread.

Union Health Service is a staff-model HMO. After several years of operation, the physician staff formed an association, which serves primarily as a bargaining unit with the plan's administration. Over time, the plan has gone from employing part-time to full-time primary care physicians. In recent years, the plan has instituted controls over inpatient utilization. The plan has limited geographic accessibility with one primary site and one satellite. It recognizes the need to expand, so it is considering affiliation with existing groups or establishing small clinics on its own.

Anchor, a staff model, employs a staff of primary care physicians who all hold teaching appointments at Rush Medical College and have staff appointments at Rush-Presbyterian-St. Luke's Medical Center. The decision to have the staff physicians hold teaching appointments at the medical college and staff privileges at the medical center has facilitated recruitment. Physicians are basically on the payroll of the medical center and the HMO pays either all or a portion of their salary. This assisted the HMO with staffing during periods when full-time staff for the HMO were not required. Now the HMO has a full-time physician staff. Initially, the HMO received some opposition from the primary care physicians affiliated with the medical center, but specialists were supportive. Utilization controls are a relatively recent part of Anchor's program. At first, a small and dedicated staff provided cost-effective medical care in response to informal controls and peer pressure. With growth in the physician staff and less ideological reasons for practicing in a prepaid plan, formal controls have become necessary. Recently, the plan has been assessing various physician incentive plans. Physicians have formed a physicians association, partially as a result of a growing rift between management and physicians. Anchor has been rapidly expanding the number of their delivery sites. Each site is staffed by primary care physicians employed by the plan.

Michael Reese Health Plan started as a group model. When the plan was organized, a number of physicians affiliated with the Michael Reese Hospital formed a medical group and contracted with the plan. Other primary care physicians opposed the plan. However, a physician leader at the hospital urged the plan to form the HMO through the medical staff and board. After years of operation, the hospital offered to sell the health plan to the physician group. They refused, and the health plan hired its own physician staff. At this point, the opposition from the physicians at the hospital surfaced again. The health plan was viewed as competing with private practitioners affiliated with the hospital. The health plan has faced staffing and space problems until recently. For several years, the health plan experienced difficulties with controlling inpatient utilization. Instituting utilization control procedures and hiring an active and effective medical director largely eliminated this problem. More recently, the health plan has experimented with incentives to increase physician performance and reward utilization control. Over the past several years, the health plan has expanded its clinic sites, primarily in the southern and southeastern metropolitan areas.

Medical services for NorthCare were rendered by the NorthCare Medical Group, which was formed with the health plan to deliver services under an exclusive contract. Initially, the physicians of the medical group served some fee-for-service patients as well as members of the HMO. Eventually, they converted to an entirely prepaid model. The initial contractual arrangement between the health plan and the medical group specified a "pass through" of the expenses of the medical group to the health plan. Under the agreement with PruCare, the medical group receives a capitation for physician services with incentives to control inpatient utilization. PruCare has invested significant funds into the expansion of the health plan from its northern focus to throughout the metro area.

Chicago HMO initially purchased physician services from the Chicago Center Hospital (formerly Roosevelt Hospital), and it used the hospital's outreach clinics as delivery sites. Physicians staffing these clinics were salaried by the hospital. The HMO has moved since then toward a network model by affiliating with small (2 to 3 person) medical groups. The health plan has expanded the number of delivery sites significantly.

Intergroup was the first network model in the Chicago area. Initially, the health plan affiliated with existing multispecialty medical groups. As a result of the limited number of multispecialty medical groups in the Chicago area, the HMO has recently affiliated with primary care groups and has been moving toward hospital-focused IPA arrangements. Many of the groups affiliated with Intergroup are also affiliated with the other network model, HMO Illinois. This presents some marketing problems, particularly to employers that offer HMO Illinois. However, utilization control is better because a group pays more attention to cost containment when a larger percentage of their practice is prepaid. These groups are, in fact, subject to two sets of control mechanisms. One disadvantage is that these groups can play one HMO against the other. Intergroup initially formed the provider network without realizing the importance of utilization controls. The HMO's first major task was attracting medical groups, and it feared that stressing utilization controls would have made this task more difficult. Although there were always some controls imposed, medical groups are more willing now to accept controls and to play an active role in their implementation. Intergroup had the majority of its first delivery sites in Chicago with several in the suburban areas. Over time, they have aimed at filling in the delivery network. Their most recent activities have focused on adding providers in the suburban areas.

As noted above, HMO Illinois is also a network model. It affiliates with several of the medical groups that are affiliated with Intergroup. Over time, HMO Illinois has focused on filling in their delivery network. Like Intergroup, its main focus has been on suburban areas. Since 1979, recruitment of physician groups into the HMO has changed. Rather than the HMO seeking out groups, medical groups have been seeking out the HMO. In addition, physicians have approached the HMO for assistance in forming groups to affiliate with the HMO. The addition of new groups to the HMO is market driven, that is, new groups are added in areas that are prime marketing targets. HMO Illinois attempts to put new medical groups and satellites of existing group into areas not served currently by other HMOs.

New network HMOs are developing with hospitals as their focus. Over time, Rush-Presbyterian-St. Luke's has realized that Anchor must use less expensive community hospitals for the majority of its primary care inpatient services and use the medical center for tertiary inpatient care. Michael Reese Hospital, which initially saw its health plan as a feeder for the hospital, has now learned that suburban members do not want to travel to the hospital in Chicago. Recently, the hospital has recognized that the plan must use less expensive community hospitals. Chicago HMO has increasingly used other hospitals because Chicago Center Hospital does not offer all of the HMO's needed inpatient services.

Until recently, hospitals in Chicago have generally not been willing to make financial arangements with HMOs that specify reimbursement less than charges. As HMO market shares increased, though, several HMOs negotiated discounts with hospitals interested in capturing a portion of the market. Several hospitals have affiliated with HMOs as provider groups offering both physician and inpatient services.

MARKETING DEVELOPMENT

Marketing is one of the most critical aspects of HMOs. HMOs have the ability to offer the traditionally separate products of insurers and providers as an integrated package. The HMO's traditional product involves two customers—an employer (purchaser) and an employee (consumer).

HMO marketing is a two step process. The first step involves convincing the employer to offer the HMO's services, usually as an option to the traditional health insurance plan. The second step involves convincing the employee to enroll in the HMO plan.

The traditional targets of HMO marketing efforts have been the largest employer groups and public sector employers because the HMO can realize economies of scale in their marketing activities. When a market matures, however, HMOs begin to look at customer groups that they ignored in the past, even individuals.

Very few markets have reached such a level of maturity. A mature market is usually characterized by the following factors: 1) the largest employers all offer one or more HMOs, 2) many employers offer multiple HMOs, 3) penetration in the largest employers approaches high levels (50 to 75 percent), and 4) competition on the basis of access and price among HMOs reaches acute levels.

In mature markets, HMOs begin to focus efforts on smaller employers. While these employers are less knowledgeable about HMOs, they are currently experiencing the largest increases in premiums of any size of employer. In addition, these smaller employers use insurance brokers to a large extent for their health insurance needs. To gain acceptance in this market, HMOs must focus on educating both the small employers and the health insurance brokers. In short, different market segments require different marketing approaches.

As markets mature, HMOs also begin offering their products to public programs, such as Medicare and Medicaid. Some HMOs have been quite successful with the Medicare program, but few HMOs are involved in the Medicaid program at this point. Again, HMOs must tailor their marketing approaches to these programs. The needs of these markets are different from the commercial group market, and the ways of accessing them are also different.

In mature markets, HMOs also examine ways to "feed" their various programs. An example of this is marketing to college students or Medicare spouses. The HMO hopes that these segments will develop a relationship with the HMO, so when they become eligible for coverage, they will "graduate" into the HMO's program.

An important factor affecting HMO marketability is the synchrony between the HMO product and the type of product that the market demands. HMOs historically offered comprehensive coverage for physician and hospital services without copayments or deductibles. Historically, HMOs have offered only this one product. If the market demands a relatively scant package of benefits, though, it will be difficult for an HMO to sell its product. In areas where there is great diversity in the levels of employee health benefits offered by employers, HMOs may also have a more difficult time marketing their product. The comprehensive benefit package offered by most HMOs may be too expensive compared to other health plans offered by employers.

HMOs are increasingly involved in new product development. This is particularly true in mature markets. As HMOs reach out to different market segments, they are finding that these new customer groups require different products. Some HMOs are offering additional health services, such as dental and vision services.

There is also a trend toward increasing benefit flexibility; that is, HMOs are more willing to tailor benefit packages to the requirements of the purchaser. Along this line, HMOs are developing benefit packages that include copayments and deductibles. These low-option benefit packages are attractive to smaller employers. These efforts also seem to be in step with the general market trend toward greater employee cost sharing.

HMOs are also adapting their product lines in response to competition from a vast array of alternative delivery systems currently being developed. Preferred provider organizations are especially causing concern among HMOs. Therefore, some HMOs are developing their own extended access programs that offer the advantage of not limiting the HMO member's access to a specified group of providers.

Competition is also coming from fee-for-service insurers who are incorporating cost containment strategies in their health benefit packages, making them more cost competitive. Some HMOs are marketing their cost containment technologies to employers. Finally, some HMOs are marketing themselves as third-party administrators for self-insured employer groups.

In the development of a market for HMOs, that is, in reaching out to the potential purchasers and consumers of the HMO's product, education has always played an important role. Education must be aimed at both the purchaser and consumer. There are also different educational requirements in different markets. For example, in markets where there is a large geographic expanse or a heterogeneous population, it is more difficult to acquaint employees with HMOs.

Employers play a chief role in introducing employees to HMOs, so the support of the employer is initially critical to the HMO's marketing program. In the early 1970s, a tremendous amount of education was necessary to overcome the reluctance of employers to offer HMOs. Employers have since become more familiar with the HMO concept.

There remain, though, significant differences in the knowledge of small and large employers regarding HMOs. Large employers, with a staff of professional health benefits administrators are quite knowledgeable about HMOs. Larger employers were also the first target of HMO marketing efforts. As a result, HMOs are still rather foreign to smaller employers. One factor that has significantly increased the knowledge and interest of all employers about HMOs has been escalating health care costs. HMOs have been identified by employers as a strategy to contain costs while maintaining a high level of benefits.

Federal qualification played an important role in overcoming the inertia of employers during the depressed economic times in the middle to late 1970s. In addition, some HMOs sought federal qualification to tap into federal grants and loans. HMOs are becoming qualified for competitive purposes. Many national companies have a policy that they will offer only federally qualified HMOs. In addition, many employers perceive federal qualification to be a "Good Housekeeping seal."

As employers in a community begin to offer HMOs in their benefit packages, an interesting phenomenon occurs. Rather than emphasize the general benefits of the HMO concept, HMOs begin to compete against each other by accentuating the differences between them. Competition begins initially in terms of accessibility and then in terms of price.

Advertising takes on an important role in developed markets as HMOs attempt to differentiate themselves. Advertising is a means of communicating with both purchaser and consumer. It is one of the most important means of reaching the consumer.

Advertising must be tailored to the particular customer groups to which it is aimed. Customer groups have differing levels of knowledge and awareness about HMOs. The employee of the large business group usually knows about HMOs, so advertising is used as a means to create familiarity with a particular HMO. For employees of smaller groups, advertising must serve an educational purpose.

Another factor that becomes important in mature markets is retention. Brand-name loyalty and promotional activities are aspects of efforts to enhance retention.

When an HMO market is approaching maturity, HMOs also explore ways to expand geographically. This can be through the addition of delivery points within their geographic area or through expansion to a new health care market. Some HMOs are investigating the prospects of establishing national networks to attract national employers.

Minneapolis-St. Paul

In the early 1970s, the Twin Cities market was primed for HMO marketing efforts. There was strong support for the HMO concept among leading employers. HMOs were offered initially not as cost containment but as a "better value" for employers interested in expanding benefits. Although HMO premiums were generally higher on introduction than indemnity-based health insurance, larger employers were willing to invest higher premium costs in HMOs because they liked the concept and hoped for a payoff later in cost containment. The majority of small employers had generally been satisfied with their fee-for-service health insurance coverage, so they delayed offering HMOs until the middle to late 1970s.

From 1970 to 1975, HMOs were offered by the small number of large and supportive private sector employers and by the majority of large public employers. During this period, the HMOs marketed to different market segments generally defined by their delivery sites or by preexisting relationships with employer groups.

HMO marketing efforts suffered from 1974 to 1977 as a result of economic recession and of the lack of clarity regarding employer obligations under the federal HMO act. In 1976, SHARE Health Plan drew attention to HMOs when it became federally qualified. They took advantage of mandating procedures that required employers to offer HMOs to their employees. Because SHARE was relatively unknown and had limited geographic accessibility, and, employers say, because they wanted to make their own decisions, employers who were mandated generally offered several HMOs besides SHARE. This marked the beginning of a period of extensive growth for HMOs in the Twin Cities. It also marked the beginning of HMO competition.

From 1977 to 1980, HMO market share rose sharply, fueled by employers offering multiple HMOs and by the geographic expansion of the HMOs. Some employers attained HMO penetrations greater than 50 percent, and the overwhelming majority of the largest employers offered one or more HMOs. HMO competition based on price and other factors increased. Since 1980, HMOs in the Twin Cities have increasingly stressed their differences, often by advertising. HMOs are also developing new products.

Group Health Plan, which stresses that it is the largest and oldest HMO in the Twin Cities and the upper midwest, also stresses the benefits of their "one stop" medical care. In recent years, Group Health Plan has marketed to the following market segments: individual, Medicare (cost contract), Medicaid, and small and large employer groups. Group Health has developed an attractive product for small employers. It involves offering the employer a combination of indemnity and HMO policies. This enables the small employer to deal with one vendor and still offer its employees a dual option. If employees use Group Health physicians, they receive full comprehensive benefits; if they don't, they receive lesser indemnity benefits with copayments and deductibles. Group Health Plan is also involved with several other HMOs nationwide, offering their network to major national employers with employees in the cities where the HMO affiliates are located. Recently, Group Health Plan has started to advertise, often emphasizing its extensive dental program.

Coordinated Health Care initially confined its limited marketing efforts to public sector employers in Ramsey County. The strategy was to break even with enrollment from public sector employers then go into the private market. A dedicated marketing staff was not hired until they entered the private market some years later. Marketing was difficult because the sponsoring hospital had a public hospital image, there was limited accessibility, the public believed the plan was confined to Ramsey County workers (thus, the name change), and the HMO entered the market behind two more successful programs. Now Coordinated Health Care markets itself as distinct because it has federal qualification, because their service area includes part of western Wisconsin, and because its size allows it to provide personal service.

Marketing for MedCenter Health Plan was first done under contract with Northwestern National Life Insurance Company. MedCenter pursued employers with managerial, professional, and technical workers. Since the health plan's delivery sites were located in the suburban areas of Minneapolis, it was convenient to these workers. The health plan's marketing strengths include its affiliation with the well-known and prestigious St. Louis Park Medical Center and its education program. The health plan has done little advertising and has increasingly marketed its products to small employers. It has also participated in the Twin Cities Medicare Capitation Demonstration Project, with which it has had limited success.

Nicollet-Eitel Health Plan was first marketed by Aetna insurance agents. However, there were few incentives for the agents to sell the HMO, and they were not experienced at selling a prepaid product. Eventually, the plan's marketing was brought inside. The plan had other marketing problems, including the number and location of its delivery sites and the image of the hospital. Over time, the health plan has expanded its delivery network. Nicollet-Eitel is also involved with the Medicare demonstration project. They have had limited success marketing the program.

SHARE was the first, and for a long time, the only federally qualified HMO in the Twin Cities. As discussed earlier, SHARE's attempts to take advantage of the federal mandating process may have helped other HMOs in the Twin Cities as much as it did SHARE. In 1979, SHARE began to expand by affiliating with an existing group practice and by establishing new delivery sites. It was the first HMO to serve the Medicare population, and until it joined the Medicare demonstration project recently, it held a cost contract with the Health Care Financing Administration. Now SHARE has a risk contract and has been successful enrolling senior citizens. SHARE's other marketing efforts include: marketing to small employers and individuals, telemarketing, and advertising. SHARE's service area includes the Twin Cities and northern Minnesota.

HMO Minnesota stresses the breadth of its service area in its marketing. It has a balanced delivery system, located throughout the metro area. This geographic dispersion leads to a balanced risk selection. In its sales strategy, HMO Minnesota compares closed and open panel HMOs and emphasizes the differential selection. HMO Minnesota also emphasizes that a primary care physician coordinates the member's care. They stress that this enables the health plan to provide excellent, cost-effective care. HMO Minnesota works with brokers. It markets to small groups and is interested in marketing to individuals. Like other HMOs involved in the Medicare demonstration project, it has had limited success marketing the program.

HMO Minnesota has been tailoring benefit packages more to the needs of employers. They start with a basic package and allow the employer to add benefits incrementally. Some of their benefit packages have copayments on illnesses and injuries, but all preventive care is paid completely. The cost sharing provisions and the data about costs and utilization that the plan will provide to employers have been attractive to many businesses. The health plan operates in the Twin Cities and throughout Minnesota, and it has become more aggressive in its advertising.

Physicians Health Plan was initially marketed through a subsidiary of the St. Paul Companies. Like Nicollet-Eitel's efforts, this strategy was unsuccessful because the brokers didn't understand the HMO product and there was no financial incentive to sell the HMO. Eventually, the plan internalized their marketing efforts. The plan offers a variety of health benefit packages. Some have copayments included. Cost sharing is important to compete with insurers that offer less expensive benefits and to protect the HMO from adverse selection. Physicians Health Plan has successfully marketed to small employers, who usually offer only the HMO and terminate their indemnity coverage. The health plan has the largest delivery network of any of the HMOs, including an IPA of dentists. The plan stresses that it is the only "pure" IPA model in the Twin Cities. Recently, the plan became federally qualified.

Physicians Health Plan is offering many options in service, including a preferred provider contract that allows employees to use providers not affiliated with the health plan for less comprehensive coverage. Physicians Health Plan offers preadmission certification to employers to help them control health care costs in their self-insured plans, and it provides employers with cost and utilization data. They also offer a Medicare benefit on a "cost plus" basis (a Medicare supplemental). A variation of this program allows seniors to select a low cost program if they are willing to use specified providers. The health plan has advertised aggressively for several years.

Chicago

It has been noted that employers in Chicago were generally unfamiliar with the HMO concept in the early 1970s. Chicago did not have HMO information brokers, such as InterStudy and the TCHCDP. Some organizations sponsored HMO forums before 1973, but there was little interest by the employers in attendance. During this period, employers in Chicago seemed satisfied with their health insurance programs. Employers were not interested in expanding employee health benefits, and they were not interested in competitive reform. Besides, HMO premiums were higher than those offered by conventional insurers. The early supporters of HMOs in Chicago believed in the preventive aspect of HMOs. Chicago employers did not accept the cost containment premise of HMOs, so they were unwilling to invest in high premiums in hope of later payoff.

Before 1973, there were a few employers receptive to the HMO concept. These included several financial institutions, utilities, and some public sector employers. Early marketing efforts in Chicago concentrated on explaining the HMO concept. HMOs had little success with most employers because of the high premium differentials and lack of geographic accessibility. After the passage of the federal HMO law, employers' resistance set in. Employers did not know what they were responsible for under the HMO regulations and tried to "put the HMOs off." After several HMOs in Chicago became federally qualified, the mandating battle between qualified HMOs began. Some HMOs sent mandating packages to employers by registered mail. Many observers claimed that this use of the mandate provisions retarded HMO development in Chicago for many years. It created an atmosphere of antagonism and animosity that lasted for several years. Following this period, HMOs engaged in cooperative education efforts, focusing on the general concept.

Finally, in the late 1970s and early 1980s, employers in Chicago began embracing HMOs in response to rapidly escalating health benefit costs. For the first time, HMO premiums were equal to or lower than insurance premiums. HMOs have also greatly expanded their delivery networks, so their services are more accessible. HMOs in Chicago have experienced intense growth since 1980. Intense competition is now emerging among HMOs, which are finally attempting to differentiate themselves.

Union Health Service is the oldest prepaid health plan in Chicago. In many cases, union members receive comprehensive outpatient care through the health plan, but their hospitalization is self-funded. Union Health Service also offers an HMO, but it has not received many members under this program because of the lack of delivery sites. It is offered by major private and public sector employers that have a policy of offering all HMOs. In addition, its union connection provides it with access to other public sector employers. Over the past few years, Union Health Service has noticed increasing interest in its program from union trust funds facing the same escalating costs as others. Union Health Service sees its growth coming from its HMO and trust fund programs.

Anchor Organization for Health Maintenance was initially opened as an outpatient clinic for employees. Later it affiliated with Blue Cross-Blue Shield's Co-Care program. Anchor was marketed by this program for several years. During this period, Anchor received a grant to develop an internal marketing program. Anchor is currently enrolling as many employer groups as possible and has the largest client base of any of the HMOs in Chicago. They are selective in their enrollment. If the premium differential is large, they will not offer their program. Their affiliation with a prestigious medical center and the quality of their medical group are important marketing points. The health plan has increasingly used advertising, primarily mass mailings, and it employs a special person to cultivate union accounts. The health plan also has a cost contract to enroll Medicare beneficiaries.

CNA Insurance was initially interested in Intergroup because they saw the possibility of cross-fertilization of group accounts, but this did not work out. In the early days, Intergroup would not market to any group that offered the other network plan, HMO Illinois. Now Maxicare/Intergroup competes directly with HMO Illinois. Maxicare differentiates itself from its competitors by the service it provides to enrollees and employers. Maxicare has a number of provider groups and sites that are not in the HMO Illinois network. Maxicare/Intergroup stresses its health education and has dispatched service representatives to each of its major affiliated medical groups to help members use the HMO effectively. The plan is part of Maxicare's national HMO network and it has a national accounts manager for employers in the network's other service areas. Recently, the plan engaged a broker development program. Maxicare/Intergroup also operates in southern Illinois.

HMO Illinois is the successor of Illinois Blue Cross-Blue Shield's Co-Care program. Initially, marketing for HMO Illinois focused on converting Co-Care accounts. Following this, the HMO focused on selling the HMO to existing Blue Cross accounts. Now, the HMO markets to all employers, and Blue Cross representatives offer the HMO to employers they contact. The Blue Cross-Blue Shield affiliation is important or detrimental depending on the employer. HMO Illinois is part of the national Blue Cross-Blue Shield Association's HMO network. The plan works actively with labor unions in the Chicago area, and it will tailor benefit packages to the employer's needs. HMO Illinois operates throughout Illinois.

Michael Reese Health Plan initially served hospital employees. It did not have a full-time marketing staff. Instead, financial solvency came first. The health plan hit breakeven very early with enrollment from the medical center. Overcrowding at facilities and a lack of local hospital locations have been major marketing problems for the health plan. Michael Reese Health Plan is now constructing a new central clinic site, and it is expanding into new areas in the metro area. Location is the main factor differentiating Michael Reese from Anchor and Prucare. Southern delivery locations and the affiliation with Michael Reese Hospital and Medical Center are major selling points.

Marketing NorthCare was difficult at first because of limited geographic access. The health plan had locations only in the northern metro area. In addition, the publicized lack of financial stability hurt its marketing. Prucare has rectified both of these problems, and the health plan has rapidly expanded. Prucare is extremely market and service sensitive. It differentiates itself from its competitors by emphasizing the quality of its medical group and facilities. While Prucare does offer its product to different market segments, e.g., Medicare beneficiaries, its primary goal is expanding its delivery sites.

Chicago HMO's marketing to Medicaid recipients in the central city was done by community workers going door-to-door. Later, the Illinois Department of Public Aid allowed mailings to recipients. After several years, Chicago HMO became federally qualified, and they offered services to private employers. Its central city location and image as a "welfare" HMO caused difficulty marketing to private employers. The first employers to offer the plan had a policy of offering all HMOs. Later, Chicago HMO redirected its marketing efforts to people in its service area, i.e., blue-collar and medically underserved urban dwellers. In other words, they focused on a segment not traditionally served by HMOs. Chicago HMO's marketing is directed at the consumer. In recent years, the health plan has dealt successfully with unions and expanded its delivery network to serve them. In addition, the health plan is having great success with small employers, who have generally been neglected by other HMOs. Chicago HMO continues to serve the Medicaid population.

SUMMARY

This analysis of four aspects of HMO development in two markets shows important differences, but these differences result largely from different environments rather than from the organization and operation of the HMOs themselves.

The formation of the seven HMOs in the Twin Cities must be viewed as a whole. Their development is interrelated. The early HMOs provided an example for others to follow and the incentive for others to compete. In Chicago, the HMOs were more independent and isolated in their initiation and formation. In Minneapolis-St. Paul, multispecialty group practices were important early sponsors. In Chicago, individual unions, hospitals, and carriers sponsored the first HMOs. Several developing HMOs in the Twin Cities contracted administrative and management services from outside. In Chicago, the HMOs for the most part performed these services themselves.

In the Twin Cities, the HMOs' medical delivery systems were based largely on existing multispecialty groups with service and communication appropriate to HMOs. In addition, two large IPAs were initiated by the Hennepin and Ramsey County medical societies. Now in the early 1980s, the overwhelming majority of physicians in the Twin Cities metro area are affiliated with one or more HMOs. In Chicago an established system did not exist. Staff models were the predominant model, and they have grown slowly. The two network models in Chicago have been limited by the scarcity of multispecialty groups and the unfamiliarity and resistance of solo practitioners. Only a small percentage of physicians in Chicago are affiliated with an HMO.

Dramatic differences were found in the market for HMO services in the two areas. Employers' awareness and concern seem to be the key. In the Twin Cities, the market developed rapidly in the 1970s because employers' interest was essentially strong, responsive, and reinforcing just when the HMOs were developing and beginning to market to employers. The market is now mature and enrollment is leveling off. In Chicago the market developed slowly in the 1970s because employers were mostly unaware, unresponsive, and, in fact, negative to HMO marketing. In the 1980s, in part because of HMO's own marketing efforts, and largely because of the nationwide concern about escalating health benefit costs and the awareness of alternatives, the Chicago market is developing more rapidly.

This examination of past and present development, management, and marketing of HMOs suggests some expectations for the future. Effective management and sponsorship has been seen to be very important. Although there will always be local HMOs, national HMO management and development firms will play an increasingly important role in developing new HMOs and managing existing ones. These national firms have great financial resources by virtue of their access to financial markets. These organizations are acquiring not only financial resources but also management expertise and administrative resources.

Interesting coalitions can be expected to form between providers in the sponsorship of HMOs. Hospitals and physicians will join forces in the development of HMOs and other alternative delivery systems. National multihospital firms are likely to play an increasingly important role in alternative delivery system development. Indemnity insurers, who are not already in the HMO industry, may increasingly develop cost containment methodologies and confine their involvement in alternative delivery system development to the area of third-party administration and preferred provider arrangements.

Great diversity is likely in HMO medical delivery systems as they adapt their delivery systems to the requirements of their service area. Hybrid models, which mix the best aspects of the various traditional HMO models, will be commonplace. Control technologies will continue to be developed. However, when HMOs approach optimal cost efficiency, they will look toward fully integrating and controlling all aspects of their production technologies. Vertical and horizontal integration is likely to occur to fully rationalize their delivery systems. HMO operations will become increasingly bureaucratized and formalized. HMOs will also scrutinize their cost structures and pricing policies.

HMO marketing can be expected to present combinations of current prepaid products with increasingly flexible benefits and possibly a cafeteria-style product line. These new product developments will go together with marketing efforts to new groups, such as small employers, and Medicare and Medicaid recipients. HMOs are also likely to diversify their products and to develop product synergies. There will be increased attention to cost containment techniques, preferred provider arrangements, multiple employer trusts, and programs for worker's compensation.

Conclusion

This study demonstrates how health maintenance organizations developed in two different metropolitan areas during a time when rising expenditures for personal health services caused great concern. This study established a baseline of more than ten years' experience with fifteen HMOs in two large market areas. Although HMOs developed more rapidly in the Twin Cities than in Chicago, the issue, we found, was not one of success or failure. It is the different social, political, and economic environments, and the initiatives and responses in the two communities that caused the market to mature earlier in Minneapolis-St. Paul than in Chicago.

Why do more than 25 percent of the residents in Minneapolis-St. Paul receive their health care through HMOs compared with only 4 percent of the residents in Chicago? In the last chapter, it was noted that when the HMOs of the two communities were compared historically what had appeared superficially to be marked differences between them reflected not variation in the organization or operation of the HMOs themselves, but rather differences in their stages of development. When corresponding stages are compared, the contrasts between communities are not significant. Thus, the issue to be explained is not success or failure but differential growth. Because HMOs were established in both market areas at nearly the same time and their internal behavior and characteristics were similar, the question becomes why was development accelerated in the Twin Cities? The com-

---

The conclusion was written by Claire H. Kohrman, Research Project Analyst.

munity context was clearly crucial. Thus, the analysis of the seven sectors in each community, reflected in the preceding chapters, contributes to our understanding. Each sector has had its unique role to play. Now, they must be considered together for an overall understanding. While a number of aspects of the individual sectors are shown to be necessary for HMO development, none alone is sufficient to guarantee their success. No amount of available capital, motivated providers, eager consumers, or creative marketing can by itself account for the differential development of HMOs in the two markets.

The development of HMOs as well as other aspects of health care in the two metropolitian areas can be described in the context of well-known indicators of health system performance: access, quality, and cost. We both measured (to the extent possible) and interviewed about these issues as we searched for a cause of the community differences.

Although the study sought a cause, it found instead a set of conditions, a series of actions, and a network of interactions that only *together* provide an explanation. That is, analysis of the interviews with those immersed in the sectors of the community and familiar with the health care market development in the 1970s and early 1980s, reveals three fundamental categories for explaining the differential development of HMOs:

Preexisting environment, i.e., social, political, and economic context as well as the perceived state of the delivery system, *before* the period of HMO activity considered in this study;

Initiatives or actions regarding HMOs; and

Responses in the community which, in fact, reflect the interaction of the actions or events with the preexisting environment, and with the current environment. (The ever-changing environment is itself a consequence of all three of these parameters.)

PREEXISTING ENVIRONMENT

Minneapolis-St. Paul

Invariably, in all of the earlier chapters, authors have referred to the homogeneity and progressiveness in the Twin Cities.

It remains only to say that this combination of social homogeneity, political progressivism, and economic stability reflected in every sector of the Minnesota analysis provides not only a facilitating environment but also a primary cause of the accelerated development of HMOs. For example, one way in which the progressive and homogeneous characteristics of the medical sector were manifest was in the high incidence of preexisting multispecialty group practice. Thus, the form of medical practice, to which HMOs needed only add the prepayment mechanism, was already well-known and respected. Furthermore, those physicians who had been associated with innovations in the past could be expected to adopt new innovations most quickly (Coleman, et al., 1966).

Among employers there was already established a history of responsible and successful community leadership, including the "5 % Club" in which corporations taxed their financial, social, and managerial resources in the interest of community growth and well-being.

Hospital administrators exemplified the homogeneity, cooperation, and communication patterns within sectors. In addition, the field researchers noted, the Twin Cities hospital administrators were more like, for example, employers and insurers in the Twin Cities than like hospital administrators in Chicago.

The preexisting similarities, cooperative history, and networks *between* the sectors, as well as within the sectors, and at the highest levels of leadership (exemplified by the Citizens League) provided ideal conditions for the support and spread of innovation (Burt, 1980).

Also in the environment were the community perceptions of the performance of the then available health care system—its accessibility, its quality, and its cost. Throughout the interviewing in the Twin Cities, there was uniform pride expressed in the quality of health care available in the Twin Cities. Furthermore, all sectors, including consumer groups, felt that all citizens of Minneapolis-St. Paul had access to good health care. In fact, the unique or unanimous concern was with cost, and in this case, each sector had its own perspective on the problem of rising health care cost. Because there was a widely shared perception among consumers, payers, and providers about health care delivery in their metropolitan area, there was also a preexisting readiness to agree on solutions.

Chicago

In Chicago, in the early 1970s, the social, political, and economic environment did not provide a foundation for the support or diffusion of a new idea in health care delivery. Although certain individuals made isolated efforts to promote HMOs, the absence of centralized nonpolitical civic leadership, the emphasis in Chicago on social, political, and economic differences, and the lack of communication networks, even within the sectors, inhibited the acceptance, support, or diffusion of HMOs.

Physicians outside of university medical centers practiced almost exclusively as solo practitioners, and the medical centers had a long history of competition for resources and patients. Although resources in the Twin Cities and Chicago appeared superficially to be similar—that is, the per capita income was similar—in Chicago, resources were very unevenly distributed among a heterogeneous population largely through an adversarial political process. Where in the Twin Cities there has been a perception of plenty, in Chicago there has been a perception of scarcity. Furthermore, the boundaries of ethnic and racial, urban and suburban neighborhoods were sharply defined and consequently not conducive to the citywide spread of new ideas.

Perceptions of the health care delivery system differed widely in Chicago among payers, consumers, and providers. Although payers were concerned with efficient use of health care dollars, the consumers and providers saw quality and access as the most important problems. The absence of consensus on the nature of the problem provided an unlikely environment for common solutions.

National

The environmental factors influencing HMO development that have been discussed have been largely local. Certain national influences, like feasibility study grants for HMOs and the federal qualifying regulations, were noted. In the 1980s, there has been increased national awareness of health care costs and health care policy. This awareness is part of each community's environment. Because, as was just noted, the HMOs' market development of these two communities is at different stages, increased national activity has different effects in each community. In Minneapolis-

St. Paul, where local efforts have already educated the community, a mature market has developed, and the larger employers have been enrolled; there is little effect from the national attention being given procompetition solutions such as HMOs. However, in Chicago, where there has been little local initiative and the large employers have not been extensively enrolled, the national attention given to cost and health care delivery alternatives now supplements local support. Thus, it has played an important role in the accelerated growth of HMOs there.

INITIATIVES

Although the prexisting environment has been shown to be powerful, the initiatives and responses concerning HMOs are also important factors which contribute to an explanation of their different development in the two markets being studied here. The actions regarding HMOs were initiated for different reasons, by different groups, with different influence in the two communities.

Because cost, not access or quality, was the concern in the Twin Cities, it was payers—influential corporate employers and some insurers—who raised the issue and formed the influential Twin Cities Health Care Development Project (TCHCDP). The actions and findings of the TCHCDP were widely reported, and they raised awareness of prepaid health care in the community.

At approximately the same time, physicians at the prestigious St. Louis Park Medical Center were aware of the growing concerns about cost and of the abundance of physicians in their area. Eager to be ahead of possible regulation, they began to experiment with prepayment for a small part of their clinic population. In addition, national health policy advisor, Paul Elwood, from InterStudy, vigorously advocated national, as well as local, support of HMOs as a cost-saving, competitive health policy alternative.

In Chicago, early actions were initiated not in response to cost, but largely in response to concerns about access and quality. They were initiated by consumers and providers, not payers. Homemakers, schooled by earlier cooperative and religious activities, proposed and sponsored NorthCare to improve access to health care for themselves and their families. In another part of the city, unions at Rush-Presbyterian-St. Luke's and later at Michael Reese pressured the hospitals to offer access to prepaid care for the hospital workers.

RESPONSES

These similar actions by committed individuals and organizations in the two communities evoked different results. In the Twin Cities, the action brought responses that multiplied in the densely networked environment. When St. Louis Park developed its experimental MedCenter Health Plan, it was widely known and carefully observed. It soon elicited both enrollees and competitors. In Chicago, though, when Anchor and Michael Reese Health Plan were opened, most of the health care community knew nothing about them, or they ignored them because they considered them unimportant in their market or community. NorthCare, when introduced in the northern suburb of Evanston, was considered more of a curiosity or human interest story than a significant institution, relevant to the very large, fragmented city of Chicago to its south.

There is excellent communication and responsiveness not only between sectors in the Twin Cities but also within sectors. For example, when SHARE, the only federally qualified HMO, mandated employers, the employers communicated among themselves both informally and formally, and most responded by offering not only SHARE but also a selection of other HMOs—an important step in their distribution and growth.

In Chicago, when employers were first mandated by federally qualified HMOs, the employers, largely isolated from each other, reported that they did not know how to respond. They dragged their feet, then passively made the HMO available to their employees.

In the Twin Cities, responsiveness was further enhanced by managerial and material resources not available in Chicago. For example, when HMOs approached Twin Cities hospitals, the administrators had not only the incentive to negotiate but also a cooperative relationship with their medical staff and the support of their hospital trustees.

In summary, one can see that the social, economic, and political environment, as well as the health care concerns, together have had the most powerful influence on the development of

HMOs—richly facilitating and reinforcing their development and impact in the Twin Cities, and blunting or inhibiting their development and impact in Chicago. In the 1980s, Chicago may depend more on the impact of national health policies and escalating health care costs to alter entrenched local systems and to facilitate the growth of HMOs. In the 1970s, Minneapolis-St. Paul benefited from its abundant resources and an established cooperative pattern in its community. It has itself provided a model for health care delivery as it has facilitated the development and growth of health maintenance organizations.

Epilogue

This study demonstrates that the development of competitive HMO options needs a community acceptance and support, even though some of the capital may come from the outside, as in Chicago. It will be recalled that the Twin Cities wished to depend on home capital and initiation largely because of the cohesive nature of that metropolitan area.

Although HMOs in the Twin Cities were developed largely to reduce the cost of medical care, after more than ten years of development in the Twin Cities, it is not possible to determine conclusively if competition lowers costs. Providers have found ways to improve and expand services competitively within existing cost structures, and the Twin Cities experience suggests that hospital utilization and expenditures may drop. Twin Cities respondents active in the Citizens League and the Metropolitan Health Board anticipate that the transformation of the health services delivery system will take from ten to fifteen years. This is a sobering but mature judgment given the usual propensity of Americans for quick-fix solutions. Quick-fix solutions are clearly inappropriate for something as ponderous and complicated as a health services delivery system, which is constantly and intensely interacting with providers, patients, insurers, employers, and regulatory agencies. The health services enterprise is fundamentally different from other goods and services in that its customers are sick by and large, and the providers are necessarily and inherently expensive. It still remains to be seen if the consumers are willing to settle for the lowest-cost delivery system or what may be regarded as a reasonably priced one. It may be that consumers will opt for a higher expenditure than employers or government are willing to match. In that case, consumers would perforce have to pay more for more expensive and presumably more desirable HMOs and the battle for more funding from employers and government would continue.

Already in both the Twin Cities and Chicago there is evi-

The epilogue was written by Odin W. Anderson, Principal Investigator.

dence that employers are turning to self-insurance, which is increasing as deductibles and co-insurance are rising and benefit ranges are being pared. Although the Twin Cities are homogeneous with a very small poor population, Chicago is heterogeneous and has a very large concentration of poor people. HMOs were not designed to serve the poor without subsidy from one source or another. They were designed to be efficient methods of financing and delivering services to a stable, employed group. Chicago informants did not tend to see HMOs as a helpful broad-based alternative. The Twin Cities informants did not share this concern, understandably so, since the population is much more homogeneous—ethnically, educationally, and economically. It will be recalled that one Chicago respondent with experience in the Twin Cities said that he would send any member of his family to any hospital in the Twin Cities area, but not in Chicago. Perhaps, the two-tiered and possibly even three-tiered system is universally inevitable in delivery systems, considering the difficulties of one-class service. Perhaps a two-tiered system is so inevitable that there will eventually emerge luxury HMOs and "adequate" HMOs, varying according to premium cost. Even though this practice would go against the grain of American belief in equity, another option, a universal health insurance system, has its own problems of equity.

No HMOs in the Twin Cities have failed. One was financially troubled in Chicago until it was bought out by a major insurance company when the original sponsors realized that they could not operate it like a community service agency and expect to recover deficits from the community.

In essence both Chicago and the Twin Cities have the same health services delivery structure, which is supposed to be in the process of transformation, i.e., free-standing hospitals (with many in multiple units), privately practicing physicians with hospital affiliations, and a variety of funding sources—employers, employees, government, and insurance agencies. These similar characteristics provide similar avenues for containing costs. The extent to which each market area will be penetrated by HMOs remains to be seen. Although it is likely that the Twin Cities will eventually have a greater market penetration than Chicago, it is apparent that the Twin Cities has been an easier market to penetrate than Chicago. A market penetration of 20 percent in Chicago might well be regarded as a greater achievement than 30 percent in the Twin Cities. Chicago is clearly at a take-off point, and the Twin Cities area is in a period of maturation. HMOs in the Twin Cities are beginning to collide with each other and to regroup internally to contend with the new and tougher market conditions there.

Both market areas have evolved during the last fifteen years or so under an umbrella of certificate-of-need laws and hospital rate regulations, but with somewhat different results. The Minnesota certificate-of-need law, together with the recommendations of the Citizens League and cooperation from the hospitals, had some effect on the supply of hospital beds. As for rate review of hospitals, Minnesota depended on hospital cooperation whereas Illinois' rate review agency was set up but has since been abandoned. A clear demonstration of the cooperation between the public and private sectors in the Twin Cities is that Minnesota is ready to abandon its certificate-of-need regulation because of the perception that HMOs and competition preclude the necessity for the regulation of supply.

What seems to be emerging in both of the market areas and, indeed, throughout the United States generally is a retreat from overall health planning. Each medical care complex is establishing its turf and feeling out its respective boundaries.

FUTURE RESEARCH

As the HMOs acquire an increasing share of the market, what are the subsequent research questions that should be addressed, building upon the baseline established by this study in the two market areas?

1. Is there adverse selection, i.e., do HMOs get the "healthier risks" and, therefore, are they able to have relatively low premiums? Is the whole traditional group insurance concept, which protected itself from self-selection, being shattered?
2. Will there be less concern about adverse selection and cost shifting if a large proportion of the population is enrolled? If Medicare and Medicaid recipients are enrolled?
3. If there is adverse selection, what are the public policy implications when some elements of the population, such as the sicker and more aged ones, are left with higher costs than the healthier and younger population?
4. What are the differences in physician practice patterns in dif-

ferent organizational contexts? Are there quality implications? What changes in physicians' decisions occur?

5. In the long run how much shifting is there from plan to plan during open enrollment periods and what are the characteristics of that shifting?
6. Is the hospital case mix changing toward sicker patients?
7. Given the lower use of hospitals what happens to the service mix in the spectrum of services? Does the distribution of medical complaints brought to the physician's office change?
8. Does the greater attention to the bottom line result in longer delays in getting appointments, shorter consultations, or increased out-of-plan use?
9. How large will the mainstream health services market be, and why do people remain in the mainstream market?

The most general concerns out of the above list are physicians' practice pattern and patient self-selection. It is important to gain some insight into what a well-considered, cost-conscious health services delivery system will cost in terms of adequacy, quality, and convenience, and then to consider who is left out if the group insurance concept is eroded.

In the meantime, the United States is trying to transform its delivery system so that a large portion of it can be highly structured along HMO lines and a large portion will also remain more or less "loose-jointed" and give the American people a choice with minimum concern for equity. Choice will presumably give the consumer some leverage on the medical care system that was not there before. It is hoped that the American public will be knowledgeable enough to know what choices to make. This will be the ultimate test of the viability of the concept of consumer sovereignty.

References

Introduction

Anderson, Odin W.
1972 Health Care: Can There Be Equity? New York: John Wiley and Sons.

Anderson, Odin W. and Joanna Kravits
1968 Health Services in the Chicago Area—A Framework for Use of Data. Research Series 26. Chicago: Center for Health Administration Studies, University of Chicago.

Banfield, Edward C.
1961 Political Influences. New York: Free Press.

Blegen, Theodore C. (ed.)
1975 Minnesota: A History of the State. Minneapolis: University of Minnesota Press.

Christianson, Jon B. and Walter McClure
1979 "Competition in the Delivery of Medical Care." New England Journal of Medicine. 301 (October 11): 812–818.

Citizens League
1976 "The Citizens League Itself: Report on its Achievement of a Record of Cumulative Effectiveness in the Twin Cities Area." Reprinted from the National Civic Review (July).

Citizens League
1977 "More Care About the Cost in Hospitals." Citizens League Report. Citizens League Committee on Hospitals in the Twin Cities (September 16).

Cope, Lewis
1971 Minneapolis Tribune (April 22).

Cope, Lewis
1979 Minneapolis Tribune (April 12).

Elazar, Daniel J.
1970 Cities of the Prairie: The Metropolitan Frontier and American Politics. New York: Basic Books.

Enthoven, Alain C.
    1980 Health Plan. Menlo Park, CA: Addison-Wesley.

Gibson, Geoffrey, et al.
    1970 Emergency Medical Services in the Chicago Area. University of
          Chicago: Center for Health Administration Studies.

Gieske, Millard L.
    1979 Minnesota Farmer-Laborism: The Third Party Alternative. Min-
          neapolis: University of Minnesota Press.

Gleason, Bill
    1970 Daley of Chicago: The Man, The Mayor, and the Limits of Con-
          ventional Politics. New York: Simon and Schuster.

Greenstone, J. David and Paul E. Peterson
    1973 Race and Authority in Urban Politics: Community Participation
          and the War on Poverty. New York: Russell Sage Foundation.

Harrigan, John J. and William C. Johnson
    1978 Governing the Twin Cities Region: The Metropolitan Council in
          Comparative Perspective. Minneapolis: University of Minnesota
          Press.

Hauser, Philip M. and Evelyn M. Kitagawa (eds.)
    1953 Local Community Fact Book for Chicago, 1950. Chicago: Uni-
          versity of Chicago Press.

Herman, Edith
    1974 Chicago Tribune (May 29).

ICF, Inc.
    1980 Case Study Report on the Competitive Impact of HMOs in Chi-
          cago. Washington, DC: U.S. Government Printing Office, Con-
          tract No. OHMO-DHHS 282-79-0094-GH.

Janowitz, Morris
    1967 The Community Press in an Urban Setting. Second edition. Chi-
          cago: University of Chicago Press.

Karlen, Harvey M.
    1958 The Governments of Chicago. Chicago: Courier Publishing.

Kilian, Michael, et al.
    1979 Who Runs Chicago? New York: St. Martin's Press.

Kotulak, Ronald
    1972 Chicago Tribune (March 1).

Luft, Harold S.
    1981a Health Maintenance Organizations: Dimensions of Perfor-
          mance. New York: John Wiley and Sons.

Luft, Harold S.
1981b The Operations and Performance of Health Maintenance Organizations: A Synthesis of Findings from Health Services Research. USDHHS-PHS-NCHSR Contract No. 233-79-3016.

Mayer, Harold M. and Richard C. Wade
1969 Chicago: Growth of a Metropolis. Chicago: University of Chicago Press.

Metropolitan Council—Metropolitan Health Board
1981 "The Health Care System in Transition: Problems and Progress in the Twin Cities Metropolitan Area." Report Prepared for the Council's 1981 State-of-the-Region Conference. Publication No. 18-81-017 (March 18).

Minneapolis Star
1972 (April 31).

Minneapolis Tribune
1980 (September 21).

Minneapolis Tribune
1981 (June 7).

Morone, James A.
1982 The Dilemma of Citizen Representatives: Democracy Planning and Bureaucracy in Social Health Politics. Ph.D. Dissertation. University of Chicago.

Nye, Russell B.
1959 Midwestern Progressive Politics: A Historical Study of its Origins and Development, 1870–1958. East Lansing, MI: Michigan State University Press.

Pearre, James
1976a Chicago Tribune (February 21).

Pearre, James
1976b Chicago Tribune (April 15).

Royko, Mike
1971 Boss: Richard J. Daley of Chicago. New York: Dutton.

Schmid, Calvin F.
1937 Social Sage of Two Cities: An Ecological and Statistical Study of Social Trends in Minneapolis and St. Paul. Minneapolis Council of Social Agencies.

Shortell, Stephen M. and Arnold D. Kaluzny (eds.)
1983 Health Care Management: A Text in Organization Theory and Behavior. New York: John Wiley and Sons.

Simak, Clifford
1974   Minneapolis Tribune (March 15).

Slovut, Gordon
1971   Minneapolis Star (April 21).

Slovut, Gordon
1973   Minneapolis Star (April 28).

Uphoff, Mary Jo and Walter Uphoff
1980   Group Health: An American Success Story in Prepaid Health Care. Minneapolis: Dillon Press.

Wolfe, Shiela
1972   Chicago Tribune (February 24).

Wolinsky, Fredric D.
1980   "The Performance of Health Maintenance Organizations: An Analytic Review." Milbank Memorial Fund Quarterly: Health and Society, 58:4 (Fall), 537–587.

Zelten, Robert A.
1979   "Alternative HMO Models." Issue Paper No. 3. University of Pennsylvania, National Health Care Management Center (April).

Chapter 1: Minneapolis-St. Paul and Chicago

Berki, Sylvester E. and Marie L. Ashcraft
1980   "HMO Enrollment: Who Joins What and Why." Milbank Memorial Fund Quarterly/Health and Society 58 (Fall): 588–632.

Berki, Sylvester E., et al.
1978   "Enrollment Choices in Different Types of HMOs" Medical Care 16 (August): 682–697.

Christianson, Jon B.
1980   "Can Business Stimulate Economic Competition in Health Care?" Business and Society (Winter): 15–22.

Goldberg, Lawrence G. and Warren Greenberg
1981   "The Determinants of HMO Enrollment and Growth." Health Services Research 16:4 (Winter):421–438.

ICF, Inc.
1980   Case Study Report on the Competitive Impact of HMOs in Chicago. Washington, DC: U.S. Government Printing Office.

Keller, Polly
1981   "A Population Ecology Model of the Distribution of Organiza-

tional Forms: The Case of Health Maintenance Organizations."
Dissertation, Stanford University.

Luft, Harold S.
1981 Health Maintenance Organizations: Dimensions of Performance. New York: John Wiley and Sons.

McNeil, Richard Jr. and Robert F. Schlenker
1975 "HMOs, Competition, and Government." Milbank Memorial
Fund Quarterly 53:2 (Spring):195–224.

Morrisey, Michael A. and Susan Ashby
1981 "An Empirical Analysis of HMO Market Share." Revised ver-
sion of a paper presented at annual meetings of the American
Public Health Association (October, 1980).

Yedidia, Avram
1959 "Dual Choice Programs." American Journal of Public Health,
49:11 (November):1475–1480.

Chapter 2: HMOs and Regulators

Goldberg, Lawrence G. and Warren Greenberg
1981 "The Determinants of HMO Enrollment and Growth." Health
Services Research 16:4(Winter):421–438.

Luft, Harold S.
1981 The Operations and Performance of Health Maintenance Organizations: A Synthesis of Findings From Health Services Research USDHHS-PHS-NCHSR Contract No. 233-79-3016.

Mackie, Dustin L.
1981 "An Overview of HMOs From The Federal Perspective." in
Dustin L. Mackie and Douglas Decker, Eds., Group and IPA
HMOs. Rockville, MD: Aspen.

McNeil, Richard, Jr. and Robert E. Schlenker
1975 "HMOs, Competition, and Government." Milbank Memorial
Fund Quarterly 53:2 (Spring):195–221.

Minnesota Department of Health
1982 "Voluntary Price Reporting Under Chapter 614 of Minnesota
Laws 1982" (December 21).

Strumpf, George B.
1981 "Historical Evolution and The Political Process." in Dustin L.
Mackie and Douglas Decker, Eds., Group and IPA HMOs. Rockville, MD: Aspen.

Uphoff, Mary Jo and Walter Uphoff
1980   Group Health: An American Success Story in Prepaid Health Care. Minneapolis: Dillon Press.

Chapter 3: HMOs and Consumers

Aday, Lu Ann, Ronald Andersen, and Gretchen V. Fleming
1980   Health Care in the United States: Equitable for Whom? Beverly Hills: Sage Publications.

Citizens League
1981   "Paying Attention to the Differences in Prices: A Health Care Cost Strategy for the 1980s." Citizens League Report.

Harrelson, E. Frank, and Kirk Donovan
1975   "Consumer Responsibility in a Prepaid Group Health Plan." American Journal of Public Health, 65:10 (October):1077–1086.

Lou Harris & Associates, Inc.
1980   American Attitudes toward Health Maintenance Organizations. New York: Lou Harris & Associates, Inc.

Luft, Harold S.
1981a Health Maintenance Organizations: Dimensions of Performance. New York: John Wiley and Sons.

Luft, Harold S.
1981b The Operations and Performance of Health Maintenance Organizations: A Synthesis of Findings from Health Services Research. USDHHS-PHS-NCHSR Contract No. 233-79-3016.

Mercer, Lyle
1973   "The Role of the Member in the Group Health Cooperative of Puget Sound" in U.S. Health Maintenance Organization Service, Selected Papers on Consumerism in the HMO Movement. Washington, DC: USGPO, Department of Health, Education and Welfare Publication No. HSM 73-13012, July.

Minneapolis Star
1978   "How the Twin Cities Cut Health Care Costs." Editorial (October 17).

New York Times
1978   (November).

Uphoff, Mary Jo and Walter Uphoff
1980   Group Health: An American Success Story in Prepaid Health Care. Minneapolis: Dillon Press.

Chapter 4: HMOs and Hospitals

American Hospital Association
1980   Hospital Statistics: Data from the American Hospital Association 1979 Annual Survey. Chicago, Illinois: American Hospital Association.

Appel, Gary L.
1982   "HMOs—The Minneapolis Experience." Luncheon address to The Chicago Hospital Council Symposium "Prepaid Health Plans—An Alternative to Current Delivery Systems." (November 3, 1982).

Appel, Gary L. and David Aquilina
1982   "Hospitals Won't Compete on Price Until Spurred by Buyers' Shopping." Modern Health Care (November): 108–110.

Aquilina, David and Gary L. Appel
1983   "HMOs' Real Competitive Role." Hospitals (September 1):89–92.

Blau, Peter
1964   Exchange and Power in Social Life. New York: John Wiley and Sons.

Chandler, Alfred
1962   Strategy and Structure: Chapters in the History of The American Industrial Enterprise. Cambridge, MA: MIT Press.

Christianson, Jon B.
1981   "The Competitive Approach to Health Care Reform: Implications for Hospital Mangement." Health Care Management Review 6 (Fall):7–15.

Citizens League
1981   "Paying Attention to the Differences in Prices: A Health Care Cost Strategy for the 1980s." Citizens League Report.

Dorman, Noel
1982   "Competition and the Hospital Industry: The Promise vs. The Risks." Princeton, NJ: HRET Report No. 4 (March).

Downs, A.
1967   Inside Bureaucracy. Boston: Little Brown.

Fink, Frederick S. and John H. Trimmer
1981   "Operating and Financial Implications of Prepaid Plans On Hospitals." Topics in Health Care Financing (Fall): 57–67.

Freeman, John and Michael T. Hannan
   1983 "Niche Width and the Dynamics of Organizational Popula-
        tions." American Journal of Sociology 88 (6): 1116–1145.

Goldsmith, Jeff
   1981 Can Hospitals Survive? Homewood, IL: Dow Jones-Irwin.

Goldsmith, Jeff
   1983 "Hospitals Aim PPOs at Own Workers." Modern Healthcare
        (June):132–133.

Group Health Association of America, Inc.
   1981 "Hospital Contracting in Group Practice HMOs." Proceedings
        Of the Medical Directors Conference, Medical Directors Divi-
        sion, Washington, D.C. (June 12–13).

InterStudy
   1983 National HMO Census 1982.

Johnson, Richard L.
   1981 "Alternative Delivery Systems to Diversify Hospital Revenues."
        Topics in Health Care Financing (Fall).

Kralewski, John, et al.
   1982 "Patterns of Interorganizational Relationships Between Hospi-
        tals and HMOs." Inquiry 19 (Winter): 357–362.

Kuntz, Esther F.
   1983 "Aggressive Payers Push Twin Cities Hospitals to the Wall for
        Discounts." Modern Healthcare (July): 68–70.

Luft, Harold S.
   1978 "How Do Health Maintenance Organizations Achieve Their
        Savings: Rhetoric and Evidence." New England Journal of
        Medicine 298 (June 15): 1336–1343.

Mason, Scott and Mara M. Melum
   1979 "Cooperative Hospital Arrangements: The Twin Cities Health
        Systems and Shared Services Organizations, American Hospital
        Association (August).

Maykovich, Minako
   1980 Medical Sociology. Sherman Oaks, CA: Alfred Publishing Com-
        pany.

Melum, Mara M. (ed.)
   1980 The Changing Role of the Hospital: Options For the Future. Chi-
        cago: American Hospital Association.

Pfeffer, Jeffrey and Gerald R. Salancik
   1978 The External Control of Organizations: A Resource Dependence
        Perspective. New York: Harper & Row.

Seermon, Lynn
1981 "HMO-Hospital Relations" Center for Health Administration Studies. Unpublished.

Thompson, James D.
1967 Organizations in Action. St. Louis: McGraw-Hill.

Zelten, Robert A.
1979 "Alternative HMO Models." Issue Paper No. 3. University of Pennsylvania, National Health Care Management Center (April).

Chapter 5: HMOs and Physicians

Adams, David R. and A. Leslie Richardson
1983 "Affecting Legislation on the State Level." Medical Group Management 30 (March/April):34–36.

American Medical Association (AMA)
1982 Medical Groups in the U.S., 1980. Chicago: American Medical Association.

American Medical Association (AMA)
1981 Reference Guide to Policy and Official Statements. Chicago: American Medical Association.

Anderson, Odin W.
1968 "The Medical Profession and the Public: An Examination of Interrelationships." Michigan Medicine (April).

Becker, Howard S., et al.
1961 Boys in White: Student Culture in Medical School. Chicago: University of Chicago Press.

Berki, Sylvester E. and Marie L. Ashcraft
1980 "HMO Enrollment: Who Joins What and Why." Milbank Memorial Fund Quarterly/Health and Society 58:(588–632) Fall.

Boehm, William F., M.D.
1976 "Prepayment Group Practice: An Insider's Viewpoint. Chicago Medicine 79 (June 12):601–604.

Bosk, Charles L.
1979 Forgive and Remember: Managing Medical Failure. Chicago: University of Chicago Press.

Brown, Lawrence D.
1983 Politics and Health Care Organization: HMOs as Federal Policy. Washington, DC: Brookings Institution.

Chicago Medical Society
1970 Chicago Medicine (March 28).

Chicago Medical Society
1971 "Council Gives Go-Ahead to the Creation of a Foundation for Medical Care." Chicago Medicine 74 (May 8):341.

Chicago Medical Society
1981 Chicago Medicine (December 7).

Chicago Medical Society
1982 Chicago Medicine (November 7).

Coleman, James, et al.
1966 Medical Innovation: A Diffusion Study. Indianapolis: Bobbs-Merrill.

Ellwood, Paul M., Jr. and Linda Ellwein
1981 "Physician Glut Will Force Hospitals to Look Outward." Hospitals, 55 (January 16).

Enthoven, Alain C.
1980 "How Interested Groups Have Responded to a Proposal for Economic Competition in the Health Services." American Economic Review 70 (May):142–148.

Fitzmaurice, Bertrand T.
1959 "Our Doctor Sponsored Prepaid Plans in Washington: A Factor in Our Future." Northwest Medicine 58 (December):1707–1710.

Flexner, Abraham
1910 Medical Education in the United States and Canada. A Report to the Carnegie Foundation for the Advancement of Technology. Carnegie Foundation Bulletin No. 4 New York.

Foldes, Steven S.
1983 "Competition, HMOs and Changing Physician Behavior: A Critique of Public Policy in the Health Services Industry." Presentation to Center for Health Administration Studies Workshop (April).

Freeman, Howard, et al.
1979 Handbook of Medical Sociology. Englewood Cliffs, NJ: Prentice Hall.

Freidson, Eliot
1970 Profession of Medicine. New York: Dodd, Mead.

Freidson, Eliot
1975 Doctoring Together: A Study of Professional Social Control. New York: Elsevier Scientific.

Fuchs, Victor
1974 Who Shall Live? Health, Economics, and Social Choice. New York: Basic Books.

Goldberg, George A. and Warren Greenberg
1977 The HMO and Its Effects on Competition. Washington, DC: Federal Trade Commission, Bureau of Economics.

Goode, William
1957 "Community within a Community." American Sociological Review (22):194–199.

Group Health Association of America
1980 Group Health News (April).

Hennepin County Medical Society.
1974 Hennepin County Medical Society Bulletin 45 (May): 108.

Lou Harris & Associates, Inc.
1982 Medical Practice in the 1980's: Physicians Look at Their Changing Profession. New York: Lou Harris & Associates, Inc.

Luft, Harold S.
1981a Health Maintenance Organizations: Dimensions of Performance. New York: John Wiley and Sons.

Luft, Harold S.
1981b The Operations and Performance of Health Maintenance Organizations: A Synthesis of Findings from Health Services Research. USDHHS-PHS-NCHSR Contract No. 233-79-3016.

Meier, Gerald B. and John Tillotson, M.D.
1978 Physician Reimbursement and Hospital Use in HMOs. Excelsior, MN: InterStudy.

Minneapolis Star
1978 (May 3).

Minneapolis Star
1980 (February 25).

Minnesota Medical Association
1981 Minnesota Medicine (December).

Ramsey County Medical Society
1983 Ramsey County Medical Society Bulletin President's Page 77 (September).

Shouldice, Robert and Katherine Shouldice
1978 Medical Group Practice and Health Maintenance Organizations. Washington, DC: Information Resources Press.

Starr, Paul
    1982 The Social Transformation of American Medicine. New York: Basic Books.

Stevens, Rosemary
    1971 American Medicine and the Public Interest, New Haven: Yale University Press.

U.S. Department of Commerce, Bureau of the Census
    1982 County and City Data Book. Washington, DC: U.S. Government Printing Office.

U.S. Department of Commerce, Bureau of the Census
    1981 Statistical Abstract of the United States 1981. Washington, DC: U.S. Government Printing Office.

Chapter 6: HMOs and Insurers

Anderson, Odin W.
    1975 Blue Cross Since 1929: Accountability and the Public Trust. Cambridge, MA: Ballinger.

Carroll, Marjorie S. and Ross H. Arnett III
    1981 "Private Health Insurance Plans in 1978 and 1979: A Review of Coverage, Enrollment, and Financial Experience." Health Care Financing Review (September): 55–87.

Enthoven, Alain C.
    1980 "How Interested Groups Have Responded to a Proposal for Economic Competition in the Health Services." American Economic Review 70 (May):142–148.

Health Insurance Association of America
    1969 "Health Care Delivery in the 1970s" Recommendations of the Subcommittee on Health Care Delivery of the Committee on Medical Economics. Chicago: Health Insurance Association of America.

Health Insurance Association of America
    1982 Source-Book of Health Insurance Data: 1981–1982. Washington, DC: Health Insurance Association of America.

Koncel, Jerome A.
    1980 "Private Health Insurance Looks at HMOs." Hospitals 54 (August 16):137–142.

Munts, Raymond
    1967 Bargaining for Health: Labor Unions, Health Insurance, and Medical Care. Madison, WI: University of Wisconsin Press.

Provence, Marc E.
1981 "Insurance Carriers and the Business of HMOs." University of
      Washington HMO Technical Assistance Project Occasional Pa-
      pers Series (September).

Sheps, Cecil G. and Daniel L. Drosness
1961 "Prepayment for Medical Care." New England Journal of Medi-
      cine 246 (March 9):390–396.

Somers, Anne R. and Herman M. Somers
1961 Doctors, Patients and Health Insurance. Washington, DC: The
      Brookings Institution.

U.S. Department of Commerce, Bureau of Labor Statistics
1981 Area Wage Surveys. Washington, DC: U.S. Government Printing
      Office.

Woodward, Albert
1978 "The U.S. Health Insurance Industry." International Journal of
      Health Services 8 (3):491–507.

Chapter 7: HMOs and Employers

Berki, Sylvester E. and Marie L. F. Ashcraft
1980 "HMO Enrollment: Who Joins What and Why: A Review of the
      Literature." Milbank Memorial Fund Quarterly/Health and So-
      ciety 58 (Fall):588–632.

Ellwood, Paul M., et al.
1981 "Competition: Medicine's Creeping Revolution." Presented to
      the Sixth Private Sector Conference, Duke University Medical
      Center (March 23).

Enthoven, Alain C.
1978 "Shattuck Lecture—Cutting Cost without Cutting the Quality of
      Care." New England Journal of Medicine 298 (June 1):1229–
      1238.

Ginsburg, Paul B.
1981 "Altering the Tax Treatment of Employment-Based Health
      Plans." Milbank Memorial Fund Quarterly 59 (2):224–255.

Juffer, Jane
1982 "Firms Find Recession a Good Time to Reduce Employee Bene-
      fit Costs." Wall Street Journal (August 25):21.

Lou Harris & Associates, Inc.
1980 Employers and HMOs: A Nationwide Survey of Corporate Em-

ployers in Areas Served by Health Maintenance Organizations. New York: Lou Harris & Associates, Inc.

Luft, Harold S.
1978 "How Do Health Maintenance Organizations Achieve Their Savings: Rhetoric and Evidence." New England Journal of Medicine 298 (June 15):1336–1343.

Morrisey, Michael A.
1983 "Corporate Health Benefits and the Indexing of the Personal Income Tax." Journal of Health Politics, Policy and Law 7 (Winter):846–854.

Munts, Raymond
1967 Bargaining for Health: Labor Unions, Health Insurance and Medical Care. Madison, WI: University of Wisconsin Press.

Rushefsky, Mark E.
1981 "A Critique of Market Reform in Health Care: The 'Consumer Choice Health Plan'." Journal of Health Politics, Policy and Law 5 (Winter):720–741.

Sapolsky, Harvey M., et al.
1981 "Corporate Attitudes toward Health Care Costs." Milbank Memorial Fund Quarterly 59 (4):551–585.

Sehnert, Keith W. and John K. Tillotson
1978 How Business Can Promote Good Health for Employees and Their Families. Washington, DC: National Chamber Foundation 4.

U.S. Chamber Survey Research Center
1981 Employee Benefits, 1981. Washington, DC: Chamber of Commerce of the United States.

U.S. Department of Commerce, Bureau of the Census
1981a Statistical Abstract of the United States, 1981. Washington, DC: U.S. Government Printing Office.

U.S. Department of Commerce
1981b Survey of Current Business. Cited in U.S. Chamber Survey Research Center, Employee Benefits, 1981. Washington, DC: Chamber of Commerce of the United States.

Wilensky G. R. and Amy K. Taylor
1982 Tax Expenditures and Health Insurance: Limiting Employer-Paid Premiums." Public Health Reports 97 (September-October):438–444.

Chapter 8: HMOs and Organized Labor

Business Week
1977 "Dwindling Benefits Fuel a UMW Strike Threat: Management Refuses to Reopen Contracts on Health and Pension Issues." (July 25).

Business Week
1983 "Trying to Curb Health Care Costs at the Bargaining Table." (September 19):73–76.

ICF, Inc.
1980a Case Study Report on the Competitive Impact of HMOs in Chicago. Washington, DC: U.S. Government Printing Office.

ICF, Inc.
1980b Case Study Report on the Competitive Impact of HMOs in Philadelphia. Washington, DC: U.S. Government Printing Office.

Kirkland, Lane
1975 "Labor's Point of View on HMOs." Public Health Reports (March-April):104–105.

Kovner, Anthony R.
1977 "HMO and the United Auto Workers." Health Maintenance Organizations: Presentations from the 1976 Guest Lecture Series, Training Program in HMO Management. Philadelphia: Leonard Davis Institute of Health Economics, University of Pennsylvania: 217–226.

Luft, Harold S.
1981 Health Maintenance Organizations: Dimensions of Performance. New York: John Wiley and Sons.

Mabry, Bevars D.
1979 "Bargaining Power and Changes in Fringe Benefits." Review of Social Economy (April):25–36.

Munts, Raymond
1967 Bargaining for Health: Labor Unions, Health Insurance, and Medical Care. Madison, WI: University of Wisconsin Press.

Sapolsky, Harvey M., et al.
1981 "Corporate Attitudes toward Health Care Costs. Milbank Memorial Fund Quarterly 59 (4):551–585.

Seidman, Bert
1976 "The Role of Organized Labor in the Development of Prepaid Group Practice." Collective Bargaining Issues. Washington, DC: U.S. Government Printing Office.

Shelton, Jack K.
    1979 "Community HMO Built by Ford." Hospitals (August 16):79–
          80.

United States Council on Wage and Price Stability
    1976 The Complex Puzzle of Rising Health Care Costs. Washington,
          DC: U.S. Government Printing Office.

Uphoff, Mary Jo and Walter Uphoff
    1980 Group Health: An American Success Story in Prepaid Health
          Care. Minneapolis: Dillon Press.

Chapter 9: HMOs: A View from Inside

Kimberly, John R., et al.
    1980 The Organizational Life Cycle. San Francisco: Jossey-Bass Pub-
          lishers.

Lewis, Charles E.
    1977 "Health-Services Research and Innovations in Health-Care
          Delivery." New England Journal of Medicine. 297 (8): 423–427.

Luft, Harold S.
    1981a Health Maintenance Organizations: Dimensions of Perfor-
          mance. New York: John Wiley and Sons.

Luft, Harold S.
    1981b The Operations and Performance of Health Maintenance Orga-
          nizations: A Synthesis of Findings from Health Services Re-
          search. USDHHS-PHS-NCHSR Contract No. 233-79-3016.

Morrisey, Michael A. and Susan Ashby
    1981 "An Empirical Analysis of HMO Market Share." Revised ver-
          sion of a paper presented at annual meetings of the American
          Public Health Association (October, 1980).

Starr, Paul
    1982 The Social Transformation of American Medicine. New York:
          Basic Books.

Uphoff, Mary Jo and Walter Uphoff
    1980 Group Health: An American Success Story in Prepaid Health
          Care. Minneapolis: Dillon Press.

Wolinsky, Fredric D.
    1980 "The Performance of Health Maintenance Organizations: An
          Analytic Review." Milbank Memorial Fund Quarterly: Health
          and Society, 58:4 (Fall), 537–587.

Zelten, Robert A.
1979 "Alternative HMO Models." Issue Paper No. 3. University of
Pennsylvania, National Health Care Management Center (April).

Conclusion

Burt, Ronald S.
1973 "The Differential Impact of Social Integration on Participation
in the Diffusion of Innovations" Social Science Research 2 (August):125–144.

Coleman, James S., Elihu Katz, and Herbert Menzel
1966 Medical Innovation: A Diffusion Study Indianapolis: Bobbs-
Merrill.

Appendix A

Methodology

INTRODUCTION

To understand the factors affecting the introduction and growth of HMOs and their impact on the health care system, a methodology comprised of three distinct data collection approaches was formulated. A broad-based methodology was required to adequately understand HMO development and impact at several levels of analysis: individuals, health care organizations, and the health care system at large. The three data collection approaches used included: 1) a contextual market area analysis; 2) interviews with health care and community elite; and 3) HMO organizational case histories. These approaches render a data base of both qualitative and quantitative information which was used in the subsequent analyses. This data base was comprised of contextual, attitudinal, and organizational information. These types of data were complementary and, when used in combination, provided a rich source of data to understand HMOs.

A HISTORICAL AND COMPARATIVE FOCUS

The methodology for this study was both longitudinal and comparative: All three data collection approaches embody these attributes.

By design, this methodology incorporated a historical perspective. An important objective of this study was to capture the dynamic process of HMO development. Important research questions in the study focused on the *development* of HMOs within

---

Appendix A was written by Terry E. Herold and Ellen M. Morrison.

health care markets. The study focused on questions regarding both the introduction as well as subsequent growth of HMOs. Furthermore, it was important to view the HMOs' impact over time, as their impact was likely to differ depending when it was measured.

This research focused on Minneapolis-St. Paul and Chicago, where the health care systems and community structures are quite different. The HMO developmental experiences in these two areas have also been quite different. By viewing HMOs in these two quite different cities, the effects of contextual variables on HMO development can be precisely specified. Since many of the contextual characteristics varied between these two cities, insights into the types of effects produced by different levels of these variables can be gained. A comparative approach provided a perspective on the generality of the research findings.

Each of the three data collection approaches are discussed below. The technique used to collect data and how data contributed to understanding HMO development and impact are also discussed.

CONTEXTUAL MARKET AREA ANALYSIS

Recognizing that the context in which HMO development occurred may affect the course of that development as well as the potential impact of HMOs, detailed information on the health care system and health care market area was compiled for the Chicago and Minneapolis-St. Paul SMSAs.

HMOs are viewed as part of the larger health care system. The health care system provides health care resources required for their operation, such as labor, facilities, and financing. The availability of these resources affects HMO development.

The metropolitan area also serves as the potential market for the HMO's services. Understanding the market area in terms of population trends, socioeconomic and demographic characteristics, and employment and industrial characteristics defines the potential market for the HMO's services.

The potential for HMOs to affect the whole health care system may be measured in terms of their share of the health insurance market and the volume of services that they must purchase from other health care purchasers and providers. Information on the health insurance market share and the health care expenditures and utilization of various insurers and providers defines potential impact.

A data base, comprised of the contextual information specified above, was compiled for the Chicago and Minneapolis-St. Paul SMSAs for the period from 1950 to 1980. This data was collected mostly from secondary, existing data sources; such as census publications; health insurance industry publications; local, state, and regional regulatory and planning agencies; and health industry trade association publications. Estimates of sources and destinations of health care finances have also been constructed.

Based on existing research of the market area and health system correlates of HMO development, individual variables from the data base were analyzed with respect to their ability to facilitate or inhibit HMO development. Taken as a whole, these variables indicated the predisposition and potential of the metropolitan area for HMO development. Information from this data base was also used as contextual background data in the analyses of the other two data bases—interviews with health care and community elite, and the HMO case histories.

INTERVIEWS WITH HEALTH CARE AND COMMUNITY ELITE

The analysis of HMO development and impact had to consider the complexity of the health sector and the multiplicity of interests. Various groups have strong interests and large decision making roles in the health care system. The attitudes and perspectives of these groups toward HMOs were likely to affect the development and success of HMOs.

An important aspect of this research was to evaluate the impact of HMOs on various other parties in the health care system. This research assessed the range as well as the degree of HMO impact.

To understand the impact of various parties in the health care system on HMO development as well as the impact of HMOs on these various parties, face-to-face, semi-structured interviews were conducted with opinion leaders in the health care system and local community.

Preparation

In the early stages of the project, staff members conducted two analyses which provided information used to guide the overall investigation. First, staff members identified the key actors in the HMO arena. These actors include both individuals and organizations who interact with and/or influence HMOs. Second, staff members conducted an extensive review of HMO research and media coverage. This analysis identified the relevant issues and events which shape HMO development and growth. This section describes the developmental work.

The development of any organization requires resources and support from many sources. A new health care organization like an HMO requires inputs from its members, from other actors in the health care system, and from the community. Actors in the health care system and the community comprise the health care organization's environment.

During the planning stages of this study, staff members identified categories (sectors) of individuals and organizations which comprise the HMO's environment. Earlier research provided a framework for the identification of these sectors (Anderson and Kravits, 1968). The environment of a health maintenance organization consists of the following sectors:

1. Regulators
2. Consumers
3. Hospitals
4. Physicians
5. Insurers
6. Employers
7. Organized Labor

It was stated above that organizational development is shaped by actors within an organization as well as those in its environment. Therefore, in addition to the sectors which comprise the HMO's environment, the HMOs themselves comprise an important sector.

In addition to identifying key sectors, staff members conducted a thorough review of published research and literature on HMOs. The purpose of this review was to familiarize project staff with research findings on HMOs, attitudes toward HMOs, and local events and issues that had shaped HMO development.

The comprehensive literature review included: 1) past and

current research on HMO emergence, development, and operation; 2) case studies of HMOs; and 3) research on HMO marketing and performance. Project staff also reviewed literature on the adoption and diffusion of innovations, community decision making, organizations, competition in health care, insurance, and the health care system in general. Literature sources ranged from academic publications to trade association and professional publications. In addition, the staff consulted health services researchers in other institutions regarding HMO research in progress. Contact with other researchers was maintained and review of current research, editorials, and journal articles continued throughout the study.

Project staff also compiled briefing books for Minneapolis-St. Paul and Chicago. These books, comprised of selected newspaper articles, chronicle local events and issues relevant to HMO development, personnel, operation, performance, and environment. Newspapers also served as sources of information on community and health care influentials. Such information proved useful both for the selection of respondents and for the preparation of interviewers.

The majority of the newspaper articles examined were dated from 1970 to 1981. Project staff considered it important to cover HMO-related issues and events in the period preceding and coincident with major HMO activity. Because HMOs are a recent development, media coverage of HMO-related issues was limited to the period following 1970. The passage of HMO-enabling legislation at the state and federal levels in the early 1970s, and the subsequent growth of HMOs, attracted a high degree of media attention during this period. Media coverage of HMO activity increased in both metropolitan areas as the number and size of HMOs increased. In Minneapolis-St. Paul and in Chicago, only one HMO was established before 1970. Six of the seven HMOs in the Twin Cities and six of the eight HMOs in Chicago became operational between 1970 and 1981.

In examining newspaper coverage of HMOs, project staff reviewed the indexes of the major Twin Cities newspapers. Articles falling under the selected index headings were scanned by at least two staff members and marked for selection using the following criteria:

1. Reference to state and local issues and events only, unless national events had specific local relevance,

2. Reference to local HMOs' development personnel, operation, or performance, or to interactions between other sectors of the community and HMOs, and/or
3. Reference to legislative or regulatory changes influencing HMOs and consumer or health care provider stances on HMOs.

This procedure, with appropriate modification of key words, was also followed for the major Chicago newspapers. In total 273 articles from Minneapolis-St. Paul and 527 articles from Chicago were on file.

Interview process

Much of the information used for subsequent analyses was gathered from focused interviews with community and health care influentials. The interview process consisted of a series of steps: 1) the selection of informants, 2) the design of the interview protocol, 3) the interview itself, and 4) the analysis of the responses. Each step was important to the study and the validity of its findings. This section describes the methods used in each of these steps.

One goal of the study was to understand the role of the community and the health care market in HMO development in the two study sites. An important strength of the interview process was that it was "self-adjusting," that is, sensitive to environmental variation. The interview methodology was designed to incorporate additional informants and questions as the research team gathered data, analyzed the complexities of each study site, and recognized the need for additional information. Similar qualitative methodology was used by other researchers (Glaser and Strauss, 1967; Schatzman and Strauss, 1973).

Selection of informants

HMO development and growth are affected by the attitudes and behaviors of influential social actors in the community and the health care system. Social actors have been classified as individuals, organizations, or collectivities (Laumann and Knoke, 1980). An organization is a group of individuals that possesses legal authority to engage in certain transactions as a unitary actor. The organizations most commonly referred to are formal ones like HMOs, hospitals, medical societies, corporations, unions, etc. A collectivity is a group of loosely-organized aggregates that lack the formal organization of corporate bodies to act authoritatively as a unitary actor. Examples of collectivities include occupational aggrégates (physicians, hospital administrators), representative decision-making bodies (state legislatures and county and city governing bodies), and interest groups (Gray Panthers, NOW, Association of Health Care Consumers). A key attribute of a collectivity is the existence of multiple interest factions within its membership, necessitating collective decision-making through negotiation and compromise.

Within each of the sectors targeted for study, project staff selected informants who were influential individuals, or representatives of influential organizations or collectivities. "Influence" was gauged by the real or potential impact a social actor had on HMO development and growth. In both study sites, actors exerted influence on HMO development by virtue of their noninvolvement as well as their involvement. Because the study examined factors that both enhance and inhibit HMO growth, direct involvement in HMO development was not the only measure of influence.

Drawing on previous research on community decision making, a multi-method approach was developed to select community and health care influentials. Four sets of complementary criteria were employed for selection of influentials:

1. *Positional Criteria:* Individuals were selected who occupied central positions in organizations that had functions or interests in one or more of the identified sectors.
2. *Decisional Criteria:* Individuals were selected who were often mentioned in press reports or in other published, secondary sources. Many individuals identified through this method were also identified through positional criteria. However, this method was able to discover individuals who did not occupy formal positions in organizations but were consequential in decision making. Actors mentioned in the media were more likely to be consequential rather than marginal.
3. *Reputational Criteria:* A panel of judges, selected because of their specialized knowledge about the community or the health care field, nominated individual and collective actors who had reputed influence in one or more of the identified sectors.

4. *Relational Criteria:* Influentials selected using positional, decisional, or reputational criteria were asked to name other individuals with whom they interacted on issues or whom they perceived to have influence in one or more of the identified sectors.

A flexible combination of these sets of criteria was used to develop a list of selected respondents. In each site, an initial list was drafted from the recommendations of the panel of judges. These panels were asked to recommend individuals who, by virtue of their position or activities, had reputed influence in one or more of the identified sectors. Panel members were also asked to name influential positions and organizations, even if the name of the current incumbent or representative was unknown. Project staff appended to this initial list the names of individuals or organizations who appeared in the newspaper briefing books. This method was particularly helpful in identifying and gathering information on the members of influential organizations, as well as tracking the emergence of informants around particular events or issues. Review of newspaper and journal editorials was useful for identifying individuals who favored or opposed HMO development. Special attention was paid to the size and character of their constituencies and their perceived professional or community standing, to gauge the relative weight of their opinions.

The list of selected influentials was modified further as a result of taped interviews with general informants. These informants included researchers, newspaper reporters, journalists, and consultants. These general interviews served multiple purposes. For example, the taped interviews provided feedback regarding interview structure, style, and content. Second, these interviews provided useful information regarding the historical and political character of the community and health care system. Informants were also probed at length for recommendations of influentials. These recommendations were considered with those of the panel of judges.

In a small number of cases, the informants selected were replaced. During initial phone conversations with potential interviewees, staff members screened the individuals for their length of tenure and their role in the organization. Staff members also informed potential respondents of the goals of the interview so that individuals could screen themselves. In some cases either the staff member requested the individual to recommend a more appropriate respondent, or individuals realized that they were not an appropriate respondent and recommended a replacement. In a few cases, another respondent was recommended because of time or travel constraints.

Interviews were conducted first with the influentials selected by positional, decisional, and reputational criteria. During these interviews, respondents were asked to recommend individuals with whom they interacted on issues relevant to HMOs or whom they perceived to have influence in one or more of the identified sectors. Respondents were asked to recommend actors within their own sectors as well as within other sectors and the community at large. These recommendations were logged and discussed with other project members for possible inclusion on the list. Selection criteria for recommended influentials included:

1. Multiple recommendations.
2. Recommendation as an influential or appropriate representative in a state, county, or local organization hypothesized by the staff to have a real or potential impact on HMOs. Examples of such individuals were the director of benefit design in a large corporation, a hospital president, and the governor's assistant for health policy.
3. Recommendation as an influential or appropriate representative of an organization who could add to the understanding of each metropolitan area. Examples include individuals and representatives from different geographic regions of the metropolitan area; organizations reflecting ethnic, political, or other focused interests; and individuals or organizations of national reputation that are based in the metropolitan areas.

The number of interviews varied across sectors and metropolitan areas. The initial lists in each site contained ten or more potential informants per sector. The lists were modified using all of the methods described above. Interviews in each sector continued until they no longer contributed new information. In a sense, the number of interviews conducted in the different sectors and metropolitan areas represents one finding. Larger number of interviews do not necessarily suggest greater importance of a sector but rather its complexity or diversity. For example, in the Twin Cities, fewer interviews were conducted than in Chicago in most sectors. This reflected the size of the metropolitan area, the more institutionalized communitywide networks of communication, a greater homogeneity of response, and the tendency toward consensus in Minneapolis-St. Paul. Conversely, the greater number of interviews conducted in Chicago reflects fewer institutionalized communitywide networks of communication, greater heterogeneity of responses and activities, and a greater number of isolated responses and activities that required investigation.

An interesting variation in sector interviews across metropolitan areas further clarifies the self-adjusting feature of the methodology. The union and employer sectors were examined as one sector in the Twin Cities. Information gathered from the panel of judges and from others suggested that those sectors operate together. As a result, only four interviews with union officials were conducted. In Chicago, however, it became clear in the early stages of the project that unions had a distinct and complex set of interactions with HMOs, employers, and other sectors. The self-adjusting methodology led project staff to consider unions as a separate sector and to interview more extensively in Chicago.

Protocol design

Interview protocols were designed to guide the collection of information. The interviews illuminated 1) the role which the various actors played in promoting or opposing HMOs, 2) the environmental and organizational obstacles facing HMOs, and 3) the level of support needed for successful HMO development. In addition, the interviews yielded qualitative information about the impact of HMOs on various groups in the health care system and about the overall performance of the health care market.

Given the diversity of roles and perspectives of the people selected for interviewing, the interview protocols required flexibility to capture as much information as possible from each respondent. On the other hand, given the comparative nature of the study and the large number of interviews, the protocols also required structure to allow for meaningful comparisons and analyses. The study employed several methods to enhance both the depth and comparability of the interview data.

The study employed a semi-structured interview protocol. This is defined as an

> . . . interview guide . . . a list of questions or issues to
> be explored in the course of an interview. [It] is pre-

> pared in order to make sure that basically the same
> information is obtained from a number of people by
> covering the same material ... It provides topics or
> subject areas within which the interviewer is free to
> explore, probe and ask questions that will elucidate
> and illuminate that particular subject ... It provides
> a framework within which the interviewer [can] de-
> velop questions, sequence those questions and make
> decisions about which information to pursue in
> greater depth (Patton, 1980).

The use of such an interview protocol design required that
the staff develop a set of general questions and topics to be addressed in each interview. The design also required the interviewers to be knowledgeable about the scope and content of the
research project. Interviewers were often required to use this
knowledge to make decisions about appropriate questions to pursue during the interviews. The semi-structured format offered a
framework to systematize the collection of information and, giv-
en the training of the staff, a means to explore certain issues in
depth. This format is explained more fully below.

In the first stage of protocol development, the staff identified
the parameters that the interviews would follow. These parameters were determined using information gathered in the prepara-
tory stages of the project. The following interview parameters
were identified:

1. Range of questions: questions would address the respondents' attitudes and activities concerning HMOs. The protocols would be designed to adapt to respondents who had no
   previous HMO involvement as well as those actively involved in HMOs.
2. Time frame: questions would address historical developments and changes in support, involvement, and impact over
   time. Questions would also assess present status and anticipated developments.
3. Level of response: questions would address the respondent
   as an individual, as a representative of an organization, and
   as a member of a collectivity. For example, a hospital administrator would be asked about his or her own perceptions and
   behavior, the response of his or her hospital, and the response of the hospital industry in that community.
4. Interview flexibility: respondents would be probed about

their knowledge of events and issues beyond the structured protocol. This method would increase greatly the staff's understanding of the history and political character of both metropolitan areas.

5. Comparability: a general set of questions would be asked of all respondents, both within and across sectors.

After the interview parameters were determined, the staff drafted a generic list of questions that could be modified, as necessary, for each sector and each metropolitan area. These questions were first arranged by these major topic areas:

1. Patterns of communication, power, and decision making in each sector
   - How do groups and organizations in the sector communicate or interact with one another?
   - What is the decision-making structure within the respondent's organization?
   - Who are the influential actors in the sector?
   - How are decisions made and implemented in each sector?
2. Support for and opposition to HMOs
   - Which actors have supported or opposed the development of HMOs? Why?
   - What are the perceived advantages and disadvantages of HMOs among the various actors?
   - What are the major health care concerns and issues confronting these actors and how do HMOs affect them?
   - How has the level of support for or opposition to HMOs changed over time? Why?
3. Involvement and experience with HMOs
   - What is the level of the actors' involvement with HMOs? Why are they involved or not involved?
   - What factors are considered in the decision to become involved with HMOs?
   - What are the perceived costs and benefits associated with HMO involvement?
   - Are the HMOs differentially attractive? How? Why?
   - How has the involvement of these actors with the various HMOs changed over time? Why?
4. Impact of HMOs
   - Have the HMOs succeeded or failed? In which ways? Why?
   - How have HMOs affected the actors? How have the actors responded?

- How have HMOs affected the overall health system? How have they affected health care costs, quality, access, and competition?
- Are some HMOs more effective in containing costs than others?
- How have the HMOs influenced each other?
- How has the impact of HMOs changed over time?

Using the above guidelines, the staff drafted one general protocol and seven sector-specific protocols for the Minneapolis-St. Paul market area. These eight protocols were merged to form a sequence of interview questions. Trial interviews were conducted with staff members who had some knowledge of the appropriate sector to streamline the protocols before beginning the field work. Field work began by pretesting the protocols with general informants. While interviewing in the Twin Cities, the protocols changed very little. As field work progressed, responses were analyzed and questions reexamined and modified as appropriate.

The protocols developed for the Twin Cities were modified for use in the Chicago market area. These modifications were suggested by background information on Chicago and by data gathered in the Chicago pretest interviews. For example, questions regarding reasons for the high HMO market share in Minneapolis-St. Paul elicited rich and elaborate responses. In contrast, questions regarding reasons for the low HMO penetration in Chicago often elicited little response and required further probing by the interviewer. In Chicago, HMOs had apparently not yet gained sufficient visibility and salience to cause respondents to ponder the reasons for their development. Similarly, a question about competition in the Twin Cities, where competition in health care is a frequent subject of newspaper articles, drew interested, often animated, responses from Twin Cities respondents. Chicago respondents appeared to have given less thought to the concept of competition in their own area.

Protocol implementation

Field work began after the interview protocol was completed. Interviews in the Minneapolis-St. Paul area were conducted between May and October, 1982. Chicago interviews were conducted between October, 1982 and April, 1983.

The project staff encountered little difficulty in gaining access to informants. Staff members successfully reached informants by telephone to request interviews and to brief them about the study. When an informant could not be reached directly, an appointment was scheduled and a brief description of the study was mailed to his or her office. In Minneapolis-St. Paul, 100 percent of the selected influentials agreed to be interviewed. In Chicago, more than 97 percent of the selected influentials agreed to participate.

Although slight, the difference in participation rates between the sites may reflect two factors affecting interviewer access. The first factor is HMO market share. Because of the high HMO market share in Minneapolis-St. Paul, many Twin Cities informants were familiar with HMOs and comfortable with the nature of the interview. Indeed, many respondents expressed pride in the HMO activity and were eager to share their views. As a result of the low HMO market share in Chicago, fewer Chicago informants were familiar with HMOs. Staff members often had to convince informants that personal involvement with HMOs was not required to answer the interview questions.

The second factor is respondents' perceptions of the University of Chicago. Although HMOs are the subject of much research in the Twin Cities, observation by an externally based group, especially by an institution as prestigious as the University of Chicago, was perceived by many respondents as an honor. In Chicago, however, the staff met with mixed feelings about the University. Some respondents reacted positively, while others reacted negatively due to perceptions of being selected out of convenience or due to perceptions that the university is a national rather than a community-invested institution. The latter perception was particularly notable among local consumer and community representatives.

Roughly 97 percent of the interviews were recorded on tape, yielding four hundred hours of recorded information. The remainder could not be recorded because of technical difficulties or respondent refusal. These interviews were summarized in notes made during and after the interview. The lengths of the interviews ranged from thirty to ninety minutes. The majority lasted approximately one hour.

During the interview, project staff briefly described the study, explained the interview parameters, and then proceeded with the questions. Respondents were first asked about their professional and personal background, as appropriate. This background information helped the interviewer to ask the questions most relevant to the respondent's experience. Most of the interview questions were drawn from the general and sector-specific protocols. However, if the respondent's name had appeared in the press or if others had mentioned the respondent in connection with a particular issue or event, the basic protocol was expanded accordingly to cover these instances.

At the conclusion of the interview, respondents were asked to raise new issues. This gave the informant the freedom to further expand the interview structure. Certain sector-specific patterns emerged from these responses. For example, consumers were more likely to discuss issues of patient satisfaction; physicians more likely to discuss quality of care; and hospital administrators were more likely to discuss issues of regulation and competition.

Analysis of the interviews

The interviews were examined for both general and sector-specific information. A number of interviews were seen by all of the staff. These included interviews with central figures in the community or health care system who had a general understanding of their city and whose comments were particularly illuminating. The content of these interviews helped staff members gain an understanding of the character of the two metropolitan areas and the important issues and events within each. For the purpose of the final analysis, however, staff members divided up the responsibility for interviews by the seven sectors. The assignment of responsibility for a specific sector was based on the staff's interests and experience.

Within each sector, staff members used several methods to analyze the interview data. The responsible staff members listened intensively for five to twenty days to all the interviews from the particular sectors. During this period, staff members identified 1) patterns in the data, 2) supportive evidence of these patterns, 3) exceptions, and 4) key responses. At the same time, staff members conducted focused literature reviews for their particular sectors. These reviews supplemented the broad review completed during the developmental stages of the research, and called attention to issues and events relevant to each sector and its interactions with HMOs. Staff members then prepared written reports, which synthesize the interview analysis and focused literature review about each sector.

HMO ORGANIZATIONAL CASE HISTORIES

The way HMOs are structured and how they operate may affect their development and ultimately their impact on the health care system. To document the development of HMOs, organizational case histories were conducted for the fifteen HMOs (seven in the Twin Cities; eight in Chicago). Information was collected on HMO structure, operation, and performance from their inception to 1980.

Preparation

An essential part of the methodology for the case histories was forging a working relationship with the HMOs. Several factors affected the development of such a relationship. HMOs in both areas brought into the research relationship a set of attitudes toward research and researchers that had to be overcome to a certain extent. In the Twin Cities, HMOs have been the center of attention for many years. Consequently, they have had many demands for data from a variety of research organizations. Twin Cities HMOs explained that they were inundated by requests for information to be used in research. In addition, another important factor affecting the development of working relationships with HMOs in the Twin Cities was that this research team was comprised of outsiders, that is, from an institution outside the Twin Cities metropolitan area.

In Chicago, HMOs have also been the center of much attention in recent years but for different reasons than the HMOs in the Twin Cities. While research interest in the Twin Cities has been in why HMOs have been so "successful," in Chicago the interest has been in why HMOs have been so "unsuccessful," particularly in their marketing efforts. Several HMO executives in Chicago felt that they had received undue adverse publicity from several previous research studies. In addition, HMOs in Chicago were concerned that invidious comparisons had been drawn between HMO development in Chicago and Minneapolis-St. Paul in the past and that the current study would draw similar comparisons.

It must also be understood that HMOs are businesses operating in very competitive markets. As such, HMOs were reluctant to open their operations to researchers who might unveil proprietary information. Interestingly, the information that HMOs considered proprietary varied widely.

With that background, the steps in developing the research relationship were virtually the same in both areas. Introductory letters were written to the executive directors of the HMOs describing the general research objectives. These letters explained the importance of their involvement, input, and cooperation in the study. In Chicago, after the general letters were sent, project staff discussed the study and answered questions at a meeting of the Illinois Association of HMOs, a federation of HMOs principally from the Chicago metropolitan area. An endorsement of the study's objective and methodology was obtained from this group.

Following the introductory letters, project staff met with HMO directors on an individual basis to answer their questions and enlist their cooperation. During these meetings, the directors were asked to appoint a contact person at the HMO with whom project staff could work.

This process resulted in the development of excellent working relationships with all of the HMOs in the two areas. Overall, the HMOs displayed a high level of cooperation with the study. No HMO refused to participate in the study.

Data collection

Each case history was comprised of longitudinal data on HMO organization and operation. These histories document the HMO's introduction into the health care market as well as its subsequent growth and development. They also document the performance of the HMO over time in terms of enrollment, finance, and utilization.

Data collection for the case histories was conducted in three phases. In the first phase, information was collected from existing sources. An exhaustive review of the HMO literature provided many articles and books about HMOs in the two areas. Another valuable source of information was newspaper articles. Major newspapers in the two areas were searched for information relevant to the HMOs and their environment from 1970 to the present.

Documents from regulatory agencies provided a rich source

of information on HMO development and performance. Information filed in the state application for a certification of authority to operate provided detailed information on the early history and organization of the HMOs. Provider contracts and applications for service area expansions also provided useful information. Reports on HMO operations and finance filed annually with the state regulatory agencies were a primary source of information on the enrollment, utilization, and financial performance of the HMOs.

Readily available, existing information was also requested from the HMOs themselves. Marketing materials, newsletters, and consultants' reports were among the types of information that were obtained from the HMOs.

After all this information was inventoried, assessed, and compared to a predefined requisite data set, the HMOs were approached to provide additional data to fill in the "gaps." This comprised the second phase of the data collection effort.

A prospectus describing the objectives of the HMO case history, including areas of research interest, data requirements, and time frame, was mailed to the HMO representatives soliciting their review and comment. Later, a meeting was scheduled with the contact person to determine data availability and access. During this meeting, issues of confidentiality, data use, additional data sources, and arrangements for collecting the data were discussed. In addition, the availability of certain items considered proprietary were negotiated. Following this, the actual data collection from the HMOs commenced.

Data collection from the HMO was accomplished in two principal ways: either 1) the HMO contact person compiled the requested data or 2) project staff were given access to the data and they abstracted the required information. Examples of data obtained directly from the HMOs include group account data, hospital-specific utilization data, governing board meeting minutes, and organizational charts.

The final phase in the data collection for the HMO case histories involved interviews with informants. Additional data deemed necessary, after the previous data collection efforts, were collected through semi-structured interviews with HMO founders and operational personnel. The nature and process of these interviews were similar to those described in the section on interviews with health care and community elite. Interviews with founders focused on the early history of the HMO, e.g., precipitants for development, planning, sponsorship, and developmental issues. Interviews were also conducted with the chief executive officers (or chief operating officers) and the marketing directors of each HMO. Additional operational personnel, such as physician leaders or provider relations personnel, were interviewed in certain HMOs. Interviews with operational personnel focused on recent developments in HMO management, operations, and marketing.

Analysis

The information obtained from the various data sources was organized into case records for each of the HMOs. The case record served to organize the data from the diverse sources into a common format. The record was divided into three sections: 1) introduction and early development, 2) development of the administrative, medical delivery, and marketing structures, and 3) HMO performance. Information on the financial performance of the HMOs, which was obtained from reports submitted by HMOs to regulatory agencies and from HMO financial statements were standardized to minimize discrepancies resulting from a lack of generally accepted financial reporting standards among HMOs.

Analyses of the HMO case records focused on the patterns of development across the fifteen cases. These analyses focused on common problems and the range of solutions devised to address these problems. Analyses also investigated the adaptation of the HMOs to their environments and the organizational and operational correlates of HMO performance.

References

Anderson, Odin W. and Joanna Kravits
  1968 Health Services in the Chicago Area: A Framework for Use of Data. Chicago: Center for Health Administration Studies, University of Chicago.

Coleman, James
  1974 Power and the Structure of Society. New York: Norton.

Glaser, Barney G. and Anselm Strauss
  1967 Discovery of Grounded Theory: Strategies for Qualitative Research. Chicago: Aldine Publishing.

Laumann, Edward O. and David Knoke
  1980 "The Social Organization of National Policy Domains. Proposal to the National Science Foundation.

Patton, M. W.
  1980 Qualitative Evaluation Methods. Beverly Hills: Sage Publications, Inc.

Schatzman, L. and Anselm Strauss
  1973 Field Research: Strategies for a Natural Sociology. Englewood Cliffs: Prentice-Hall, Inc.

Appendix B

Employee Health Benefits in Chicago: A Survey of Major Metropolitan Chicago Employers

INTRODUCTION

Employers occupy an important position in the health care industry because they finance the health care of their employees through health benefits. Private employers, through employee health benefits, pay for approximately one-fifth of the total national health care bill (U.S. Chamber Survey Research Center, 1981). Historically, businesses have not actively managed health care costs; they have simply paid the bills. In recent years, health care costs, rising at nearly twice the rate of general inflation, have become salient for employers. However, now with the continued escalation of health care costs, employers are not only managing their employee health benefits but are increasingly involving themselves in activities designed to directly affect the organization and delivery of health care services. In addition, employers are rapidly becoming aware of their potential leverage in the health care industry.

METHODOLOGY AND DATA COLLECTION

The Center for Health Administration Studies conducted a survey of major employers, both public and private, in the Chi-

Appendix B was written by Ellen M. Morrison based on a report by Terry E. Herold.

cago metropolitan area from January through June 1983. Private sector employer respondents were selected from the 1980 edition of *Metropolitan Chicago Major Employers*, published by the Chicago Association of Commerce and Industry. Since employers offering HMOs were of primary interest in this survey, they were identified using HMO lists of commercial group accounts, and they were disproportionately sampled (although only 25 percent of employers in the association's directory were identified as offering an HMO, purposive sampling resulted in a 50 percent representation of these firms). Firms were then stratified according to the following characteristics (in order of priority):

1. Size—250–500 employees, 500–1000 employees, 1000 and more employees;
2. Type—Manufacturing, Non-manufacturing;
3. Primary Worksite Location—Chicago, Suburban; and
4. Headquarters Location—Chicago SMSA, Outside Chicago SMSA.

An additional purposive sample of the largest public sector employers was drawn, resulting in a final sample of 301 employers distributed as follows: HMO, 132; nonHMO, 155; public, 14. In all analyses, percentages were weighted appropriately to adjust for differential sampling.

The survey instrument, a 23-item questionnaire, was pretested on a purposive sample of employers, then mailed to the health benefits administrators of all those selected. Both mail and telephone follow-up methods were used for non-respondents. Nine employers selected in the sample had gone out-of-business or could not otherwise be located and were therefore excluded from the sample. Non-respondents and employers indicating that they did not wish to participate in the survey were sent a one-page questionnaire containing the most important questions.

No substantive changes were made in the questionnaire following the pretest. Therefore, responses from the pretest were pooled with the private and public survey data. The combined response rate for all categories of employers was 62 percent.

CHARACTERISTICS OF THE EMPLOYEE HEALTH BENEFITS MARKET

Using survey responses, we may extrapolate some general characteristics of the employee health benefits market in Chicago. Estimates of the trends in health insurance and HMO market shares, penetration rates, and employer contributions are presented below.

Market share is commonly expressed as a proportion of all *employees* in the market area enrolled in a particular health insurance plan. Self-insured plans led the employee health benefits market in Chicago with 38 percent of the market in the survey. Blue Cross-Blue Shield plans accounted for approximately one-third of the market (32 percent). The remaining portion was occupied by indemnity plans (18 percent) and HMO plans (10 percent). It should be noted that Blue Cross-Blue Shield and indemnity companies were involved in administering many of the self-insured plans. Blue Cross-Blue Shield displayed the largest mean enrollment per employer (4,292), followed by self-insured (1,319), indemnity (1,030), and HMOs (390).

Another perspective on the employee health benefit market is provided by examining the proportion of *employers* who offered the various types of health insurance plans. Self-insured plans again led the market, being offered through the largest percentage of surveyed employers (55 percent). While HMOs accounted for the smallest share of the market in terms of enrollees (10 percent), they ranked second in the proportion of employers that offer them to employees (40 percent). Indemnity plans were offered by 35 percent of the employers in Chicago, and Blue Cross-Blue Shield was offered by only 16 percent of the employers.

Survey responses indicate that a significant percentage of Chicago employers pay the total premium for employees' single health care coverage (69 percent of surveyed employers). Approximately one-third of the surveyed employers reported paying 100 percent of the health insurance premium for family coverage. Level dollar contributions across health plans, proposed by researchers to promote competition and employee cost awareness, are not common in Chicago (11 percent for single, 24 percent for family coverage among surveyed employers). However, benefit redesign programs, which increase employee cost sharing, are gaining popularity. Over 80 percent of surveyed employers who had implemented higher coinsurance and deductibles and higher employee premium contributions had implemented these programs since 1980.

Trends in employee health insurance show an increasing acceptance of alternatives to Blue Cross-Blue Shield and indemnity plans since 1970. Approximately one-half of surveyed employers offering Blue Cross-Blue Shield or indemnity plans offered this coverage to their employees prior to 1970. Twenty-nine percent of the employers offering self-insurance and only one percent of the employers offering HMOs began offering them before 1970. As cost containment gained importance in the late 1970s and early 1980s, both self-insurance and HMOs became increasingly popular. Fifty-eight percent of the employers offering HMOs first offered them between 1980 and 1983. Over half of the surveyed employers reported offering HMOs and self-insurance as cost containment strategies. Other cost containment strategies reported include coordination of benefits/subrogation, claims review, pre-admission testing, second surgical opinion programs, and long-term disability review. As a cost containment strategy, HMOs were rated as very effective by 13 percent of surveyed employers, and as moderately effective by 35 percent.

Forty percent of the surveyed employers reported offering one (19 percent) or more (21 percent) HMOs. Four of the seven HMOs accounted for nearly equal shares of the total number of health plans offered by employers: Anchor, 13 percent; HMO Illinois, 13 percent; Maxicare/Intergroup, 16 percent; and Prucare, 13 percent. Michael Reese Health Plan was offered less frequently, 9 percent, and Chicago HMO and Union Health Services accounted for only 1 percent of all health plans offered.

HMO marketing is a two-step process. Once an HMO convinces employers to offer its service, the HMO must convince employees to enroll in its plan. HMO penetration rate is defined commonly as the percent of the total number of employees eligible for health benefits who have enrolled in an HMO. In general, HMO penetration rates for employers in Chicago were low. Many factors explain this phenomenon, of which the most important are consumer preference, employer support, and price. In 42 percent of the Chicago firms in which HMOs were offered, the HMO penetration rate was 10 percent or less. In 11 percent of the firms, the HMO penetration rate was over 50 percent.

The employee health benefits market in Chicago, as estimated from survey responses, has changed in the past decade. Going into the 1970s, Blue Cross-Blue Shield and indemnity plans held solid market positions. In the early 1980s, employers sought alternatives to traditional insurance to contain costs. HMOs are perceived by many employers as viable cost containment alternatives. HMOs are challenged to market a quality product to employees as well as to demonstrate cost effectiveness to a receptive employer community.

CHARACTERISTICS OF EMPLOYERS

Characteristics and attitudes of employers are critical determinants of the types of employee health benefit plans offered and how they are offered. Clearly, different employers require different employee health benefits. Employer attitudes are particularly important in the decision to offer multiple health plans and to offer alternative health plans like HMOs.

Trends in attitudes and behavior among surveyed employers are presented within the context of the employer characteristics used to organize respondents: size, type, primary worksite location, headquarters location, and public vs. private. In addition, differences in attitudes are presented between employers who offer HMOs and those who do not. Within each category, only significant findings pertinent to HMO acceptance and growth are reported.

Size of employer

Researchers have found that larger employers are more likely to offer HMOs (Harris, 1980). Results from this survey corroborate this finding. While approximately one-third of the employers with workforces of less than 1000 employees offered HMOs, 55 percent of the employers with over 1000 workers offered HMOs. Larger employers were also more likely to offer more than one HMO. Larger employers were more familiar with the HMO concept, and they were more likely to encourage employees actively to join an HMO, whether or not they currently offer HMOs. They encouraged HMOs despite their concern that multiple choice health plans created more paperwork, administrative difficulty, and problems due to adverse selection. Also, the survey showed that larger employers were more likely to implement cost containment strategies and were less likely to pay 100 percent of the premium for employees' single coverage.

Type of employer

Respondents from manufacturing firms agreed that multiple choice of health plans created more paperwork and administrative difficulty. Manufacturing firms most likely paid 100 percent of employees' premiums for single coverage and most often reported HMO penetration rates less than 5 percent. These low penetration rates may be due to the confounding variable of white collar/blue collar workforces. Although, the level of workforce unionization is not correlated with the likelihood of offering HMOs, the more white collar workers employed, the more likely HMOs will be offered.

Primary worksite and headquarters locations

Firms with headquarters in the Chicago SMSA were more likely to offer HMOs than those with headquarters located elsewhere. Significant differences appeared between firms within the Chicago SMSA. Firms with primary worksite locations in the suburbs were more likely to pay 100 percent of their employees' premiums for single and family coverage. Firms with primary worksite locations in Chicago proper are more likely to offer HMOs and to offer more than one HMO.

Public vs. private firms

Bearing in mind that public employers surveyed were selected purposively, important differences in attitudes and behavior appeared between public and private sector respondents. Public sector employers were more likely to report high health benefit costs and to have implemented cost containment strategies. The largest percentage of HMOs' market shares comes from public employers. While only 40 percent of the private sector firms offered HMOs, 92 percent of the public firms did so. Also, public sector firms were more likely to offer more than one HMO and more likely to encourage employees to join. Employees' response to this encouragement is dramatic; 75 percent of the public sector respondents reported HMO penetration rates greater than 15 percent.

HMO firms vs. nonHMO firms

Survey results indicate that experience with HMOs enhances positive perceptions of HMOs. Although this variable interacts with the other employer characteristics, definite patterns appeared that distinguish the attitudes of HMO firms from non-HMO firms. HMO firms were more likely to rate HMOs as better than traditional insurance in terms of cost (total cost, cost to employee, cost containment and administrative cost) and of health improvement and level of coverage. NonHMO firms were more likely to rate traditional insurance as better than HMOs in terms of convenience (location of doctor's office and hospitals).

SUMMARY

Responses from this survey reflect a changing employee health benefits market in Chicago. Cost containment is becoming more important to employers, and employers are becoming more receptive to alternatives in health care coverage. Large employers, public employers, employers headquartered in Chicago, and employers with primary worksite locations in Chicago proper are more likely to offer and promote HMOs to their employees. However, these characteristics often overlap, so the potential for future HMO expansion is great. Employer promotion of HMOs to employees; HMO marketing, which would increase penetration within firms already offering HMOs; and HMO expansion into the smaller, private, and suburban firms, could dramatically increase HMO market penetration in Chicago.

References

Chicago Association of Commerce and Industry
    1980   1980 Metropolitan Chicago Major Employers. Chicago: Chicago Association of Commerce and Industry.

Lou Harris & Associates, Inc.
    1980   Employers and HMOs: A Nationwide Survey of Corporate Employers in Areas Served by Health Maintenance Organizations. New York: Lou Harris & Associates, Inc.

Suburban Health Systems Agency
    1981   To Join or Not to Join: A Study of Employee and Employer Per-

ceptions of Health Maintenance Organizations. Oak Park, IL: Suburban Health Systems Agency.

U.S. Chamber Survey Research Center
1981 Employee Benefits, 1981. Washington, DC: Chamber of Commerce of the United States.

Index

Center for Health Administration Studies
Graduate School of Business
Division of Biological Sciences
The University of Chicago
Research Series

RS #1 —*The Behavioral Scientists and Research in the Health Field—a questionnaire survey*, Odin W. Anderson, Ph.D., and Milvoy Seacat. 1957. 15 pp.

RS #2 —*An Examination of the Concept of Medical Indigence*, Odin W. Anderson, Ph.D., and Harold Alksne. 1957. 14 pp.

RS #3 —*The Prescription Pharmacist Today*, Wallace Croatman and Paul B. Sheatsley. 1958. 27 pp.

RS #4 —*The Public Looks at Hospitals*, Eliot Freidson and Jacob J. Feldman. 1958. 24 pp.

RS #5 —*Public Attitudes Toward Health Insurance*, Eliot Freidson and Jacob J. Feldman. 1958. 18 pp.

RS #6 —*The Public Looks at Dental Care*, Eliot Freidson and Jacob J. Feldman. 1958. 16 pp.

RS #8 —*Health Research Opportunities in Welfare Records—a preliminary report on illness and economic dependency*, Herbert Notkin, M.D., M.P.H. 1958. 20 pp.

RS #9 —*Comprehensive Medical Insurance—a study of costs, use, and attitudes under two plans*, Odin W. Anderson, Ph.D., and Paul B. Sheatsley. 1959. 105 pp.

RS #11—*Measuring Health Levels in the United States, 1900–1958*, Odin W. Anderson, Ph.D., and Monroe Lerner. 1960. 38 pp.

RS #12—*An Examination of the Concept of Preventive Medicine*, Odin W. Anderson, Ph.D., and George Rosen, M.D., Ph.D., 1960. 22 pp.

RS #13—*Hospital Use and Charges by Diagnostic Category—a report on the Indiana study of a Blue Cross population*, Monroe Lerner. 1960. 32 pp.

RS #18—*Proprietary Nursing Homes—a report on interviews with 35 nursing home operators in Detroit, Michigan*, Thomas E. Mahaffey. 1961. 44 pp.

RS #19—*Hospital Use by Diagnosis—a comparison of two experiences*, Monroe Lerner. 1961. 46 pp.

RS #21—*An Analysis of Personnel in Medical Sociology*, Odin W. Anderson, Ph.D., and Milvoy S. Seacat. 1962. 8 pp.

RS #22—*Syphilis and Society—problems of control in the United States, 1912—1964*, Odin W. Anderson, Ph.D. 1965. 62 pp.

RS #23—*People and Their Hospital Insurance—comparisons of the uninsured, those with one policy, and those with multiple coverage,* Ronald Andersen and Donald C. Riedel, Ph.D. 1967. 37 pp.

RS #24—*Hospital Use—a survey of patient and physician decisions,* Odin W. Anderson, Ph.D., and Paul B. Sheatsley. 1967. 215 pp.

RS #25—*A Behavioral Model of Families' Use of Health Services,* Ronald Andersen, Ph.D. 1968. 106 pp.

RS #26—*Health Services in the Chicago Area, a framework for use of data,* Odin W. Anderson, Ph.D., and Joanna Kravits. 1968. 133 pp.

RS #27—*Medical Care Use in Sweden and the United States,* Ronald Andersen, Ph.D., Björn Smedby, Med. Lic., and Odin W. Anderson, Ph.D. 1970. 174 pp.

RS #28—*The Relationship Between Administrative Activities and Hospital Performance,* Duncan Neuhauser, Ph.D. 1971. 115 pp.

RS #29—*Ambulatory Use of Physicians' Services in Response to Illness Episodes in a Low-Income Neighborhood,* William C. Richardson, Ph.D. 185 pp.

RS #30—*Patterns of Dental Service Utilization in the United States: A Nationwide Social Survey,* John F. Newman, Ph.D., and Odin W. Anderson, Ph.D. 127 pp.

RS #31—*A Model of Physician Referral Behavior: A Test of Exchange Theory in Medical Practice,* Stephen Shortell, Ph.D. 200 pp.

RS #32—*Access to Medical Care in the U.S.: Who Has It, Who Doesn't,* Lu Ann Aday, Ph.D., Gretchen V. Fleming, Ph.D., Ronald M. Andersen, Ph.D. 1984.

RS #33—*HMO Development: Patterns and Prospects,* Odin W. Anderson, Ph.D., Terry E. Herold, A.M., Bruce Butler, M.B.A., Claire Kohrman, M.A., Ellen M. Morrison, M.A. 1984.

A price list and copies of RS #1 through #31 can be obtained directly from the Center for Health Administration Studies, University of Chicago, 1101 East 58th Street, Chicago, IL 60637. RS #32 and #33 can be purchased through Pluribus Press, Inc., 160 East Illinois Street, Chicago, IL 60611.